Mental Illnesses: Therapy and Implications

Mental Illnesses: Therapy and Implications

Edited by **John Dalvi**

FOSTER
A C A D E M I C S

New Jersey

Published by Foster Academics,
61 Van Reypen Street,
Jersey City, NJ 07306, USA
www.fosteracademics.com

Mental Illnesses: Therapy and Implications
Edited by John Dalvi

International Standard Book Number: 978-1-63242-275-0 (Hardback)

Printed in the United States of America.

Contents

Preface

This book has been a concerted effort by a group of academicians, researchers and scientists, who have contributed their research works for the realization of the book. This book has materialized in the wake of emerging advancements and innovations in this field. Therefore, the need of the hour was to compile all the required researches and disseminate the knowledge to a broad spectrum of people comprising of students, researchers and specialists of the field.

This book emphasizes on the therapeutic aspects of mental illness. It is important to assess mental illness seriously, to comprehend its nature, predict its long-term outcome and treat it with specific rather than generic treatment, such as pharmacotherapy. Community-wide and cognitive-behavioral approaches are essential methods and should be incorporated to decrease the severity of symptoms of mental illness. Unfortunately, those who should benefit the most by the combination generally refuse treatment or show poor devotion to treatment maintenance. Mental illness cannot be treated with one single kind of treatment method. Individual, community and socially-oriented treatments along with latest distance-writing technologies will allow a more effective and unified approach to fight mental illness world-wide. This book contains three sections namely: pharmacotherapy, implications and conclusion.

At the end of the preface, I would like to thank the authors for their brilliant chapters and the publisher for guiding us all-through the making of the book till its final stage. Also, I would like to thank my family for providing the support and encouragement throughout my academic career and research projects.

Editor

Part 1

Pharmacotherapy

Ultrastructural Distinctions Between Treatment Responders and Non-Responders in Schizophrenia: Postmortem Studies of the Striatum

Rosalinda C. Roberts[1], Joy K. Roche[1],
Shahza M. Somerville[2] and Robert R. Conley[3]
[1]*Department of Psychiatry and Behavioral Neurobiology*
University of Alabama, Birmingham, Birmingham, AL
[2]*Technical Resources International, Bethesda, MD*
[3]*Department of Neuroscience , Lilly Technology Center, Indianapolis, IN*
USA

1. Introduction

1.1 Schizophrenia

Schizophrenia (SZ) typically manifests itself in early adulthood with psychotic symptoms (hallucinations, delusions, disorders of thought or speech, grossly disorganized behaviour), cognitive impairments and in some, negative symptoms. This illness affects 1% of the population worldwide (APA, 1994). Risk factors for schizophrenia suggest both a developmental and genetic basis. Neuropathology and abnormalities in multiple neurotransmitter systems have been reported throughout the brain (Harrison 1999; Powers 1999). However, there is no diagnostic pathology that identifies the brains of SZ subjects.

1.2 Treatment response/resistance

Antipsychotic drugs (APDs) act primarily to relieve positive symptoms with little or no effect on negative (i.e. social withdrawal, anhedonia, avolition) and cognitive symptoms (McEvoy 2006). Not all patients respond to treatment and in those who do, only psychotic symptoms are usually improved (Conley & Kelly 2001; Meltzer 1997). Treatment response to APD is best defined along a gradient, one end of which is characterized by no response (TNR) also referred as "treatment resistant". The reported rate of treatment response can vary from 25 to 70% (Brenner, et al., 1990). The reason for treatment resistance (or nonresponse) is poorly understood but appears to have a biological basis (Altamura et al., 2005; Beerpoot et al., 1996; Sheitman and Lieberman, 1998). A relationship between pathophysiology in SZ and the degree of treatment response has been shown in several neuroimaging studies (Arango et al., 2003; Rodriguez et al., 1997; Staal et al., 2001). MRI studies have shown that treatment nonresponsive SZ subjects have greater cortical atrophy in certain regions (Mitelman et al., 2005), smaller putamen volumes (Mitelman et al., 2009) and larger cerebral ventricles than do treatment responsive SZs (Bilder et al. 1994; Staal et al., 2001; Stern et al., 1993). SPECT shows differential values for cerebral perfusion, an index of neuronal activity (Gemmell et al., 1990; Turkington et al., 1993), in treatment responsive vs. resistant SZ subjects (Rodriguez et al., 1997). APD naïve SZ subjects who eventually respond to treatment have elevated dopamine release compared to those subjects who do not eventually respond (Abi-Dargham et al. 2000). Importantly, treatment resistance does not occur because of a failure of D_2 receptor blockade by APDs as these treatment resistant subjects show a 95% blockade of striatal D_2 receptors following typical APD treatment (Coppens et al., 1991). Neurobiological differences between treatment response and treatment resistance in SZ are rarely studied at the microscopic level in postmortem tissue, but provide a strategy for trying to link psychosis with particular neuropathology (Roberts et al., 2009; Somerville et al., 2011b). Although numerous neuroimaging studies suggest a biological basis to treatment response/resistance, to our knowledge, only our postmortem studies have addressed this issue (Roberts et al., 2009; Somerville et al., 2011b).

The striatum is rich in dopamine receptors and all known effective APDs block dopamine D_2 receptors (Creese, et al., 1976; Lahti et al., 2003; Seeman et al., 1975). Dopamine modulation depends on many factors such as receptor subtype and location (Cepeda et al., 2001; Onn et al., 2000; West and Grace, 2002), the concentration of ambient dopamine and the activity state of the spiny neuron (Cepeda & Levine, 1998). Brain imaging studies show that the striatum of subjects with SZ displays augmentation of presynaptic dopamine function, indicating an increase in dopamine synthesis capacity and/or an increase in presynaptic dopamine stores (Abi-Dargham et al., 1998, 2000; Breier et al., 1997; Dao-Castellana et al., 1997; Hietala et al., 1995, 1999; Laruelle et al., 1996, 1999). Specifically, there is an increase in the release of dopamine (Abi-Dargham et al., 1998; Laruelle et al., 1996, 1999) and in the density and occupancy of dopamine D_2 receptors (Abi-Dargham et al., 2000; Wong et al., 1986). Patients with SZ with high dopamine release are far more responsive to APDs than those patients who have dopamine levels lower than or comparable to that of healthy volunteers (Abi-Dargham et al., 2000). In addition, dopamine D_2 receptor density in the caudate nucleus is higher in the unaffected monozygotic twins of SZ subjects compared to unaffected dizygotic twins and healthy control twins (Hirvonen et al., 2005). The studies suggest that dopamine transmission dysfunction confers a genetic risk for schizophrenia.

1.3 Striatal pathology in schizophrenia

The striatum of subjects with schizophrenia shows several pathological abnormalities in vivo (Buchsbaum & Hazlett, 1998) and in postmortem tissue (Harrison, 1999; Powers, 1999). Grossly, the striatum of neuroleptic-naïve schizophrenia subjects is smaller than normal, but upon antipsychotic treatment with several but not all drugs, the striatum enlarges (Brandt & Bonelli, 2008; Chakos et al., 1994). Surface deformation mapping results have shown localized volume decreases in both the caudate nucleus and putamen in neuroleptic free patients; such changes were most pronounced in the associative striatum (Mamah et al., 2007). Moreover, affective flattening was correlated with abnormalities in the anterior putamen (Mamah et al., 2007). Also, the unaffected siblings of schizophrenia patients showed intermediate changes between that of controls and their ill siblings (Mamah et al., 2008). Offspring of schizophrenia patients also have smaller caudate nuclei (Rajarethinam, et al., 2007). Taken together, these data suggest that gross morphological changes in the caudate nucleus and/or putamen may be a core feature of the illness or confer a risk factor. Consistent with the imaging data, results from microscopy show a 10% decrease in cell

Ultrastructural Distinctions Between Treatment Responders and Non-Responders in Schizophrenia: Postmortem
Studies of the Striatum

5

number in the caudate nucleus and putamen (Kreczmanski et al., 2007). Neurochemical
deficits include decreases in 1) uptake sites for glutamate and GABA (Simpson et al., 1992),
2) excitatory amino acid transporter 3 and vesicular glutamate transporter 1 (VGlut1)
(Nudmamud-Thanoi et al., 2008), 3) enkephalin (Kleinman et al., 1985) and neurotensin
receptors (Lahti et al., 1998) and 4) fewer interneurons that express acetylcholine (Holt et al.,
1999). Several studies have implicated mitochondrial abnormalities in subjects with
schizophrenia (Ben-Shachar, 2002; Ben-Shachar & Laifenfeld, 2004; Kung and Roberts, 1999;
Prince et al., 1999; Somerville et al., 2011a,b). These include genetic, metabolic, structural,
and enzymatic alterations, many of which occur in the basal ganglia (Ben-Shachar, 2002).
Many of the postmortem pathological findings in the striatum in schizophrenia have been
conducted at the ultrastructural level by Uranova and colleagues and us. Uranova and
colleagues (1996, 2001, 2007) have found abnormalities in oligodendrocytes, myelin sheaths,
astrocytes and synapses in the caudate nucleus and other regions. Our work has
concentrated on synaptic organization, and anatomical indicators of synaptic function.
Initially, we found that the size of striatal dendritic spines was smaller in schizophrenia
subjects, a change that could impact synaptic efficacy (Roberts et al., 1996). Later we found
more synapses in the caudate nucleus in a mixed cohort of schizophrenia patients (Roberts
et al., 2005a). When examining the patch and matrix compartments, these synaptic changes
were specific to the caudate matrix and putamen patches (Roberts et al., 2005b). The types of
synapses that were increased in density were morphologically similar to glutamatergic
inputs from cortex or thalamus or possibly serotonergic inputs.

1.4 Striatal connectivity

Knowledge of striatal circuitry has evolved over the decades from the idea of parallel
segregated pathways (Alexander et al., 1986; DeLong & Wichmann, 2007) to functional
connectivity (motor, limbic and associative) (Haber et al., 2000), patch/ matrix
compartments (Gerfen 1984; Graybiel & Ragsdale 1978) and an integration of these circuits
(Graybiel 2005; Joel & Weiner, 2000). Figure 1 illustrates a "simplified" diagram of striatal
connections, the details of which are reviewed in our recent paper (Perez-Costas et al., 2010).
Striatal patch and matrix compartments process different circuitry and subserve different
functions, though there is evidence of cross-talk between these compartments (Bennett &
Bolam 1994; Walker et al 1993). Striatal patches have connections to limbic brain regions
(Cote et al. 1995; Gerfen 1984; Levesque & Parent 1998; Parent & Hazrati 1993) and abnormal
circuitry therein could play a role in psychosis. This compartmentalization has been
demonstrated with a variety of immunohistochemical markers (Graybiel & Ragsdale, 1978).
Graybiel and Ragsdale (1978) defined these anatomically distinct compartments as
striosomes (patches) and extrastriosomal matrix (matrix), though the presence of these
compartments is less clear in ventral striatal areas in primate (Holt et al., 1997; Prensa et al.,
1999a,b). These compartments differ from each other in several ways including the content
of neurotransmitters, peptides and receptors (Graybiel & Ragsdale, 1978; Holt et al., 1997;
Joel & Wiener, 2000), neuronal organization (Penny et al., 1988; Walker et al., 1993),
connectivity (Gerfen 1984), developmental schedule (Graybiel & Hickey, 1982; van der Kooy
and Fishell, 1987), and behavioral function (White & Hiroi, 1998). Moreover, the patches and
matrix themselves are each inhomogeneous, with the patches having a belt and core (Holt et
al., 1997; Prensa et al., 1999), and the matrix containing matrisomes, which are areas of focal
afferents and efferents (Graybiel et al., 1991). Most medium spiny neurons have their local
axon arborizations and dendritic trees located in the matrix or the striosomes, following

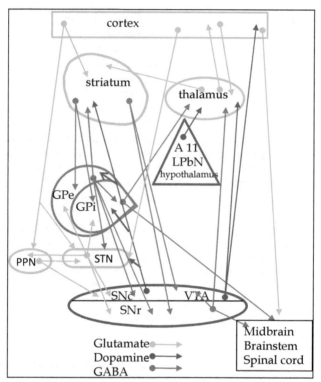

Fig. 1. Diagram of striatal connections.
Connections are shown by arrows: green for excitatory, red for inhibitory, and purple for dopamine. Abbreviations: A11, dopamine cell group #11; LPbN, lateral parabrachial nucleus; GPe/GPi: globus pallidus external/internal; PPN, pedunculopontine nucleus; STN, subthalamic nucleus; SNc/r; substantia nigra pars compacta/reticulate; VTA, ventral tegmental area.

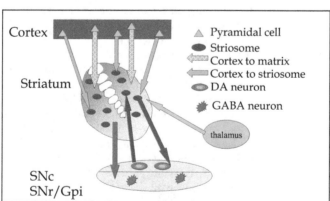

Fig. 2. Diagram of striosomal connections
Simplified diagram of striosomal organization. Abbreviations: same as in Figure 1.

Ultrastructural Distinctions Between Treatment Responders and Non-Responders in Schizophrenia: Postmortem
Studies of the Striatum

7

strictly compartmental boundaries (Penny et al., 1988). However, at least in primates, there
are also medium spiny neurons that do not respect these boundaries and have dendrites
crossing from one compartment to the other (Walker et al., 1993; Yung et al., 1996), allowing
cross-talk between compartments. Finally, ultrastructural analysis has shown that in the
human striatum the matrix and striosomes have marked differences in the frequency of
various types of synapses (Roberts and Knickman, 2002).

1.5 Striatal synaptic organization

In various mammalian species (Chung et al. 1977; Hassler et al. 1978; Pasik et al. 1976;)
including human (Roberts and Knickman, 2002), the majority of synapses in the striatum form
asymmetric synapses, characteristic of excitatory synaptic transmission. The terminals forming
these synapses originate predominantly from neurons in the cortex (Kemp & Powell 1971a, b,
c), with less extensive inputs arising from the thalamus (Kemp & Powell 1971a, b, c; Raju et al.
2006; Sadikot et al. 1992; Smith et al. 1994) and the raphe (LaVoie & Parent, 1990). Symmetric
synapses, typical of inhibitory synaptic transmission, originate from several sources including
striatal interneurons (DiFiglia & Aronin 1982; DiFiglia 1987; Ribak et al. 1979), collaterals of
striatal projection neurons (Hutcherson & Roberts 2005; Pickel et al. 1980; Somogyi et al. 1981;
Wilson & Groves 1980) and dopaminergic nigrostriatal neurons (Freund et al. 1984; Kubota et
al. 1987a,b; Kung et al. 1998; Pickel et al. 1981). Experimental manipulations used in animal
models to trace connectivity and circuits are not an option when studying human tissue.
However, by examining the morphological characteristics of synapses, such as symmetry and
postsynaptic target, it is possible to make educated speculations as to the origin of the neurons
forming particular synapses in the human based on what is known in other species.
The main striatal targets of dopaminergic inputs are the medium spiny projection neurons
(Freund et al., 1984; Kubota et al., 1987a). It has long been known that glutamatergic
afferents and dopaminergic inputs converge on the same spines of these cells (Bouyer et al.,
1984; Smith et al., 1994). Most thalamic inputs, except those from centromedian and
parafascicular complex, also end on dendritic spines and therefore could also be modulated
by dopaminergic afferents (Raju et al., 2006; Sadikot et al., 1992; Sidibe and Smith, 1999;
Smith et al., 2004). This suggests that a major function of dopaminergic inputs to the
striatum is the regulation of the glutamatergic pathways. Figure 3 is a schematic diagram.

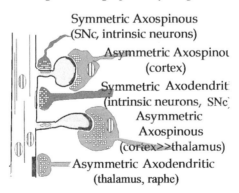

Symmetric Axospinous
(SNc, intrinsic neurons)

Asymmetric Axospinou
(cortex)

Symmetric Axodendrit
(intrinsic neurons, SNc)

Asymmetric
Axospinous
(cortex>>thalamus)

Asymmetric Axodendritic
(thalamus, raphe)

Fig. 3. Schematic illustration of synaptic connections on a medium spiny neuron.
Synapses are identified by symmetry (thickness of the postsynaptic density) and target (spine,
dendrite). Green terminals are glutamatergic, while red terminals are GABAergic and also
contain various peptides. The location of the neurons that form the synapses shown is indicated.

1.6 Study goals

The purpose of the present study was to compare the synaptic organization in striatal patch and matrix compartments in different subgroups of SZ, divided by treatment resistance or treatment response. We hypothesized that SZ subjects that were psychotic (off drug or poor responders) would have different alterations than treatment responsive SZ subjects. We examined striatal striosomal and synaptic organization at the electron microscopic level in postmortem striatum. These results have been presented in preliminary form (Roberts et al., 2007). We also include the results of two of our previous studies (Roberts et al., 2009; Somerville et al., 2011b) that examined treatment response/resistance and discuss the implications of all findings taken together.

2. Methods

2.1 Postmortem brain samples

Postmortem human brain tissue was obtained from the Maryland Brain Collection (MBC). The tissue was collected with family permission within 8 hours of death from subjects with schizophrenia (SZ) (n=14) and normal controls (NC) (n=8) (Table 1). The NCs had no history of central nervous system or neurological diseases and were matched to the SZ subjects for age, gender, postmortem interval and race when possible. Drug therapy, duration of illness and other medical details were obtained from hospital charts, autopsy reports and family interviews. The diagnosis of schizophrenia was made by two research psychiatrists according to the DSM-IV criteria using the Diagnostic Evaluation After Death (DEAD) (Salzman et. al., 1983) and the Scheduled Clinical Interview for the DSM III-R (SCID) (Spitzer et. al., 1992). The diagnoses of treatment response versus treatment resistance was made according to the following criteria (Conley, 2001; Conley & Kelly, 2000) which is a modification of the Kane criteria (Kane, 1988): 1) Presence of a drug-refractory condition,

	NCs (n=8)	SZ: Treatment Responders (n=8)	SZ: Resistant & Off APDs (n=6)	df (t or F)p value
Age in years	43±17	52±11	44±10	23 (0.775) <0.474
Race	3AA, 5C	4AA, 4C	2AA, 4C	23 (0.488)<0.620
Gender	5M, 3F	5M, 3F	2M, 4F	23 (0.655) <0.530
PMI in hours	5.4±1.6	4.62±1.41	5.50±2.43	23 (0.490)<0.619
pH (n=6/group)	7.03±0.3	6.97±0.26	6.93±0.24	18 (0.341) <0.716
DSM-IV	-----	4CUT, 3 P, 1unk	3CUT, 2P, 1unk	10 (-0.09) <0.930
APD	-----	6 typ , 2 atyp	1typ, 3atyp, 2off	12 (-4.128) <0.001
Age of onset	-----	24.4±5.8 (n=5)	21.2±6.6 (n=4)	7 (0.762)<0.471
Length of illness	-----	26.2±14.1 (n=5)	28.8±1.2 (n=4)	7 (-0.356) <0.732

Table 1. Demographic information for subjects.
Demographic information is shown for the subjects used in the synapse data, which is new data presented in this chapter. The tyrosine hydroxylase and mitochondria data are from subsets of these cases and demographics have been previously described (Roberts et al., 2009, Somerville et al., 2010a). Abbreviations: PMI, postmortem interval; APD, antipsychotic drugs; typ, typical; atyp, atypical; A, African-American; C, Caucasian; M, male; F, female; CUT, chronic undifferentiated type; unk, unknown; Not all information was known for every subject, therefore, numbers in () indicate the number of subjects where the information was known.

which is defined as at least two prior drug treatment periods of adequate length and dose with no clinical improvement; 2) Persistence of illness, defined as at least a 5-year period with no period of good social or occupational function; and 3) Presence of persistent positive psychotic symptoms (e.g., hallucinations, delusions, suspiciousness, unusual thoughts) throughout the person's life. Cases were rated for presence or absence of these three items. If all are present, a diagnosis of treatment resistance is made. If item one is not present and one or no items are present from 2 and 3, a diagnosis of treatment responsive is made. These criteria identify subjects who did not respond to repeated trials of additional antipsychotic drugs but can respond to clozapine.

2.2 Tissue processing
Coronal blocks from the head of the caudate were dissected from fresh human brain and immersed in a cold solution of 4% paraformaldehyde and 1% glutaraldehyde in 0.1M phosphate buffer (PB), pH=7.4 for at least one week at 4°C. The striatum was washed in PB and cut on a vibratome at a thickness of 40μm into 6-12 series. One series was stained for calbindin immunoreactivity, while one series was stained for tyrosine hydroxylase immunoreactivity, as detailed below. Both series were embedded as detailed below.

2.2.1 Immunohistochemistry
To distinguish the patches from the matrix, we used calbindin-d-28K (Sigma), a calcium binding protein that preferentially stains the striatal matrix (Liu & Graybiel, 1992). Briefly, free floating sections (240 μm apart) were washed in PB (3 x 10 minutes), and incubated in 2% normal serum in PB for 30 minutes, followed by the primary antibody at a dilution of 1:20,000 for 60 hours at 4°C. Another series of sections (240μm apart) were processed from each case for the immunohistochemical localization of tyrosine hydroxylase (TH) as described previously (Kung et al., 1998; Roberts et al., 2009). Briefly, the sections were incubated in normal horse serum, followed by mouse anti-TH (Boehringer Mannheim,

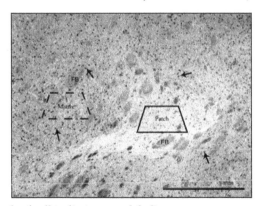

Fig. 4. Photomicrograph of calbindin immunolabeling.
Human striatum processed for calbindin immunohistochemistry to identify matrix patch compartments (defined by the darker labeling in the matrix). Note that the patch area is irregular in shape and far more lightly stained than the matrix. The trapezoids show typical areas selected for EM analysis. Arrows indicate labeled neurons. FB, fiber bundle. The scale bar = 1mm. A modification of Figure 3A in Perez-Costas et al., 2007.

Mannheim, Germany) at a dilution of 1:1,000 for 60 hours. The labeled tissue was then treated with reagents from the avidin-biotin peroxidase kit (ABC standard kit) using the recommended dilutions and times as outlined in our previous work (Roberts and Knickman, 2002; Roberts et al., 2009). Briefly, sections were then incubated in diaminobenzidine (6 mg/10 ml PB) containing 0.03% hydrogen peroxide for 5 to 10 minutes to visualize the reaction product. Controls consisted of eliminating the primary antibody but otherwise processing the tissue according to an identical protocol. Control sections did not exhibit any staining.

2.2.3 Embedding
Tissue samples were embedded using standard techniques. Briefly, the sections were rinsed in PB (3x10 minutes), immersed in 1% osmium tetroxide for 1 hour, dehydrated in ethyl alcohol, stained with uranyl acetate for 2 hours, further dehydrated in ethyl alcohol, embedded in resins on glass slides and heated at 60 °C for 72 hours. For synapse counting, at least 3 samples from different sections were randomly selected from the patches or matrix for electron microscopic analysis for each case (Figure 4). The blocks were serially thin-sectioned on an ultramicrotome at a thickness of 90nm. The average length of each ribbon was six serial sections for TH stained sections and fourteen for everything else.

2.3 Data collection and analysis
Details of the quantitative analysis of mitochondria and dopaminergic terminals have been published previously (Roberts et al., 2009; Somerville, 2011a,b). For the present analysis, in each sample, 6 photomicrographs (at a magnification of 10,000x) were taken that formed a montage. The montages were printed (final viewing magnification was approximately 25,000x), and a counting box (approximate are of 100μm^2) was drawn in each. The disector stereologic technique was utilized (Geinisman et al. 1996) and described in more detail elsewhere (Perez-Costas et al., 2007). All synapses appearing in the first montage in the series and all synapses that crossed the exclusion lines in any of the series were excluded. Any profiles that appeared for the first time in subsequent montages, that met criteria, were numbered and followed in this three-dimensional reconstruction method. All synapses were quantified and then subcategorized. Thus, we identified asymmetric axospinous (AS), asymmetric axodendritic (AD), symmetric axospinous (SS), and symmetric axodendritic (SD) synapses. Then, we combined these in various ways to tally all asymmetric synapses (AS + AD), all axospinous synapses (AS + AD), all symmetric synapses (SS + SD) and all axodendritic synapses (AD + SD). The analysis of synaptic organization was performed with the experimenter blinded to the diagnosis. Synaptic data throughout the text is the number of synapses per 10μm^3 $\pm$ standard deviation. Over 100 synapses or mitochondria were counted for each region per case and data are reported as the mean $\pm$ standard deviation.

2.4 Statistics
Group means and standard deviations for demographic data were obtained for each group or subgroup (Table 1). To determine whether the density of synapses was different between the controls, treatment responsive SZs and treatment nonresponsive SZs, an ANOVA followed by a posthoc t-test for multiple comparisons (least significant difference, LSD) was used. ANOVAs followed by the posthoc LSD t-test were used to determine if there were any group differences in age, PMI, race or gender between the three groups. Unpaired t-tests were used to compare parameters occurring between treatment responsive SZs and

treatment nonresponsive SZs (but not applicable to controls) such as age of onset, duration of illness, or antipsychotic drug use. Since there was a significant difference in APD use between the TR SZs and the TNR SZs, we performed a correlation analysis between APD and synapses in which we found significant measures. A Pearson bivariate correlation was used with a 2-tailed significance level of < 0.05. There were no correlations.

3. Results

Quantitative ultrastructural studies of postmortem human brain are rare outside of our laboratory, due in part to the difficulty in procuring the tissue so quickly after death. However, we have found the integrity of the tissue at the electron microscopic level to be quite acceptable for synapse identification and stereological analysis. Figure 5 shows examples of different kinds of synapses obtained from human postmortem striatum.

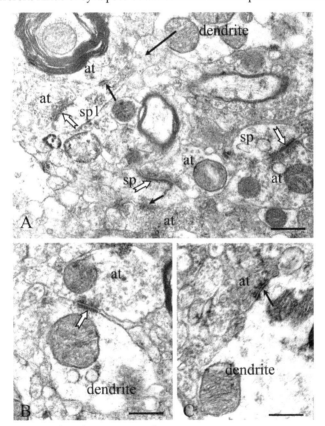

Fig. 5. Electron micrographs of postmortem human striatum.
Examples of different types of striatal synapses from control cases. Axon terminals (at) form asymmetric synapses (identified by white arrows with black borders), or symmetric synapses (black arrows). A) Several axospinous synapses are present in this field. B, C). Dendrites receive an asymmetric synapse (B) and a symmetric synapse (C). Scale bars = 0.5 μm. Figure reprinted from Figure 1 in Roberts et al., 2005b.

3.1 Striatal synaptic density

Synaptic density was determined in all three groups (controls [NCs], TR and TNR) in various regions of the striatum: caudate, putamen, patch and matrix. No matter how we divided the striatum, changes in density were found only in the asymmetric types of synapses, which signify glutamatergic inputs. In the patches (Figure 6), the data show a dichotomy in synaptic organization between TR and TNR. TNR have increased synaptic density compared to TRs or NCs for all synapses combined, asymmetric axospinous and asymmetric synapses. The density of asymmetric axodendritic synapses was increased in the TR subjects compared to both the controls and the TNR subjects. In striatal matrix (Figure 6), controls had fewer asymmetric axodendritic synapses than TR and fewer asymmetric synapses than TNR. In the matrix, controls had fewer asymmetric axodendritic synapses than TR and fewer asymmetric synapses than TNR.

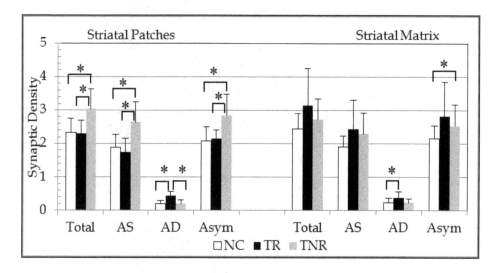

Fig. 6. Synaptic density in striatal patches and matrix.
Synaptic density (per $10\mu m^3$) is illustrated for various combinations of synapses in the patches and matrix (data combined for caudate and putamen). Total, all synapses combined, AS (asymmetric axospinous), AD (asymmetric axodendritic) and Asym (asymmetric synapses). P values are shown for LSD posthoc t-tests (*, $p<0.05$).

Synaptic density was examined in the caudate nucleus and putamen (patches and matrix combined) and differences were found here as well (Figure 7). Asymmetric axospinous synapses were higher in density in treatment non-responders significantly in the putamen, with a similar nonsignificant pattern in the caudate. The density of this type of synapse was similar between treatment responders and controls. Asymmetric axodendritic synapses were selectively elevated in the treatment responders in comparison to both controls and treatment nonresponders (Figure 7).

Ultrastructural Distinctions Between Treatment Responders and Non-Responders in Schizophrenia: Postmortem Studies of the Striatum

13

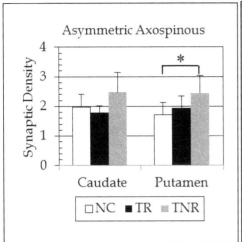 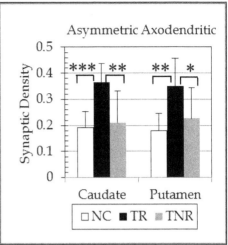

Fig. 7. Asymmetric axospinous and axodendritic synapses in caudate and putamen. Synaptic density is the number of synapses per 10 μm³. P values are shown for LSD posthoc t-tests (*, p<0.05; **, p<0.008; ***, p<0.002).

3.2 Striatal mitochondria

We have previously quantified mitochondria in cohorts of schizophrenia patients as a group and divided into various subsets (Somerville et al., 2011a,b). In a recent paper, we reported differences in mitochondrial density in SZ subjects divided by treatment response. Here we highlight the major changes we found in that study (Somerville et al., 2011b). The number of mitochondria per synapse was significantly different among groups for both the caudate

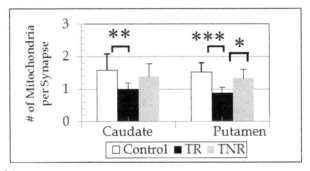

Fig. 8. Mitochondria per synapse.
Graph comparing the number of mitochondria per synapse in the caudate nucleus and putamen. ANOVA showed significant group differences for both the caudate nucleus (p<0.025) and the putamen (p<0.002). In the caudate nucleus, treatment responsive SZ subjects had fewer mitochondria per synapse than that of the NCs. In the putamen, there were significantly fewer mitochondria per synapse in treatment responsive SZ subjects compared to both NCs and treatment resistant SZ subjects. Asterisks indicate results of LSD post-hoc t-tests:* p< 0.05, ** p<0.01, ***, p<0.001. This graph is a modification of Figure 5 from Somerville et al., (2010b).

and putamen (Figure 8). Compared to controls, TR schizophrenia subjects had a 37-43% decrease in the number of mitochondria per synapse in the caudate nucleus and putamen. In the putamen, treatment responsive subjects also had decreases in this measure compared to treatment resistant subjects (34%). Our results provide further support for a biological distinction between treatment response and treatment resistance in schizophrenia.

3.3 Dopaminergic terminals in the caudate nucleus

The features of dopaminergic terminals and synapses have been described previously for normal human striatum (Kung et al., 1998) and quantified in schizophrenia (Roberts et al., 2009). Here we show the key features of those studies.

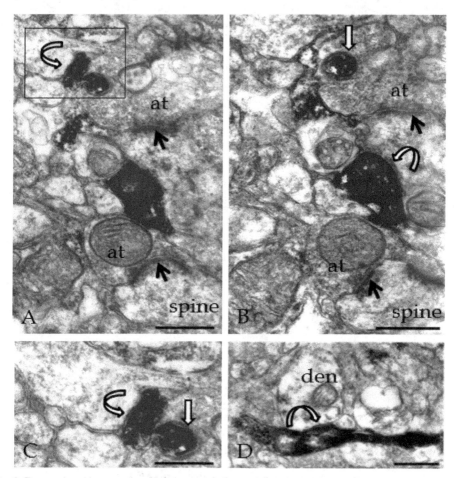

Fig. 9. Dopaminergic synapses in human caudate nucleus.
A,B) Serial sections showing several synaptic arrangements. TH-labeled axons (straight white arrows outlined in black) are adjacent to unlabeled axon terminals (at) that are forming asymmetric synapses (black arrows) with spines. TH-labeled terminals make

symmetric synapses (curved white arrows outlined in black) in both micrographs. C) Boxed
area in panel A is enlarged to show the symmetric synapse (curved white arrow outlined in
black). D) TH-labeled axon makes a symmetric synapse (arrow) *en passant* with a dendrite
(den). A modification of Figure 1, taken from Roberts et al., 2009.

Briefly, the features of TH-labeled structures were qualitatively similar between NCs and SZ
subjects. TH-labeled axons were often in close proximity to large unlabeled terminals that
formed asymmetric synapses (Figure 9A,B). Synapses were formed by TH-labeled axon
terminals (Figure 9A-C) and boutons *en passant* (Figure 9D). TH-labeled axon terminals
formed short symmetric synapses with spines and dendritic shafts (Figure 9A-D).

Next, we quantified TH-labeled axon terminals forming synapses in schizophrenia subjects
divided by treatment response or resistance (Roberts et al., 2009). The total density of TH-
labeled synapses was larger in treatment responsive SZs than either the controls or the
treatment resistant SZs (Figure 10). This represented a 43% and 51% larger density in the
treatment responsive SZs versus the controls and the treatment non-responsive SZs,
respectively. TH-labeled axodendritic synapses accounted for this difference with higher in
density in treatment responsive SZs compared to treatment resistant SZ and the controls.
This represented an 80% and 160% higher density in the treatment responsive SZ versus
controls and treatment resistant SZs, respectively. The number of TH-labeled axospinous
synapses was similar among all groups.

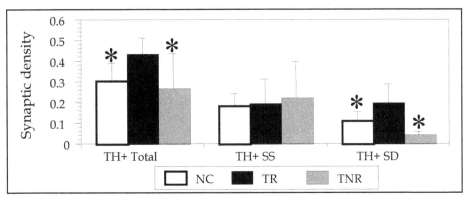

Fig. 10. Synaptic density of dopaminergic synapses in schizophrenia.
Tyrosine hydroxylase (TH) was used to identify dopaminergic synapses. Graph of the
density (per 10μm³) of TH-labeled (TH+) terminals forming synapses in controls (NC),
treatment responsive (TR) and treatment resistant (TNR) subjects. ANOVA results: TH+
Total, p<0.057; TH+ SS, p<0.888; TH+ SD, p<0.017. Total refers to all TH-labeled synapses
regardless of subtype. The density of total TH+ synapses and of TH+ symmetric
axodendritic (SD) synapses is greater in TR than NCs and TNR (*=p<0.05). A modification
of Figure 2, taken from Roberts et al., 2009.

4. Discussion

This chapter presents new data on the synaptic organization in the postmortem striatum of
treatment responsive vs. non responsive schizophrenia subjects, as well as presenting
methods and key results of two of our previous studies on dopaminergic synapses (Roberts

et al., 2009) and mitochondria (Somerville et al., 2011b) in these same subjects. We will discuss the results of each study and then a synthesis of all the results with respect to one another and what is known in the literature.

4.1 Differential organization of asymmetric synapses in TR vs. TNR

Changes in density were found only in the asymmetric types of synapses, which signify glutamatergic inputs. In the striatal patches, which process limbic information, TNR have more cortical type synapses (AS) and more glutamatergic synapses than TR and normal controls (NC). Our findings of an increased density of synapses characteristic of corticostriatal inputs in the striatal compartment that processes limbic circuitry in TNR SZ is consistent with several reports in the literature. In vivo imaging studies have shown that regional cerebral blood flow in the anterior cingulate cortex, which is involved in limbic circuitry, is elevated in normal control people given the psychotomimetic ketamine (Lahti et al. 1995; Vollenweider et al. 1997). Similarly, a direct relationship between positive psychotic symptoms and regional cerebral blood flow has been found in the hippocampus, but only when the patients are off medication (Medoff et al. 2001). These findings suggest that psychosis is associated with more activity in the cingulate and hippocampus, an interpretation that is consistent with hyperinnervation farther downstream in the striatal patches. Moreover, psychotomimetics given to animals produce increased spine density and upregulation of markers of axon sprouting (Li et al. 2003; Ujike et al. 2002), suggesting a link between psychosis and increased numbers of axospinous synapses. Thus, we interpret that the increase in density of glutamatergic type synapses in striatal patches in SZ TNR may be related to psychosis and may be an integral part of the disease. If so, the failure to normalize this anomaly may contribute to treatment resistance and persistent psychosis.

Another change which distinguished TR from TNR was the density of asymmetric axodendritic synapses, which are typical of some cortical inputs, but mostly thalamic inputs (see Introduction for references). The TR group had more of this type of synapse than that of the controls or the TNR group. These changes were present in both patches and matrix, caudate and putamen. The increase in density may be compensatory and could play a role in treatment response.

The glutamatergic system is heavily implicated in schizophrenia and examining possible aberrant circuitry or lack of plasticity may provide new insights into treatment options (Coyle 2006; Goff & Coyle 2001; Javitt 2004; Krystal 2008). Glutamate *hypofunction* has long been implicated in psychosis and schizophrenia based on the observation that psychotomimetic agents such as PCP and ketamine block NMDA receptors; however, therapeutic manipulations to restore glutamate tone have not been successful (Javitt & Zukin 1991; Javitt 2010; Kantrowitz & Javitt 2010a, b). A glutamate *hyperfunction* hypothesis has gained recent attention. There is recent MRS evidence of increased glutamate in the striatum in drug free and treated schizophrenia subjects (de la Fuente-Sandoval et al., 2009), which validates our finding of increased glutamatergic type synapses in the striatum of subjects with schizophrenia (Roberts et al., 2005a,b). Importantly for the present results, lamotrigine, which decreases glutamate release (Yuen, 1994), augments clozapine's effects in treatment resistant SZ and attenuates ketamine induced psychosis in normal controls (Dursun & Deakin 2001; Tiihonen et al. 2003). These clinical studies linking improvement in symptoms in TNR with an agent that blocks glutamate is supportive of our data showing increased glutamate type synapses only in treatment non-responders.

4.2 Mitochondria

The main results of that study (Somerville et al., 2011b) show fewer numbers of mitochondria per synapse in treatment responsive SZs vs. NCs in both the caudate nucleus and the putamen. In addition, treatment responsive SZs had significantly fewer mitochondria per synapse than that of the treatment resistant subjects in the putamen. The observation that the treatment responders have fewer mitochondria per synapse compared to treatment resistant SZs suggests a possible compensatory mechanism that may be related to the ability to respond to treatment. Mitochondria change location in response to cellular energy demands and the stage of their own life cycle. It is unclear if the decrease in number of mitochondria per synapse is a reflection of death, fewer numbers, failure of the mitochondria to move from the cell bodies of origin or overall decreased function and return to the soma. In the same cases as those in the present paper we have shown an increase in the density of synapses in the caudate nucleus and putamen patches (Roberts et al 2005a,b). Synapses need energy to form and to function properly (Wong-Riley, 1989). The decrease in density of mitochondria in terminals forming synapses may be an adaptive response to normalize overactive neurotransmission. Future studies will address if the number of mitochondria is decreased in particular populations of synapses. Based on our data, mitochondrial density at the synapse is differentially affected in SZ according to treatment response. Understanding the role that mitochondria might play in SZ could lead to better comprehension of the mechanisms of APDs to alleviate psychotic symptoms and alter brain metabolism, and what goes awry in treatment resistance.

4.3 Dopaminergic synapses

The main results of that study (Roberts et al., 2009) showed that treatment responsive SZs have more dopaminergic synapses, as identified by TH-labeled terminals, than do treatment resistant SZs or controls. These changes were specific for the axodendritic subtype of TH-labeled synapses. Several imaging studies have demonstrated enhanced dopamine release in response to an amphetamine challenge in drug free SZ subjects (Abi-Dargham et al., 1998; Breier et al., 1997; Laruelle et al., 1996, 1999; Lindstrom et al., 1999) or neuroleptic naïve SZ subjects (Laruelle et al., 1999) compared to controls. Importantly, drug free patients who eventually responded to antipsychotic drugs had elevated dopamine release compared to those subjects who never respond to treatment (Abi-Dargham et al., 2000). The higher density of dopaminergic synapses in TR SZs may explain the results of *in vivo* studies that have measured dopamine content in live patients. However, more dopaminergic synapses may not relate to higher tonic dopamine levels. There could be several other explanations for these data, including but not limited to: differential affinity for dopamine receptors, different postsynaptic mechanisms, and/or different amounts of dopamine. Differential blockade of D_2 receptors does not appear to be responsible since treatment resistant SZs have 95% D_2 receptor occupancy (Coppens et al., 1991). The results of our study suggest that one anatomical underpinning of TR may a higher density of terminals containing dopamine.

4.4 Are ultrastructural changes related to state, trait or medication?

We have previously discussed the relationship of medication on our findings (Roberts et al., 2009; Somerville et al., 2011b). Importantly for the present data sets is the potential problem that the APDs taken by subjects in the TR and TNR groups were statistically different.

However, a regression analysis of APD type and the synaptic measures in which we found differences yielded no correlations. Moreover, APDs only help positive symptoms, and studies now show that with the exception of clozapine, typical and atypical APDs alleviate positive symptoms to the same extent (Kane et al., 2008; Lieberman et al., 2005; McEvoy, 2006; McEvoy et al., 2006). Therefore, even though the SZ subgroups were composed of different numbers of subjects on typical versus atypical APDs, the possibility that the difference in results between the groups is related to medication seems unlikely.

An important issue still unresolved in these sets of experiments is if the ultrastructural features that distinguish TR from TNR are present before or at disease onset, or reflect the ability or lack thereof to respond to treatment. Since psychotomimetics induce increased spine density and upregulation of markers of axon terminals (Li et al. 2003; Ujike et al. 2002), the increase in density of glutamatergic type synapses in SZ TNR may be related to psychosis. The interpretation we favor at this time is that the increased synaptic density in TNR reflects an integral part of the disease, which these subjects fail to normalize, and this lack of plasticity contributes to treatment resistance and persistent psychosis. With regard to our findings of increased dopaminergic synapses in TR cases, but normal numbers in TNR cases, our results are consistent with the dopaminergic hypothesis of schizophrenia and what has been shown with live people who are TR. SZ subjects who eventually respond to APDs have more striatal dopamine, while those SZ who remain TNR have normal levels. It is therefore not surprising that the TNR, who have normal levels of striatal dopamine, but who are psychotic, are not helped by drugs that block dopamine. The road to psychosis for TNR may be different from those subjects who are TR, and may include glutamate abnormalities in striatum. Of the three studies reported or reviewed herein, the mitochondria data is the hardest to understand. It remains to be determined whether the TRs, who have fewer mitochondria per synapse compared to TNR and NCs, have that feature at the onset of disease or if this is a compensatory mechanism that may be related to the ability to respond to treatment.

5. Conclusion

Our previous studies has shown that compared to controls, the striatum of SZ subjects has increased synaptic density, decreased spine size, and changes in mitochondrial distribution. In the studies summarized herein, we show differential changes in ultrastructural organization that distinguish treatment responsive from nonresponsive SZ subjects. Our postmortem results are consistent with in vivo studies suggesting a biological basis to treatment response and resistance. We hypothesized that SZ subjects that were psychotic (off drug or nonresponders) would have different alterations than treatment responsive SZ subjects. Striatal synaptic organization has been worked out in animals and by identifying morphological features of the synapse, it is possible to infer connectivity and function. In the striatal patches, which process limbic information, TNR seem to have more cortical type synapses and more glutamatergic type synapses than TR and normal controls (NC). The abnormal density of corticostriatal inputs in areas that process limbic information in TNR may be an integral part of the disease, as psychosis is linked to abnormally large amounts of synapses. If so, the failure to normalize this may contribute to treatment resistance and persistent psychosis. TR subjects have normal amounts of corticostriatal type synapses and either have normal amounts at the disease onset or may have abnormally dense synapses like the TNR, but are able to normalize this measure. TRs have more synapses characteristic of thalamic inputs and dopaminergic synapses than NCs and TNRs. In addition the number of mitochondria per synapse is less than that of NCs and TNR. Increased dopamine synapses may be trait dependent as first episode SZ subjects who eventually respond to treatment have more dopamine as shown in in vivo imaging studies. Increased thalamic input and decreased mitochondria per synapse may be trait dependent as well, or may be compensatory and contribute to treatment response. Our results provide further support for a biological distinction between treatment response and treatment resistance in schizophrenia. Our data show an anatomical distinction between TR and TNR. Moreover, these data have important implications suggesting a biological basis to treatment response and resistance.

6. Acknowledgments

The authors wish to thank: 1) the members of the Maryland Brain Collection for the postmortem brain samples; 2) Drs. Adrienne Lahti and Roger Ridgeway for discussions and ideas about this line of research; and 3) Rosie Ricks for help with preparation of this manuscript. This research was supported in part by MH60744 (RCR) and MH073461 (SS).

7. References

Abi-Dargham, A., Gil, R., Krystal, J., Baldwin, R.M., Seibyl, J.P., et al. (1998). Increased striatal dopamine transmission in schizophrenia: confirmation in a second cohort. *American J Psych* 155 (6), pp. 761-767. ISSN 0002-953X.

Abi-Dargham, A., Rodenhiser, J., Printz, D., Zea-Ponce, Y., Gil, R., et al. (2000). Increased baseline occupancy of D2 receptors by dopamine in schizophrenia. *PNAS, USA* 97 (14), pp. 8104-8109. ISSN 0027-8424.

Alexander, G.E., DeLong, M.R. & Strick, P.L. (1986). Parallel organization of functionally segregated circuits linking basal ganglia and cortex. *Annual Review of Neuroscience* 9 pp. 357-381. ISSN 0147-006X.

Altamura, A.C., Bassetti, R., Cattaneo, E. & Vismara, S. (2005). Some biological correlates of drug resistance in schizophrenia: a multidimensional approach. *World J Biol Psych* 6 Suppl 2 pp. 23-30. ISSN 1562-2975.

APA. (1994) *Diagnostic and Statistical Manual of Mental Disorders. 4th ed*, American Psychiatric Press, Washington, DC.

Arango, C., Breier, A., McMahon, R., Carpenter, W.T., Jr. & Buchanan, R.W. (2003). The relationship of clozapine and haloperidol treatment response to prefrontal, hippocampal, and caudate brain volumes. *American J Psych* 160 (8), pp. 1421-1427. ISSN 0002-953X.

Beerpoot, L.J., Lipska, B.K. & Weinberger, D.R. (1996). Neurobiology of treatment-resistant schizophrenia: new insights and new models. *European Neuropsychopharmacology* 6 Suppl 2 pp. S27-34. ISSN 0924-977X.

Bennett, B.D. & Bolam, J.P. (1994). Synaptic input and output of parvalbumin-immuno-reactive neurons in the neostriatum of the rat. *Neuroscience* 62 (3), pp. 707-719.

Ben-Shachar, D. (2002). Mitochondrial dysfunction in schizophrenia: a possible linkage to dopamine. *J Neurochemistry* 83 (6), pp. 1241-1251. ISSN 0022-3042.

Ben-Shachar, D. & Laifenfeld, D. (2004). Mitochondria, synaptic plasticity, and schizophrenia. *International Review of Neurobiology* 59 pp. 273-296. ISSN 0074-7742.

Bilder, R.M., Wu, H., Chakos, M.H., Bogerts, B., Pollack, S., et al. (1994). Cerebral morphometry and clozapine treatment in schizophrenia. *J Clinical Psych* 55 Suppl B pp. 53-56.

Bouyer, J.J., Park, D.H., Joh, T.H. & Pickel, V.M. (1984). Chemical and structural analysis of the relation between cortical inputs and tyrosine hydroxylase-containing terminals in rat neostriatum. *Brain Research* 302 (2), pp. 267-275.

Brandt, G.N. & Bonelli, R.M. (2008). Structural neuroimaging of the basal ganglia in schizophrenic patients: a review. *Wien Med Wochenschr* 158 (3-4), pp. 84-90. ISSN 1563-258X.

Breier, A., Su, T.P., Saunders, R., Carson, R.E., Kolachana, B.S., et al. (1997). Schizophrenia is associated with elevated amphetamine-induced synaptic dopamine concentrations: evidence from a novel positron emission tomography method. *PNAS, USA* 94 (6), pp. 2569-2574.

Brenner, H.D., Dencker, S.J., Goldstein, M.J., Hubbard, J.W., Keegan, D.L., et al. (1990). Defining treatment refractoriness in schizophrenia. *Schiz Bull* 16 (4), pp. 551-561.

Buchsbaum, M.S. & Hazlett, E.A. (1998). Positron emission tomography studies of abnormal glucose metabolism in schizophrenia. *Schiz Bull* 24 (3), pp. 343-364 ISSN 0586-7614.

Cepeda, C. & Levine, M.S. (1998). Dopamine and N-methyl-D-aspartate receptor interactions in the neostriatum. *Developmental Neuroscience* 20 (1), pp. 1-18.

Cepeda, C., Hurst, R.S., Altemus, K.L., Flores-Hernandez, J., Calvert, C.R., et al. (2001). Facilitated glutamatergic transmission in the striatum of D2 dopamine receptor-deficient mice. *J Neurophysiology* 85 (2), pp. 659-670.

Chakos, M.H., Lieberman, J.A., Bilder, R.M., Borenstein, M., Lerner, G., et al. (1994). Increase in caudate nuclei volumes of first-episode schizophrenic patients taking antipsychotic drugs. *American J Psych* 151 (10), pp. 1430-1436.

Chung, J.W., Hassler, R. & Wagner, A. (1977). Degeneration of two of nine types of synapses in the putamen after center median coagulation in the cat. *Exp Brain Research* 28 (3-4), pp. 345-361.

Conley, R.R. & Kelly, D.L. (2001). Management of treatment resistance in schizophrenia. *Biol Psych* 50 (11), pp. 898-911.

Coppens, H.J., Slooff, C.J., Paans, A.M., Wiegman, T., Vaalburg, W., et al. (1991). High central D2-dopamine receptor occupancy as assessed with positron emission tomography in medicated but therapy-resistant schizophrenic patients. *Biol Psych* 29 (7), pp. 629-634. ISSN 0006-3223.

Cote, P.Y., Levitt, P. & Parent, A. (1995). Distribution of limbic system-associated membrane protein immunoreactivity in primate basal ganglia. *Neuroscience* 69 (1), pp. 71-81.

Coyle, J.T. (2006). Glutamate and schizophrenia: beyond the dopamine hypothesis. *Cellular and Molecular Neurobiology* 26 (4-6), pp. 365-384. ISSN 0272-4340.

Creese, I., Burt, D.R. & Snyder, S.H. (1976). Dopamine receptor binding predicts clinical and pharmacological potencies of antischizophrenic drugs. *Science* 192 (4238), pp. 481-483.

Dao-Castellana, M.H., Paillere-Martinot, M.L., Hantraye, P., Attar-Levy, D., Remy, P., et al.
    (1997). Presynaptic dopaminergic function in the striatum of schizophrenic
    patients. *Schiz Research* 23 (2), pp. 167-174.
de la Fuente-Sandoval, C., Favila, R., Alvarado, P., León-Ortiz, P., Díaz-Galvis, L., et al.
    (2009). Glutamate increase in the associative striatum in schizophrenia: a
    longitudinal magnetic resonance spectroscopy preliminary study. *Gaceta Médica de
    México* 145 (2), pp. 109-113.
DeLong, M.R. & Wichmann, T. (2007). Circuits and circuit disorders of the basal ganglia.
    Archives of Neurology 64 (1), pp. 20-24. ISSN 0003-9942.
DiFiglia, M. & Aronin, N. (1982). Ultrastructural features of immunoreactive somatostatin
    neurons in the rat caudate nucleus. *J Neuroscience* 2 (9), pp. 1267-1274.
DiFiglia, M. (1987). Synaptic organization of cholinergic neurons in the monkey
    neostriatum. *J Comparative Neurology* 255 (2), pp. 245-258.
Dursun, S.M. & Deakin, J.F. (2001). Augmenting antipsychotic treatment with lamotrigine or
    topiramate in patients with treatment-resistant schizophrenia: a naturalistic case-
    series outcome study. *J Psychopharmacology* 15 (4), pp. 297-301. ISSN 0269-8811.
Freund, T.F., Powell, J.F. & Smith, A.D. (1984). Tyrosine hydroxylase-immunoreactive
    boutons in synaptic contact with identified striatonigral neurons, with particular
    reference to dendritic spines. *Neuroscience* 13 (4), pp. 1189-1215.
Geinisman, Y., Gundersen, H.J., van der Zee, E. & West, M.J. (1996). Unbiased stereological
    estimation of the total number of synapses in a brain region. *J Neurocytology* 25 (12),
    pp. 805-819.
Gemmell, H.G., Evans, N.T., Besson, J.A., Roeda, D., Davidson, J., et al. (1990). Regional
    cerebral blood flow imaging: a quantitative comparison of technetium-99m-
    HMPAO SPECT with C15O2 PET. *J Nuclear Medicine* 31 (10), pp. 1595-1600. ISSN
    0161-5505.
Gerfen, C.R. (1984). The neostriatal mosaic: compartmentalization of corticostriatal input
    and striatonigral output systems. *Nature* 311 (5985), pp. 461-464.
Gerfen, C.R., McGinty, J.F. & young, W.S, 3rd. (1991). Dopamine differentially regulates
    dynorphin, substance P, and enkephalin expression in striatal neurons: in situ
    hybridization histochemical analysis. *J Neuroscience* 11 (4), pp. 1016-1031.
Goff, D.C. & Coyle, J.T. (2001). The emerging role of glutamate in the pathophysiology and
    treatment of schizophrenia. *American J Psych* 158, pp. 1367-1377. ISSN 0002-953X.
Graybiel, A.M. & Ragsdale, C.W., Jr. (1978). Histochemically distinct compartments in the
    striatum of human, monkeys, and cat demonstrated by acetylthiocholinesterase
    staining. *PNAS, USA* 75 (11), pp. 5723-5726. ISSN 0027-8424.
Graybiel, A.M. & Hickey, T.L. (1982). Chemospecificity of ontogenetic units in the striatum:
    demonstration by combining [3H]thymidine neuronography and histochemical
    staining. *PNAS, USA* 79 (1), pp. 198-202.
Graybiel, A.M. (1991). Basal ganglia--input, neural activity, and relation to the cortex. *Curr
    Opin Neurobiol* 1 (4), pp. 644-651. 0959-4388.
Graybiel, A.M. (2005). The basal ganglia: learning new tricks and loving it. *Current Opinion
    in Neurobiology* 15 (6), pp. 638-644. ISSN 0959-4388.

Haber, S.N., Fudge, J.L. & McFarland, N.R. (2000). Striatonigrostriatal pathways in primates form an ascending spiral from the shell to the dorsolateral striatum. *J Neuroscience* 20 (6), pp. 2369-2382.

Harrison, P.J. (1999). The neuropathology of schizophrenia. A critical review of the data and their interpretation. *Brain* 122 (Pt 4) pp. 593-624. ISSN 0006-8950.

Hietala, J., Syvalahti, E., Vuorio, K., Rakkolainen, V., Bergman, J., et al., (1995). Presynaptic dopamine function in striatum of neuroleptic-naive schizophrenic patients. *Lancet* 346(8983):1130-1131.

Hietala, J., Syvalahti, E., Vilkman, H., Vuorio, K., Rakkolainen, V., et al., (1999). Depressive symptoms and presynaptic dopamine function in neuroleptic-naive schizophrenia. *Schiz Research* 35(1):41-50.

Hirvonen, J., van Erp, T.G., Huttunen, J., Aalto, S., Nagren, K., et al. (2005). Increased caudate dopamine D2 receptor availability as a genetic marker for schizophrenia. *Archives of General Psych* 62 (4), pp. 371-378.

Holt, D.J., Graybiel, A.M. & Saper, C.B. (1997). Neurochemical architecture of the human striatum. *J Comparative Neurology* 384 (1), pp. 1-25.

Hutcherson, L. & Roberts, R.C. (2005). The immunocytochemical localization of substance P in the human striatum: a postmortem ultrastructural study. *Synapse* 57 (4), pp. 191-201. ISSN 0887-4476.

Javitt, D.C. & Zukin, S.R. (1991). Recent advances in the phencyclidine model of schizophrenia. *American J Psych* 148 (10), pp. 1301-1308. ISSN 0002-953X

Javitt, D.C. (2004). Glutamate as a therapeutic target in psychiatric disorders. *Mol Psych* 9 (11), pp. 984-997, 979. ISSN 1359-4184

Javitt, D.C. (2010). Glutamatergic theories of schizophrenia. *The Israel J Psychiatry and Related Sciences* 47 (1), pp. 4-16.

Joel, D. & Weiner, I. (2000). The connections of the dopaminergic system with the striatum in rats and primates: an analysis with respect to the functional and compartmental organization of the striatum. *Neuroscience* 96 (3), pp. 451-474. ISSN 0306-4522.

Kane, J.M., Honigfeld, G., Singer, J. & Meltzer, H. (1988). Clozapine in treatment-resistant schizophrenics. *Psychopharmacology Bull* 24 (1), pp. 62-67.

Kantrowitz, J.T. & Javitt, D.C. (2010). Thinking glutamatergically: changing concepts of schizophrenia based upon changing neurochemical models. *Clinical Schizophrenia and Related Psychoses* 4 (3), pp. 189-200. ISSN 1935-1232.

Kemp, J.M. & Powell, T.P. (1971a). The structure of the caudate nucleus of the cat: light and electron microscopy. *Philosophical Transactions of the Royal Society of London. Series B, Biological Sciences* 262 (845), pp. 383-401.

Kemp, J.M. & Powell, T.P. (1971b). The termination of fibres from the cerebral cortex and thalamus upon dendritic spines in the caudate nucleus: a study with the Golgi method. *Philosophical Transactions of the Royal Society of London. Series B, Biol Sciences* 262 (845), pp. 429-439.

Kemp, J.M. & Powell, T.P. (1971c). The site of termination of afferent fibres in the caudate nucleus. *Philosophical Transactions of the Royal Society of London. Series B, Biol Sciences* 262 (845), pp. 413-427.

Kleinman, J.E., Hong, J., Iadarola, M., Govoni, S. & Gillin, C.J. (1985). Neuropeptides in human brain--postmortem studies. *Program Neuropsychopharmacology Biol Psych* 9 (1), pp. 91-95.

Kreczmanski, P., Heinsen, H., Mantua, V., Woltersdorf, F., Masson, T., et al. (2007). Volume, neuron density and total neuron number in five subcortical regions in schizophrenia. *Brain* 130 (Pt 3), pp. 678-692. ISSN 1460-2156.

Krystal, J.H. (2008). Capitalizing on extrasynaptic glutamate neurotransmission to treat antipsychotic-resistant symptoms in schizophrenia. *Biol Psych* 64 (5), pp. 358-360. ISSN 0006-3223.

Kubota, Y., Inagaki, S., Kito, S. & Wu, J.Y. (1987a). Dopaminergic axons directly make synapses with GABAergic neurons in the rat neostriatum. *Brain Research* 406 (1-2), pp. 147-156.

Kubota, Y., Inagaki, S., Shimada, S., Kito, S., Eckenstein, F., et al. (1987b). Neostriatal cholinergic neurons receive direct synaptic inputs from dopaminergic axons. *Brain Research* 413 (1), pp. 179-184.

Kung, L. & Roberts, R.C. (1999). Mitochondrial pathology in human schizophrenic striatum: a postmortem ultrastructural study. *Synapse* 31 (1), pp. 67-75.

Kung, L., Force, M., Chute, D.J. & Roberts, R.C. (1998). Immunocytochemical localization of tyrosine hydroxylase in the human striatum: a postmortem ultrastructural study. *J Comparative Neurology* 390 (1), pp. 52-62.

Lahti, R.A., Cochrane, E.V., Roberts, R.C. & Tamminga, C.A. (1998) [³H]-Neurotensin receptor densities in human postmortem tissue obtained from normal and schizophrenic persons. An autoradiographic study. *J Neural Transmission* (105), pp. 507-516.

Lahti, A.C., Holcomb, H.H., Medoff, D.R. & Tamminga, C.A. (1995). Ketamine activates psychosis and alters limbic blood flow in schizophrenia. *NeuroReport* 6 (6), pp. 869-872.

Lahti, A.C., Holcomb, H.H., Weiler, M.A., Medoff, D.R. & Tamminga, C.A. (2003). Functional effects of antipsychotic drugs: comparing clozapine with haloperidol. *Biol Psych* 53 (7), pp. 601-608.

Laruelle, M., Abi-Dargham, A., van Dyck, C.H., Gil, R., D'Souza, C.D., et al. (1996). Single photon emission computerized tomography imaging of amphetamine-induced dopamine release in drug-free schizophrenic subjects. *PNAS, USA* 93 (17), pp. 9235-9240.

Laruelle, M., Abi-Dargham, A., Gil, R., Kegeles, L. & Innis, R. (1999). Increased dopamine transmission in schizophrenia: relationship to illness phases. *Biol Psych* 46 (1), pp. 56-72.

Lavoie, B. & Parent, A. (1990). Immunohistochemical study of the serotoninergic innervation of the basal ganglia in the squirrel monkey. *J Comparative Neurology* 299, pp. 1-16.

Levesque, M. & Parent, A. (1998). Axonal arborization of corticostriatal and corticothalamic fibers arising from prelimbic cortex in the rat. *Cerebral Cortex* 8 (7), pp. 602-613.

Li, Y., Kolb, B. & Robinson, T.E. (2003). The location of persistent amphetamine-induced changes in the density of dendritic spines on medium spiny neurons in the nucleus accumbens and caudate-putamen. *Neuropsychopharmacology* 28 (6), pp. 1082-1085.

Lindstrom, L.H., Gefvert, O., Hagberg, G., Lundberg, T., Bergstrom, M., Hartvig, P., & Langstrom, B. (1999). Increased dopamine synthesis rate in medial prefrontal cortex and striatum in schizophrenia indicated by L-(ß-11C) DOPA and PET. *Biol Psych* 46(5):681-688.

Liu, F.C. & Graybiel, A.M. (1992). Heterogeneous development of calbindin-D28K expression in the striatal matrix. *J Comparative Neurology* 320 (3), pp. 304-322.

Mamah, D., Wang, L., Barch, D., de Erausquin, G.A., Gado, M., et al. (2007). Structural analysis of the basal ganglia in schizophrenia. *Schiz Research* 89 (1-3), pp. 59-71. ISSN 0920-9964.

Mamah, D., Harms, M.P., Wang, L., Barch, D., Thompson, P., et al. (2008). Basal ganglia shape abnormalities in the unaffected siblings of schizophrenia patients. *Biol Psych* 64 (2), pp. 111-120. ISSN 1873-2402.

McEvoy, J.P. (2006). An overview of the Clinical Antipsychotic Trials of Intervention Effectiveness (CATIE) study. *CNS Spectrums* 11 (7 Suppl 7), pp. 4-8. ISSN 1092-8529

Medoff, D.R., Holcomb, H.H., Lahti, A.C. & Tamminga, C.A. (2001). Probing the human hippocampus using rCBF: contrasts in schizophrenia. *Hippocampus* 11, pp. 543-550.

Meltzer, H.Y. (1997). Treatment-resistant schizophrenia--the role of clozapine. *Current Medical Research and Opinion* 14 (1), pp. 1-20. ISSN 0300-7995

Mitelman, S.A., Shihabuddin, L., Brickman, A.M. & Buchsbaum, M.S. (2005). Cortical intercorrelations of temporal area volumes in schizophrenia. *Schiz Research* 76 (2-3), pp. 207-229. ISSN 0920-9964.

Mitelman, S.A., Canfield, E.L., Chu, K.W., Brickman, A.M., Shihabuddin, L., et al. (2009). Poor outcome in chronic schizophrenia is associated with progressive loss of volume of the putamen. *Schiz Research* 113, pp. 241-245. ISSN 1573-2509.

Nudmamud-Thanoi, S., Piyabhan, P., Harte, M.K., Cahir, M. & Reynolds, G.P. (2007). Deficits of neuronal glutamatergic markers in the caudate nucleus in schizophrenia. *J Neural Transm Suppl* (72), pp. 281-285. ISSN 0303-6995.

Onn, S.P., West, A.R. & Grace, A.A. (2000). Dopamine-mediated regulation of striatal neuronal and network interactions. *Trends in Neuroscience* 23 (10 Suppl), pp. S48-56.

Parent, A. & Hazrati, L.N. (1995). Functional anatomy of the basal ganglia. I. The cortico-basal ganglia-thalamo-cortical loop. *Brain Research Reviews* 20 (1), pp. 91-127.

Pasik, P., Pasik, T. & DiFiglia, M. (1976). Quantitative aspects of neuronal organization in the neostriatum of the macaque monkey. *Research Publications-Association for Research in Nervous and Mental Disease* 55 pp. 57-90.

Penny, G.R., Wilson, C.J. & Kitai, S.T. (1988). Relationship of the axonal and dendritic geometry of spiny projection neurons to the compartmental organization of the neostriatum. *J Comparative Neurology* 269 (2), pp. 275-289.

Perez-Costas, E., Melendez-Ferro, M. & Roberts, R. (2007). Microscopy techniques and the study of synapses, In: *Name of Book*, (Mendez-Vilas, A. & Diaz, J.), pp. 164-170, Formatex, ISBN 13: 978-84-611-9419-3, Badajoz, Spain.

Perez-Costas, E., Melendez-Ferro, M. & Roberts, R.C. (2010). Basal ganglia pathology in schizophrenia: dopamine connections and anomalies. *J Neurochemistry* 113 (2), pp. 287-302. ISSN 0022-3042.

Pickel, V.M., Sumal, K.K., Beckley, S.C., Miller, R.J. & Reis, D.J. (1980). Immunocytochemical localization of enkephalin in the neostriatum of rat brain: a light and electron microscopic study. *J Comparative Neurology* 189 (4), pp. 721-740.

Pickel, V.M., Beckley, S.C., Joh, T.H. & Reis, D.J. (1981). Ultrastructural immunocytochemical localization of tyrosine hydroxylase in the neostriatum. *Brain Research* 225 (2), pp. 373-385.

Powers, R.E. (1999). The neuropathology of schizophrenia. *J Neuropathology and Experimental Neurology* 58 (7), pp. 679-690.

Prensa, L., Gimenez-Amaya, J.M. & Parent, A. (1999). Chemical heterogeneity of the striosomal compartment in the human striatum. *J Comparative Neurology* 413 (4), pp. 603-618.

Prince, J.A., Blennow, K., Gottfries, C.G., Karlsson, I. & Oreland, L. (1999). Mitochondrial function is differentially altered in the basal ganglia of chronic schizophrenics. *Neuropsychopharmacology* 21 (3), pp. 372-379.

Rajarethinam, R., Upadhyaya, A., Tsou, P., Upadhyaya, M. & Keshavan, M.S. (2007). Caudate volume in offspring of patients with schizophrenia. *British J Psych* (191), pp. 258-259. ISSN 0007-1250.

Raju, D.V., Shah, D.J., Wright, T.M., Hall, R.A. & Smith, Y. (2006). Differential synaptology of vGluT2-containing thalamostriatal afferents between the patch and matrix compartments in rats. *J Comparative Neurology* 499 (2), pp. 231-243. ISSN 0021-9967.

Ribak, C.E., Vaughn, J.E. & Roberts, E. (1979). The GABA neurons and their axon terminals in rat corpus striatum as demonstrated by GAD immunocytochemistry. *J Comparative Neurology* 187 (2), pp. 261-283.

Roberts, R.C., Conley, R., Kung, L., Peretti, F.J. & Chute, D.J. (1996). Reduced striatal spine size in schizophrenia: a postmortem ultrastructural study. *NeuroReport* (7) pp. 1214-1218.

Roberts, R.C., Gaither, L.A., Gao, X.M., Kashyap, S.M. & Tamminga, C.A. (1995). Ultrastructural correlates of haloperidol-induced oral dyskinesias in rat striatum. *Synapse* 20 (3), pp. 234-243.

Roberts, R.C. & Knickman, J.K. (2002). The ultrastructural organization of the patch matrix compartments in the human striatum. *J Comparative Neurology* 452 (2), pp. 128-138.

Roberts, R.C., Roche, J.K. & Conley, R. (2005a). Synaptic differences in the patch matrix compartments of the striatum of subjects with schizophrenia: a postmortem ultrastructural analysis. *Neurobiology of Disease* 20 pp. 324-335.

Roberts, R.C., Roche, J.K. & Conley, R. (2005b). Synaptic differences in the postmortem striatum of subjects with schizophrenia: a stereological ultrastructural analysis. *Synapse* 56 pp. 185-197.

Roberts, R.C., Roche, J.K., Conley, R.R. & Lahti, A.C. (2007). Synaptic organization in postmortem striatum in subjects with schizophrenia: treatment responders vs. nonresponders. *Schiz Bull* 33:271.

Roberts, R.C., Roche, J.K., Conley, R.R. & Lahti, A.C. (2009). Dopaminergic synapses in the caudate of subjects with schizophrenia: Relationship to treatment response. *Synapse* 63 (6), pp. 520-530. ISSN 1098-2396.

Rodriguez, V.M., Andree, R.M., Castejon, M.J., Zamora, M.L., Alvaro, P.C., et al. (1997). Fronto-striato-thalamic perfusion and clozapine response in treatment-refractory schizophrenic patients. A 99mTc-HMPAO study. *Psych Research* 76 (1), pp. 51-61. ISSN 0165-1781.

Sadikot, A.F., Parent, A., Smith, Y. & Bolam, J.P. (1992). Efferent connections of the centromedian and parafascicular thalamic nuclei in the squirrel monkey: a light and electron microscopic study of the thalamostriatal projection in relation to striatal heterogeneity. *J Comparative Neurology* 320 (2), pp. 228-242.

Salzman, S., Endicott, J., Clayton, P. & Winokur, G. I. (1983) Diagnostic evaluation after death (DEAD).)., *National Institute of Mental Health, Neuroscience Research Branch*, Rockville, MD.

Seeman, P., Chau-Wong, M., Tedesco, J. & Wong, K. (1975). Brain receptors for antipsychotic drugs and dopamine: direct binding assays. *PNAS, USA* 72 (11), pp. 4376-4380. ISSN 0027-8424.

Seeman, P. & Lee, T. (1975). Antipsychotic drugs: direct correlation between clinical potency and presynaptic action on dopamine neurons. *Science* 188 (4194), pp. 1217-1219. ISSN 0036-8075.

Sheitman, B.B. & Lieberman, J.A. (1998). The natural history and pathophysiology of treatment resistant schizophrenia. *J Psych Research* 32, pp. 143-150. ISSN 0022-3956.

Sidibe, M. & Smith, Y. (1999). Thalamic inputs to striatal interneurons in monkeys: synaptic organization and co-localization of calcium binding proteins. *Neuroscience* 89 (4), pp. 1189-1208. ISSN 0306-4522.

Simpson, M.D., Slater, P., Royston, M.C. & Deakin, J.F. (1992). Regionally selective deficits in uptake sites for glutamate and gamma-aminobutyric acid in the basal ganglia in schizophrenia. *Psych Research* 42 (3), pp. 273-282.

Smith, Y., Bennett, B.D., Bolam, J.P., Parent, A. & Sadikot, A.F. (1994). Synaptic relationships between dopaminergic afferents and cortical or thalamic input in the sensorimotor territory of the striatum in monkey. *J Comparative Neurology* 344 (1), pp. 1-19.

Somerville, S.M., Conley, R.R. & Roberts, R.C. (2011a). Mitochondria in the striatum of subjects with schizophrenia. *World J Biol Psych* 12 (1), pp. 48-56. ISSN 1562-2975.

Somerville, S.M., Lahti, A.C., Conley, R.R. & Roberts, R.C. (2011b). Mitochondria in the striatum of subjects with schizophrenia: relationship to treatment response. *Synapse* 65 (3), pp. 215-224. ISSN 1098-2396.

Somogyi, P., Bolam, J.P. & Smith, A.D. (1981). Monosynaptic cortical input and local axon collaterals of identified striatonigral neurons. A light and electron microscopic study using the Golgi-peroxidase transport-degeneration procedure. *J Comparative Neurology* 195 (4), pp. 567-584.

Spitzer, R.L., Williams, J.B., Gibbon, M. & First, M.B. (1992). The Structured Clinical Interview for DSM-III-R (SCID). I: History, rationale, and description. *Archives of General Psych* 49 (8), pp. 624-629.

Staal, W.G., Hulshoff Pol, H.E., Schnack, H.G., van Haren, N.E., Seifert, N., et al. (2001). Structural brain abnormalities in chronic schizophrenia at the extremes of the outcome spectrum. *American J Psych* 158 (7), pp. 1140-1142. ISSN 0002-953X.

Stern, R.G., Kahn, R.S. & Davidson, M. (1993). Predictors of response to neuroleptic treatment in schizophrenia. *Psychiatric Clinics of North America* 16 (2), pp. 313-338. ISSN 0193-953X.

Stern, R.G., Kahn, R.S., Harvey, P.D., Amin, F., Apter, S.H., et al. (1993). Early response to haloperidol treatment in chronic schizophrenia. *Schiz Research* 10 (2), pp. 165-171. ISSN 0920-9964.

Tiihonen, J., Hallikainen, T., Ryynanen, O.P., Repo-Tiihonen, E., Kotilainen, I., et al. (2003). Lamotrigine in treatment-resistant schizophrenia: a randomized placebo-controlled crossover trial. *Biol Psych* 54 (11), pp. 1241-1248. ISSN 0006-3223.

Turkington, T.G., Jaszczak, R.J., Pelizzari, C.A., Harris, C.C., MacFall, J.R., et al. (1993). Accuracy of registration of PET, SPECT and MR images of a brain phantom. *J Nuclear Medicine* 34 (9), pp. 1587-1594. ISSN 0161-5505.

Ujike, H., Takaki, M., Kodama, M. & Kuroda, S. (2002). Gene expression related to synaptogenesis, neuritogenesis, and MAP kinase in behavioral sensitization to psychostimulants. *Annals of the New York Academy of Sciences* 965 pp. 55-67.

Uranova, N.A., Casanova, M.F., DeVaughn, N.M., Orlovskaya, D.D. & Denisov, D.V. (1996). Ultrastructural alterations of synaptic contacts and astrocytes in postmortem caudate nucleus of schizophrenic patients. *Schiz Research* 22 (1), pp. 81-83.

Uranova, N., Orlovskaya, D., Vikhreva, O., Zimina, I., Kolomeets, N., et al. (2001). Electron microscopy of oligodendroglia in severe mental illness. *Brain Research Bulletin* 55 (5), pp. 597-610.

Uranova, N.A., Vostrikov, V.M., Vikhreva, O.V., Zimina, I.S., Kolomeets, N.S., et al. (2007). The role of oligodendrocyte pathology in schizophrenia. *International J Neuropsychopharmacology* 10 (4), pp. 537-545. ISSN 1461-1457.

van der Kooy, D. & Fishell, G. (1987). Neuronal birthdate underlies the development of striatal compartments. *Brain Research* 401 (1), pp. 155-161.

Vollenweider, F.X., Leenders, K.L., Oye, I., Hell, D. & Angst, J. (1997). Differential psychopathology and patterns of cerebral glucose utilisation produced by (S)- and (R)-ketamine in healthy volunteers using positron emission tomography (PET). *European Neuropsychopharmacology* 7 (1), pp. 25-38.

Walker, R.H., Arbuthnott, G.W., Baughman, R.W. & Graybiel, A.M. (1993). Dendritic domains of medium spiny neurons in the primate striatum: relationships to striosomal borders. *J Comparative Neurology* 337 (4), pp. 614-628. ISSN 0021-9967.

West, A.R. & Grace, A.A. (2002). Opposite influences of endogenous dopamine D1 and D2 receptor activation on activity states and electrophysiological properties of striatal neurons: studies combining in vivo intracellular recordings and reverse microdialysis. *J Neuroscience* 22 (1), pp. 294-304.

White, N.M. & Hiroi, N. (1998). Preferential localization of self-stimulation sites in striosomes/patches in the rat striatum. *PNAS, USA* 95 (11), pp. 6486-6491.

Wilson, C.J. & Groves, P.M. (1980). Fine structure and synaptic connections of the common spiny neuron of the rat neostriatum: a study employing intracellular inject of horseradish peroxidase. *J Comparative Neurology* 194 (3), pp. 599-615.

Wong-Riley, M.T. (1989) Cytochrome oxidase: an endogenous metabolic marker for neuronal activity. *Trends in Neuroscience* (12) pp. 94-101.

Wong, D.F., Wagner, H.N., Jr., Tune, L.E., Dannals, R.F., Pearlson, G.D., et al. (1986). Positron emission tomography reveals elevated D2 dopamine receptors in drug-naive schizophrenics. *Science* 234 (4783), pp. 1558-1563.

Yuen, A.W. (1994). Lamotrigine: a review of antiepileptic efficacy. *Epilepsia* 35 Suppl 5 pp.
    S33-36. ISSN 0013-9580.
Yung, K.K., Smith, A.D., Levey, A.I. & Bolam, J.P. (1996). Synaptic connections between
    spiny neurons of the direct and indirect pathways in the neostriatum of the rat:
    evidence from dopamine receptor and neuropeptide immunostaining. *European J
    Neuroscience* 8 (5), pp. 861-869. ISSN 0953-816X.

2

Advances in the Pharmacotherapy of Bipolar Affective Disorder

Ashok Kumar Jainer, Rajkumar Kamatchi,
Marek Marzanski and Bettahalasoor Somashekar
Caludon Centre, Coventry,
United Kingdom

1. Introduction

Bipolar affective disorder is a chronic, relapsing and remitting mental illness with lifetime risk between 0.5 and 1.6% worldwide (Weissman et al. 1996). This prevalence increases to 5.5% for bipolar spectrum disorders comprising bipolar I, bipolar II and other subtypes (Reegeer et al. 2004). Bipolar disorder is a significant source of distress, disability, and loss of life through suicide (Woods 2000). It causes significant psychological and socioeconomic burden both to the patients and their carers. It remains as the sixth leading cause of disability among neuropsychiatric disorders in the world (WHO 1996). Almost 80% of the costs of bipolar disorder are indirect and only 5% is spent on drugs and another 15% on hospital charges (Dardennes et al 2006). If bipolar disorder is not treated adequately, relapses will occur more frequently with longer duration of episodes, decreased intervals between episodes and increased number of hospitalisation.

In this chapter we review the recent advances in the pharmacotherapy of bipolar affective disorder, the management of which is constantly evolving due to better understanding of its pathophysiology and introduction of new drug treatments.

2. Evolution of pharmacotherapy of bipolar disorder

The evolution of pharmacotherapy of bipolar disorder could be described in three stages: introduction of Lithium, discovery of mood stabilizing properties of anticonvulsants and development of atypical antipsychotics and other agents. Lithium carbonate has been used in the treatment of acute mania and in prophylaxis of bipolar affective disorders since 1949. First generation antipsychotics such as Haloperidol and Chlorpromazine were also helpful in the management of acute mania. However the response rate for Lithium was around 60% only, which made further search for other medications necessary. Anticonvulsants like Valproate and Carbamazepine have been introduced to the treatment of both acute phase and as maintenance therapy since the 1970's. Second generation antipsychotics began to emerge in the 1990's and numerous trials have systematically examined and proved their effectiveness. Olanzapine, Risperidone, Quetiapine, Ziprasidone and Aripiprazole have good efficacy in acute mania and some of them are also useful maintenance agents. Combinations of second generation antipsychotics with mood stabilisers have shown some advantages in comparison to monotherapy with Lithium and Valproate. Recently Lamotrigine has been investigated for both acute and prophylactic treatment of bipolar II disorder. Other agents like Topiramate and Tamoxifen have also been studied but with no convincing results.

3. Advances in the treatment of bipolar disorder

The evidence for each of these various medications and therapeutic strategies is reviewed in the treatment of acute mania and mixed episodes, bipolar depression and in maintenance therapy.

3.1 Acute mania and mixed episodes

Mania is characterised by elated, expansive mood, increased activity, pressure of speech and flight of ideas, grandiose delusions and impaired insight. In mixed episodes, both manic and depressive symptoms co-exist i.e.: a patient may be agitated and over-talkative but has severe depressive cognitions at the same time. The majority of the manic and mixed episodes require treatment in the hospital setting. Medications play an important role in their initial management.

3.1.1 Lithium

Lithium salts occur naturally in rocks, spa waters, plants and animal fluids and in the human body. It is a metal ion which is distributed widely and can penetrate cell membranes. The mechanism of action of lithium is still unclear but probably it works via second messenger systems and enhancement of 5-HT responses.

Lithium was first used by John Cade in 1949 to treat acute mania and it still has an important role in the therapy of bipolar disorder. Traditionally Lithium and anticonvulsants have been called "mood- stabilisers" to differentiate them from the first generation antipsychotics which were thought to have only anti-manic effects. The distinction has been blurred since the introduction of second generation (atypical) antipsychotics which have shown efficacy in both acute and long term treatment.

Lithium is more effective than placebo in acute mania (Bowden et al. 1994; Kushner et al. 2006; Keck et al. 2007) and nearly 50% of the symptoms improved markedly. More than 50% of patients suffer a relapse within 10 weeks of stopping lithium treatment (Suppes et al. 1991). Lithium is also effective in reducing both psychotic and depressive symptoms similar to Quetiapine (Bowden et al. 2005).

A Lithium plasma level in the range of 0.6 to 1.3mmol/L is required to obtain a therapeutic anti-manic effect (Bowden et al. 1994). The common side-effects include tremor, weight gain, polydipsia, polyuria, and worsening of skin problems. In long term, it causes renal impairment, thyroid and parathyroid problems. Lithium has a relatively slow onset of action and weak sedative property. Therefore, it is frequently necessary to add an adjunct antipsychotic or benzodiazepine in treating acute mania. The need to regularly monitor its plasma levels to prevent toxicity, as well as its side-effects makes Lithium less useful when equally effective alternatives are available.

3.1.2 Anticonvulsants

Anticonvulsants have been used in the treatment and prophylaxis of bipolar disorder since the 1970's when Sodium Valproate was first used in mania. Although various anti-convulsants have been investigated, only Valproate and Carbamazepine were found to be effective in the acute mania. Other agents have shown little or no efficacy.

Valproate

Valproate is an umbrella term used to describe the different preparations of Valproic Acid, the active component of the drugs. Various formulations like Sodium Valproate, Valproic Acid, Semisodium Valproate and Valpromide are available on the market and the most commonly used formulation is Semisodium Valproate (Depakote). The exact mechanism of action is not clear and it seems to be related to the enhancement of inhibitory neurotransmitter GABA.

The anti-manic efficacy of Valproate was first seen as early as in 1966 (Lambert et al. 1966). Subsequently its usefulness in acute mania has been investigated both as monotherapy and in combination with antipsychotics. A Cochrane review of randomised controlled trials found that Valproate is an effective treatment for acute mania and this evidence was consistent in most studies (Macritchie et al. 2003). Valproate has similar anti-manic efficacy to Lithium (Bowden et al. 1994, 2008), Haloperidol (McElroy et al. 1996) and Olanzapine (Zajecka et al. 2002).

Valproate is superior in overall outcome (both clinical and functional) compared to Carbamazepine (Vasudev et al. 2000).

Of all the anticonvulsants used in the treatment of mania, Valproate has greater efficacy in reducing manic symptoms with a response rate of 50% compared to placebo effect of 20-30%. It also has a better antimanic effect than Lithium in rapid cycling and mixed episodes. The loading dose of 20-30mg/kg body weight is more effective than slow titration regimes (Rosa et al. 2011). Gastrointestinal problems, sedation and tremor are the most commonly reported side-effects.

Carbamazepine

Carbamazepine is a dibenzazepine derivative which has been used for prophylactic treatment of bipolar disorder in patients not responding to Lithium.

Carbamazepine was found to be effective in acute mania soon after its introduction (Okuma et al. 1973). It is significantly superior to placebo and equally effective compared with antipsychotics, Valproate and Lithium as evidenced in randomised controlled studies (Weisler et al. 2004 & 2005). The onset of action is slower compared to antipsychotics and Valproate but faster than Lithium. The use of Carbamazepine in the treatment of acute mania has declined recently with the advent of other drugs. However, it may still be useful in certain subtypes of bipolar disorder which include dysphoric mania, mania co-morbid with substance misuse, mania with mood incongruent delusions and with negative family history of bipolar disorder (Post et al. 2007).

Other anticonvulsants

Oxcarbazepine is chemically related to Carbamazepine. However, its antimanic properties are not convincing (Hirschfeld and Kasper 2004). **Phenytoin** showed antimanic properties as add-on to Haloperidol in a small placebo-controlled trail (Mishory et al. 2000) but its side-effect profile and availability of better drugs makes it an unlikely choice for mania. Other agents like Topiramate, Gabapentin, Lamotrigine, Levitiracetam and Zonisamide have been tried but had no efficacy in acute mania.

3.1.3 Antipsychotics

Typical antipsychotics

Haloperidol has been used in the acute treatment of mania for several decades, but only recently significant evidence was established. A meta-analysis of various studies using

Haloperidol as comparator drug showed it was significantly better than placebo (Cipriani et al. 2006). Haloperidol has been equally effective as Olanzapine (Tohen et al. 2003), Aripiprazole (Vieta et al. 2005a), Valproate (McElroy et al. 1996), Carbamazepine (Brown et al. 1989) and Lithium (Segal et al. 1998). It is also helpful in combination therapies. Unfortunately bipolar patients are more prone to extrapyramidal side-effects of Haloperidol compared to schizophrenic patients according to naturalistic studies (Keck et al. 2000).

Chlorpromazine has equal efficacy to Lithium and Carbamazepine in acute mania (Prien et al. 1972; Okuma et al. 1979). It has been also superior to Lithium in agitated manic patients (Prien et al. 1972). Chlorpromazine can cause sedation, photo-sensitivity of the skin and liver abnormalities.

The use of typical antipsychotics such as Haloperidol and Chlorpromazine has declined over the years due to its propensity to cause extra-pyramidal side- effects in short term and tardive dyskinesia in long term treatment.

Atypical antipsychotics

The introduction of atypical antipsychotics has considerably changed the treatment of bipolar disorder. Efficacy of atypical antipsychotics has been systematically tested in numerous trials both as monotherapy and in combination with mood-stabilisers. Evidence for effectiveness of each of these drugs in acute mania is discussed below.

Olanzapine

Olanzapine is a thienobenzodiazepine derivative and one of the most extensively investigated atypical antipsychotics. It has significantly higher efficacy than placebo in monotherapy (Tohen et al. 2000, 2007, 2009). It has better outcomes than Lithium (Berk et al. 1999) and Valproate (Tohen et al. 2003b). The patients responded within a week and it was maintained. Intra muscular injection of Olanzapine is significantly superior to placebo and Lorazepam in patients with agitated mania (Meehan et al. 2001).

Olanzapine in combination with Lithium or Valproate has better results than either Lithium or Valproate alone (Tohen et al. 2002). However, in combination with Carbamazepine, it did not show any difference to placebo, probably due to Carbamazepine induced Olanzapine metabolism (Tohen et al. 2008). A more recent large study (EMBLEM - pan- European naturalistic mania study) showed good efficacy of Olanzapine as monotherapy and in combination with other medications (Vieta et al. 2008). Recommended dose for acute mania is 15mgs/day as monotherapy and 10mgs/day in combination treatment. The common side-effects include drowsiness, dizziness and weight gain. The adverse metabolic effects ranging from hyperglycaemia to diabetes and hyperlipidemia may limit its clinical use.

Risperidone

Risperidone belongs to the benzisoxazole group and has been used in the treatment of acute mania both as monotherapy and in combinations. Risperidone is significantly better than placebo (Hirschfeld et al. 2004 & Khanna et al. 2005) and has equal efficacy to Lithium, Haloperidol (Segal et al. 1998) and Olanzapine (Perlis et al. 2006). There is significant reduction in symptoms of mania as assessed by Young Mania Rating scale (YMRS).

In combination with Lithium or Valproate (Sachs et al. 2002 & Yatham et al. 2003), Risperidone has better results than Lithium or Valproate alone but failed to have the same effects with Carbamazepine. The improvements are noted as early as day 3 and most patients respond within a week. The effective dose range is from 1 to 6mgs/day.

Risperidone is well tolerated at low doses but at 6mgs/day, nearly 50% patients may develop extra pyramidal side-effects (Khanna et al. 2005).

Quetiapine

Quetiapine is a benzothiazepine, which is moderately sedative and has low risk of acute extrapyramidal side-effects. Quetiapine has been studied in the treatment of acute mania, bipolar depression and in maintenance therapy.

Quetiapine is more effective than placebo in acute mania as monotherapy and has equal efficacy to Lithium, Haloperidol and Paliperidone (Bowden et al. 2005, McIntyre et al. 2005, and Vieta et al. 2010a). It is effective across a broad range of symptoms in mania according to a systematic review (McIntyre et al. 2007).Quetiapine has also had a beneficial effect in rapid cycling bipolar disorder and there was no treatment emergent depression (DelBello et al. 2006). Quetiapine combination with Lithium or Valproate has better results than Lithium or Valproate alone (Sachs et al. 2004 & Yatham et al. 2004).

Quetiapine XL- extended release formulation also has good antimanic properties (Cutler et al. 2008). The efficacy can be noted as early as day 4 and the usual dose range is 400 – 800mgs/day. The common side-effects include somnolence, tachycardia, hypotension, dizziness and weight gain.

Aripiprazole

Aripiprazole is different from other atypical antipsychotics. It is a dopamine- serotonin system stabiliser and acts as a dopamine D2 receptor partial agonist. Aripiprazole was initially used in acute mania but now there is emerging evidence for its good effects in maintenance treatment (Keck et al. 2006; 2007).

Aripiprazole is an effective antimanic agent both as monotherapy (Sachs et al. 2006; Keck et al.2007b & Young et al.2009) and in combination with Lithium or Valproate. The combination is superior to Lithium or Valproate alone (Vieta et al. 2009a). Further, its intramuscular formulation has similar antimanic efficacy (Sanford and Scott 2008).

Aripiprazole is effective, safe and well tolerated both in bipolar mania and mixed episodes. It has rapid onset of action with improvement as early as day 4. This was proved by significant reduction in YMRS scores within few days of treatment. The dose range varies from 15 to 30mgs /day. The common side-effects include headache, somnolence and dizziness. The lack or minimal effects on weight gain, prolactin or QT interval are the main advantages compared to other atypical antipsychotics.

Ziprasidone

Ziprasidone is a benzothiazolylpiperazine derivative and has been used in both schizophrenia and bipolar disorder. It is well tolerated and has a low risk of extrapyramidal side-effects. It is effective against mania with psychotic symptoms and mixed affective states and it has been proved in double-blinded controlled trials (Vieta et al. 2009b; Greenberg and Citorme 2007). The dose range is 80- 160mgs/day and the common side-effects are somnolence, dizziness, akathisia and headache. However, the use of Ziprasidone is restricted in some countries due to its cardio-vascular side-effects such as QT prolongation and elevation of blood pressure.

Other antipsychotics

Clozapine is regarded as a last resort therapy for treatment resistant mania, refractory to both mood stabilisers and other antipsychotics. It is very effective and well tolerated which has been shown in case reports and open-labelled trials (Degner et al. 2000; Green et al. 2000; Suppes et al. 2003). Combination of Clozapine and Lamotrigine is also very helpful both in acute and maintenance treatment for refractory and rapid cycling bipolar disorders (Calabrese & Gajwani 2000; Bastiampillai et al. 2010).

Amisulpride was used in the treatment of mania before other atypical antipsychotics became available. Its efficacy is modest in acute mania (Vieta et al. 2005) and there is no additional benefit in combination with Valproate (Thomas et al. 2008). It causes hyperprolactinemia in higher doses which is usually required to treat mania.

Asenapine is another atypical antipsychotic with superior efficacy compared to placebo in the treatment of acute mania both as monotherapy (McIntyre et al. 2008) and in combination with mood-stabilisers (Calabrese et al. 2008). It causes moderate weight gain but the metabolic side-effects are unclear (McIntyre et al 2009).

Paliperidone, a derivative of Risperidone, has recently been introduced in the treatment of mania. It is superior to placebo and equally effective as Quetiapine (Vieta et al. 2010a). It is generally well tolerated. However, at higher doses, it is similar to Risperidone regarding the risk of extrapyramidal side-effects. The other side-effects include headache, somnolence, dizziness and dyspepsia. It can also cause hyperprolactinemia.

3.1.4 Other medications used in mania

Benzodiazepines are frequently used as an adjunct in acute mania, mainly due to their anxiolytic and sedative properties. Although there is some evidence suggesting their more specific antimanic action, it does not seem to be significant.

Tamoxifen, an anti-oestrogen and protein kinase C inhibitor, has some antimanic efficacy (Hah and Hallmayer 2007; Yildiz et al. 2008). However its safety in routine use is not clear.

Calcium channel blockers such as **Verapamil** and **Nimodipine** have been examined for their antimanic efficacy but have not proven to be convincingly effective. Their use in routine practice can be limited by the hypotensive effects.

3.1.5 Combination therapy in mania

Combination treatment has become common in medical practice, mainly due to the frequent partial response to monotherapy. It may be also indicated when a patient relapses on long-term treatment.

In acute mania, combination of an atypical antipsychotic with Lithium or Valproate is frequently used in clinical practice. Other combinations such as Lithium and Valproate, Lithium and Carbamazepine have also been helpful. Sometimes a triple combination (Lithium, an anticonvulsant and an atypical antipsychotic) may be needed in treatment resistant mania.

Combinations of Olanzapine, Quetiapine, Risperidone and Aripiprazole with a mood stabiliser are more effective than therapy with a single mood stabiliser (Yatham 2005; Smith et al. 2007; Ketter 2008). Combinations are also useful in long term maintenance treatment.

After an acute manic episode, psychosocial interventions may play further role to improve recovery of the patient. This could include psychoeducation focusing on importance of maintaining regular routine, prophylactic medications, monitoring mood, recognise early warnings of relapse and improve coping strategies.

Recommendations of treatment for acute mania based on currently available evidence is summarised in the Box 1.

Patients on long term maintenance treatment

1. Add an atypical antipsychotic if the maintenance agent has been a mood stabiliser
2. Increase the dose of maintenance agent
3. If still no response, different combination therapy can be tried

Patients with no long-term maintenance treatment

1. Start an atypical antipsychotic (Olanzapine, Risperidone, Quetiapine, Aripiprazole) - choice depends on side- effect profile and patient's preference
2. If no response, add Lithium or Valproate
    -   Use Lithium in less agitated patients
    -   Avoid Valproate in women of child bearing age
3. Benzodiazepines such as Lorazepam and Clonazepam can be used in agitated patients and sleep problems

Treatment resistant mania

1. Clozapine or combination of Lithium and Valproate can be tried
2. ECT to be considered

Mixed affective states

1. Treat as acute mania
2. Some evidence for Olanzapine and Aripiprazole efficacy
3. Valproate seems to be better than Lithium
4. Antidepressants to be avoided

Box. 1. Treatment of acute mania or mixed episode

3.2 Bipolar depression

People suffering from bipolar I and II disorders have more depressive episodes (67% and 94% respectively) than manic episodes (Judd et al. 2002 & 2003). However bipolar depression is a relatively new clinical concept. Bipolar depression is characterised by prolonged unstable mood, increased suicide risk, increased risk of substance misuse, higher risk of rapid cycling and increased mortality (not only by suicide but also due to cardiovascular and all causes). Most of these episodes are associated with poor outcome and higher degree of disability if not managed properly.

The treatment of bipolar depression is complex and challenging for clinicians. The evidence for various treatment options are considered below.

3.2.1 Antidepressants

The evidence for the use of antidepressants in bipolar depression is limited and diverse. The use of antidepressants was favoured earlier because of the widespread belief that they had high efficacy and the risk of switch to mania seemed to be similar to placebo (Gijsman et al. 2004). However the recent evidence suggests that their efficacy in bipolar depression is modest and their routine use is not encouraged (Sidor and McQueen 2011). Therefore antidepressants are restricted to treatment resistant depression (Vieta 2009) as an adjunct with a mood stabiliser or an antipsychotic.

3.2.2 Lithium

Lithium has modest efficacy in acute depression (Young et al. 2000; Nemeroff et al. 2001). It is used in augmentation therapy with antidepressants in both unipolar and bipolar depression.

It is as effective as a tricyclic antidepressant at serum levels above 0.8mmol/L but tolerability can be a problem at such high doses (Nemeroff et al.2001). It is also effective in combination with Valproate (Young et al. 2000). Although the evidence base for lithium monotherapy in acute bipolar depression is rather weak, its effectiveness as an antidepressant cannot be dismissed.

3.2.3 Anticonvulsants

Lamotrigine has become a recognised treatment in bipolar depression, despite its modest efficacy as proved by systematic reviews of all controlled trials (Calabrese et al. 2008; Geddes et al. 2009). It requires a slow titration, especially in combinations with Valproate and this may restrict its use in acute episodes where quick symptom relief is needed. Lamotrigine - Lithium combination is also effective in bipolar depression and there is nearly 50% reduction in symptoms (Lamlit study; van der Loss et al. 2009). Lamotrigine can cause rash in 10% of the patients and it may lead to Steven Johnson syndrome, which warrants its careful monitoring and slow titration. As a result it remains a controversial treatment option for bipolar depression.

Valproate also has modest efficacy in bipolar depression (Davis et al. 2005; Ghaemi et al. 2007; Smith et al. 2010). Smith et al reported 50% reduction in symptoms but the sample size was too small to suggest any concrete evidence.

Carbamazepine has a weak evidence base and is not a first- line agent in the treatment of bipolar depression. However it may have a role in refractory depression as proved by a crossover trail (Post et al. 1986) and is more effective in combination with Lithium than monotherapy (Kramlinger & Post 1989; Small 1990).

3.2.4 Antipsychotics

It is well recognised that both typical and atypical antipsychotics are effective in the treatment of acute mania and depression either as monotherapy or in combination with other drugs. The use of antipsychotics in bipolar depression has increased with the introduction of atypical antipsychotics and Quetiapine has been proved to be especially effective.

Quetiapine is effective as monotherapy in treating acute bipolar depression (BOLDER studies; Calabrese et al. 2005; Thase et al. 2006). It is well tolerated and the incidence of treatment emergent mania or hypomania is similar to placebo. The dose range varies between 300-600mgs/day. It is superior to Lithium and equally effective as Paroxetine in treating acute depressive episodes (EMBOLDEN studies; Young et al. 2010; McElroy et al. 2010).

Olanzapine and Fluoxetine combination was more effective than Olanzapine alone in bipolar depression (Tohen et al. 2003c). **Perphenazine**, a typical antipsychotic, added to a mood stabiliser prevented depressive episodes when used as maintenance treatment (Zarate and Tohen 2004).

3.2.5 Combination therapy in bipolar depression

Similar to acute mania, combination therapies work better than monotherapy in bipolar depression. Olanzapine- Fluoxetine combination, Lamotrigine - Lithium combination,

Lithium or Valproate and antidepressant or antipsychotic combinations have been effective. Recently a triple combination (Lithium, Lamotrigine and Paroxetine) has been used for patients who were not responding to Lithium-Lamotrigine combination. The triple combination can be useful in both acute depressive phase (van der Loss et al. 2010) and maintenance treatment (van der Loss et al. 2011).

Psychological interventions like Cognitive- Behavioural therapy (CBT), Interpersonal therapy can be used along with medications in bipolar depression. The combination of medications plus CBT may speed up the recovery process, improves the social functioning and reduces the relapses (Lam et al. 2003). Further CBT is found to be effective for patients with less than 12 previous episodes (Scott et al. 2006), indicating that psychological treatment is effective early in the course of illness.

Recommendations of treatment for acute bipolar depression based on currently available evidence is summarised in the Box 2.

---

1.   Start with a mood- stabiliser
-   Quetiapine has the best evidence followed by Olanzapine- Fluoxetine combination and Lamotrigine
-   Lithium and Valproate are considered as second- line options
2.   Add an anti-depressant if no response
-   Choice of medication depends on patient's previous response and drug side-effect profile
-   SSRI's seem to be better than other antidepressants
3.   Other combinations like Lamotrigine-Lithium, or mood stabiliser and an antipsychotic can be considered
4.   If still no response, non-pharmacological treatments like Electroconvulsive therapy or Transcranial magnetic stimulation can be tried
5.   Avoid using antidepressants as the first line treatment

Box. 2. Treatment of acute bipolar depression

3.3 Maintenance treatment of bipolar disorder

Maintenance treatment is crucially important in bipolar disorder due to its chronic and recurrent course. According to the naturalistic studies more than 50% of the patients have a relapse in a 2 - 4 year period (Tohen et al. 2003d). Prophylactic treatment prevents further relapses and reduces both morbidity and mortality. The current trend is to consider long term maintenance treatment earlier on, even after a single manic episode. The treatment should be continued for at least 2 years and in many cases indefinitely, unless risk to benefit ratio changes. Various medications used in acute phase are beneficial in maintenance treatment. The evidence for various medications used in maintenance treatment is discussed below.

3.3.1 Lithium

Lithium still remains as a cornerstone in the long-term treatment of bipolar disorder (Nivoli et al. 2010).

Lithium is more effective than placebo in preventing all relapses and especially manic relapses. Its efficacy in preventing depressive episodes is equivocal as shown in a systematic review and meta-analysis (Geddes et al. 2004). Compared with other mood stabilising agents, Lithium is less effective than Valproate and Olanzapine in preventing manic or mixed episodes and less effective than Lamotrigine in preventing depressive episodes. Its efficacy is similar to Carbamazepine in both acute and long-term treatment (Nivoli et al. 2010).

Lithium has been effective in preventing suicide, deliberate self-harm and reduces mortality from all causes in bipolar patients (Cipriani et al. 2005).

Lithium may cause renal damage and hypothyroidism in long term and so, monitoring of renal and thyroid functions is recommended every 3- 6 months.

3.3.2 Anticonvulsants

Antiepileptic drugs have been used in prophylactic treatment since the 1970's and they are moderately efficacious in preventing manic and depressive episodes. Valproate and Carbamazepine are effective in preventing manic relapses and are useful in rapid cycling disorders, whereas Lamotrigine may be useful only in preventing depressive episodes.

Valproate

Valproate monotherapy in maintenance treatment has a limited evidence base. It is superior to placebo and Lithium (Bowden et al. 2000) and similar in efficacy to Olanzapine (Tohen et al. 2003b). Nearly 50% of the patients remained relapse free at 48 weeks. Combination therapies with Quetiapine (Vieta et al. 2008) or Lithium (Geddes et al. 2010) are more effective than Valproate alone. It should be avoided as prophylactic treatment in women of child bearing age because of its teratogenic effects.

Carbamazepine

The evidence for effectiveness of Carbamazepine in maintenance treatment is not strong but it still has an important role in long-term management of bipolar disorder. It may be useful in patients not responding to other agents or not tolerating their side-effects. It is also useful in certain subtypes of bipolar disorder such as mixed affective states and those with co-morbid substance misuse (Post et al. 2007). Carbamazepine is a hepatic enzyme inducer and its interactions with other medications may be difficult to predict. In long-term use, it may cause hepatotoxicity and requires regular monitoring of liver functions. It is also teratogenic and should be used carefully in women of child bearing age.

Lamotrigine

Lamotrigine can be considered for long term treatment either alone or in combination therapy for patients who suffer more depressive than manic episodes. More than 57% of the patients remained intervention free for 18months on Lamotrigine (Goodwin et al. 2004). In combination with Lithium, it has superior efficacy than either alone, especially in preventing depression (Bowden et al. 2003 & Calabrese et al. 2003). Lamotrigine is also effective in the long term treatment of rapid cycling bipolar disorder (Calabrese et al. 2000).

3.3.3 Antipsychotics

There is good evidence for atypical antipsychotics like Olanzapine, Quetiapine and Aripiprazole in maintenance treatment of bipolar disorder.

Quetiapine is effective in preventing both manic and depressive episodes. It increases the time to relapse for any mood episode irrespective of the index episode and it is as effective as Lithium in preventing relapses (Nolen et al. 2009). In combination with Lithium or

Valproate, it is more efficient in preventing relapses than Lithium or Valproate combination with placebo (Vieta et al. 2008b). The dose varies from 300 to 800mgs/day.

Olanzapine is used both as monotherapy and in combinations with Lithium or Valproate in the long-term treatment of bipolar disorder. It is superior to placebo (Tohen et al. 2006) and reduces the incidence of both manic and depressives episodes. In comparison with Lithium, Olanzapine was better in preventing manic relapses and similar in preventing depressive episodes (Tohen et al. 2005). Olanzapine is especially effective in patients who have responded to it during an acute manic or mixed episode and in those who did not respond to other medications (Cipriani et al. 2010). The dose range is from 5 to 20mgs/day.

Aripiprazole is effective in preventing manic relapses as monotherapy (Keck et al. 2006) and the response rate is nearly 60% when it is continued for 100 weeks (Keck et al. 2007). The dose range is from 15 to 30mgs/day. The common side-effects include tremor, akathisia and dry mouth. Weight gain is similar to placebo, which will be favoured by many patients.

Depot antipsychotics can be considered as maintenance treatment in patients who have relapses due to medication non-adherence or who have failed to respond to standard treatments. The first generation depot antipsychotics used either alone or with a mood stabiliser prevent manic relapses but may increase the duration of depressive symptoms. Therefore, they are not advisable for patients who suffer frequent depressive episodes. On the other hand, **Risperidone depot either alone or with a mood stabiliser** has reduced the frequency of both manic and depressive episodes (Bond et al. 2007). There were few incidences of extrapyramidal symptoms and patient satisfaction was good. The dose range is 25 - 50mgs every 2 weeks.

3.3.4 Combination therapy in maintenance

Combination treatment should be considered when there is an inadequate response to monotherapy. At the same time, clinicians should be aware of the increased risk of side-effects during combination therapy and the ways to monitor them.

Combinations of a mood stabiliser (Lithium or Valproate) and an atypical antipsychotic (Olanzapine or Quetiapine or Aripiprazole) have been more effective than the mood stabilisers alone in reducing the frequency of episodes and delaying the time to relapse in the long term treatment (Tohen et al. 2005; Vieta et al. 2008b). Lithium and Lamotrigine combination has been effective in preventing depressive episodes (Bowden et al. 2003; Calabrese et al. 2003).

Combination of two mood stabilisers is also used in clinical practice. The combination of Lithium and Valproate was more efficacious than Valproate monotherapy and was associated with a lower risk of relapses (BALANCE trial; Geddes et al. 2010).

Psychosocial interventions play a significant role in long term maintenance treatment along with medications. The detailed descriptions of each of them are beyond the scope of this chapter. Cognitive behaviour therapy or Interpersonal Personal therapy can be used along with medications to prevent further depressive episodes. Psychoeducation to the patient about their illness and healthy lifestyle helps in relapse prevention. Patients may also benefit with advice about good sleep hygiene, regular routine and maintaining work-life balance.

Psychosocial intervention in the form of additional social support after life events and recovery from acute episode, encouraging patients to talk with their family and friends about their illness when they are well may help in relapse prevention. Family- focused therapy is associated with a 48% increase in recovery rates at 1 year and a 35%- 40%

reduction in recurrence rates over 2years (Miklowitz et al. 2003). Family therapies usually focus on psychoeducation, ways to improve communication and problem solving.

Recommendations for maintenance treatment of bipolar disorder based on currently available evidence is summarised in the Box 3.

1.	Combination treatment should be considered when there is poor response to monotherapy
2.	Choice of medication depends on the course of illness and patient's response to treatment during acute episode
3.	Quetiapine is effective in preventing both manic and depressive episodes and can be used as first line treatment
4.	Lithium, Olanzapine and Aripiprazole are more effective in preventing manic than depressive episodes
5.	Lamotrigine is more effective in preventing depressive episodes
6.	Valproate and Carbamazepine should be considered as a second choice if treatment response to other drugs was inadequate
7.	Depot antipsychotics can be considered either alone or in combination with a mood stabiliser if non- compliance with oral medications is suspected; they are also useful for patients with predominantly manic relapses
8.	Antidepressants should be avoided in the long term treatment of bipolar disorder

Box. 3. Maintenance treatment of bipolar disorder

4. Conclusions

The pharmacotherapy of bipolar disorder has expanded vastly since Lithium was first used in mania in 1949. Various treatment options are currently available; however, their effectiveness is not always satisfactory, especially in bipolar depression and long-term maintenance treatment.

Despite limitations, maintenance treatment should be considered earlier, especially if severe mania was the index episode. If the patient responds well to a medication during the acute episode, the same drug should be continued in the long-term therapy unless it is contraindicated. Combination therapy should be considered if there is no adequate response to monotherapy.

Although there are many treatment strategies currently available, management of bipolar disorder still remains a challenge for clinicians. Further research to develop new medications with different mechanisms of action is needed.

5. Acknowledgements

We would like to thank Ms. Patricia Kelly for her secretarial support in the preparation of the manuscript.

6. References

Bastaimpillai TJ, Reid CE & Dhillon R. 2010. The long-term effectiveness of Clozapine and Lamotrigine in a patient with treatment resistant rapid-cycling bipolar disorder. *Journal of Psychopharmacology* 24: 1834- 1836

Berk K, Ichim L & Brook S. 1999. Olanzapine compared to Lithium in mania: a double-blind randomised controlled trial. *International Journal of Clinical Psychopharmacology* 14: 339-343

Bowden CL, Brugger AM, Swann AC, Calabrese JR, Janicak PG, Petty F & et al. 1994. Efficacy of Divalproex vs. Lithium and placebo in the treatment of mania. The Depakote Mania study group. *Journal of American Medical Association* 271: 918-924

Bond DJ, Pratoomsri W & Yatham LN. 2007. Depot antipsychotic medications in bipolar disorder. A review of the literature. *Acta Psychiatrica Scandinavica* 116 (suppl 434): 3-16

Bowden CL, Calabrese JR, McElroy SL, Gyulai L, Wassef A & et al (Divalproex maintenance study group). 2000. A randomised, placebo-controlled 12-month trial of Divalproex and Lithium in treatment of outpatients with bipolar I disorder. *Archives of General Psychiatry* 57: 481-489

Bowden CL, Calabrese JR, Sachs G, Yatham LN, Asghar S & et al (Lamictal 606 study group). 2003. A placebo-controlled 18-month trial of Lamotrigine and Lithium maintenance treatment in recently manic or hypomanic patients with bipolar I disorder. *Archives of General Psychiatry* 60: 392-400

Bowden CL, Grunze H, Mullen J, Brecher m, Paulsson B, Jones M & et al. 2005. A randomised, double- blind, placebo- controlled efficacy and safety study of Quetiapine or Lithium as monotherapy for mania in bipolar disorder. *Journal of Clinical Psychiatry* 66: 111-121

Brown D, Silverstone T & Cookson J. 1989. Carbamazepine compared to Haloperidol in acute mania. *International Journal of Clinical Psychopharmacology* 4: 229-238

Calabrese JR & Gajwani P. 2000. Lamotrigine and Clozapine for bipolar disorder. *American Journal of Psychiatry* 157: 1523

Calabrese JR, Suppes T, Bowden CL & et al. 2000. A double-blind, placebo-controlled, prophylaxis study of Lamotrigine in rapid cycling bipolar disorder. *Journal of Clinical Psychiatry* 61: 841-850

Calabrese JR, Bowden CL, Sachs G & et al. 2003. A placebo-controlled 18-month trial of Lamotrigine and Lithium maintenance treatment in recently depressed patients with bipolar I disorder. *Journal of Clinical Psychiatry* 64: 1013-1024

Calabrese JR, Keck PE, Macfadden W, Minkwitz M, Ketter TA & et al. 2005. A Randomised, double-blind, placebo-controlled trial of Quetiapine in the treatment of bipolar I or II depression. *American Journal of Psychiatry* 162: 1351-1360

Calabrese JR, Cohen M, Zhao J & Panagides J. 2008. Efficacy and safety of Asenapine as adjunctive treatment for acute mania associated with bipolar disorder. *Proceedings of the 161th APA Conference, Washington, DC, May 3-8*

Calabrese JR, Huffman RF, White RL, Edwards S, Thompson TR, Ascher JA & et al. 2008. Lamotrigine in the acute treatment of bipolar depression: results of five double-blind, placebo-controlled clinical trials. *Bipolar Disorders* 10: 323-333

Cipriani A, Pretty H, Hawton K & Geddes JR. 2005. Lithium in the prevention of suicidal behaviour and all-cause mortality in patients with mood disorders: A systematic review of randomised trials. *American Journal of Psychiatry* 162: 1805-1819

Cipriani A, Rendell JM & Geddes JR. 2006. Haloperidol alone or in combination for acute mania. *Cochrane Database Systematic Review 3: CD004362*

Cipriani A, Rendell JM & Geddes JR. 2010. Olanzapine in the long-term treatment of bipolar disorder: a systematic review and meta-analysis. *Journal of Psychopharmacology* 24: 1729- 1738

Cutler AJ, Datto C, Nordenham A, Dettore B, Acevedo L & Darko D. 2008. Effectiveness of extended release formulation of Quetiapine as monotherapy for the treatment of bipolar mania. *International Journal of Neuropsychopharmacology* 11 (Suppl 1): 184

Dardennes R, Thuile J, Friedman S & Guelgi JD. 2006. The costs of bipolar disorder. *Encephale* 32: 18- 25

Davis LL, Bartolucci A & Petty F. 2005. Divalproex in the treatment of bipolar depression: a placebo-controlled study. *Journal of Affective Disorders* 85: 259- 266

Degner D, Belch S, Muller P, Hajak R, Adler L & Ruther E. 2000. Clozapine in the treatment of mania. *Journal of Neuropsychiatry & Clinical Neurosciences* 12: 283

DelBello MP, Kowatch RA, Adler CM, Stanford KE, Welge JA, Barzman DH & et al. 2006. A double-blind randomised pilot study comparing Quetiapine and Divalproex for mania. *Journal of American Academy of Child Adolescent Psychiatry* 45: 305- 313

Geddes JR, Burgess S, Hawton K, Jamison K & Goodwin GM. 2004. Long-term Lithium Therapy for Bipolar disorder: systematic review and meta-analysis of randomised controlled trials. *American Journal of Psychiatry* 161: 217- 222

Geddes JR, Calabrese JR & Goodwin GM. 2009. Lamotrigine for treatment of bipolar depression: Independent meta-analysis and meta-regression of individual patient data from five randomised trials. *British Journal of Psychiatry* 194: 4-9

Geddes JR, Goodwin GM, Rendell J & et al. 2010. Lithium plus Valproate combination therapy versus monotherapy for relapse prevention in bipolar I disorder (BALANCE trial): A randomised open- label trial. *Lancet* 375: 385- 395

Ghaemi SN, Gilmer WS, Goldberg JF, Zablotsky B, Kemp DE & et al. 2007. Divalproex in the treatment of acute bipolar depression: a preliminary double-blind, randomised, placebo-controlled pilot study. *Journal of Clinical Psychiatry* 68: 1840-44

Gijsman HJ, Geddes JR, Rendell JM, Nolen WA & Goodwin G. 2004. Antidepressants for bipolar depression: A systematic review of randomised controlled trials. *American Journal of Psychiatry* 161: 1537- 1547

Goodwin GM, Bowden CL, Calabrese JR, Grunze H, Kasper S & et al. 2004. A pooled analysis of 2 placebo-controlled 18-month trials of Lamotrigine and Lithium maintenance in bipolar I disorder. *Journal of Clinical Psychiatry* 65: 432- 441

Green AI, Tohen M, Patel JK, Banov M, DuRand C, Berman I & et al. 2000. Clozapine in the treatment of refractory psychotic mania. *American Journal of Psychiatry* 157: 982- 986

Greenberg WM & Citrome L. 2007. Ziprasidone for schizophrenia and bipolar disorder: a review of clinical trials. *CNS Drug Review* 13: 137- 177

Hah M & Hallmayer JF. 2008. Tamoxifen and mania: a double-blind, placebo-controlled trial. *Current Psychiatry Reviews* 10: 200-201

Hirschfeld RM & Kaspers S. 2004. A review of the evidence of Carbamazepine and Oxcarbazepine in the treatment of bipolar disorder. *International Journal of Neuropsychopharmacology* 7: 507- 522

Hirschfeld RM, Keck PE Jr, Kramer M, Karcher K, Canuso C, Eerdekens M & et al. 2004. Rapid antimanic effect of Risperidone monotherapy: a 3-week multicenter, double-blind, placebo-controlled trail. *American Journal of Psychiatry* 161: 1057- 1065

Judd LL, Akisal HS, Schettler PJ, Coryell W, Endicott J, Maser JD & et al. 2003. A Prospective investigation of the natural history of the long-term weekly symptomatic status of bipolar II disorder. *Archives of General Psychiatry* 60: 261- 269

Judd LL, Akisal HS, Schettler PJ, Endicott J, Maser J, Solomon DA, Leon AC & et al. 2002. The long-term natural history of the weekly symptomatic status of bipolar I disorder. *Archives of General Psychiatry* 59: 530- 537

Keck PE, McElroy SL, Strakowski SM & Soutullo CA. 2000. Antipsychotics in the treatment of mood disorders and risk of tardive dyskinesia. *Journal of Clinical Psychiatry* 61 (suppl 4): 33- 38

Keck PE Jr, Calabrese JR, McQuade R & et al. 2006. A randomised, double-blind, placebo-controlled 26- week trial of Aripiprazole in recently manic patients with bipolar I disorder. *Journal of Clinical Psychiatry* 67: 626- 637

Keck PE Jr, Calabrese JR, McQuade R & et al. 2007a. Aripiprazole monotherapy for maintenance therapy in bipolar I disorder: a 100-week double-blind study versus placebo. *Journal of Clinical Psychiatry* 68: 1480- 1491

Keck PE, Sanchez R, Torbeyns A, Marcus RN, McQuade RD, Forbes A. 2007b. Aripiprazole monotherapy in the treatment of acute bipolar I mania: a randomised, placebo- and Lithium- controlled study. *Program and abstracts of the 160th annual meeting of the American Psychiatric Association; May 19-24, 2007; San Diego, CA*. New Research poster 304

Ketter TA. 2008. Monotherapy versus combined treatment with second generation antipsychotics in bipolar disorder. *Journal of Clinical Psychiatry* 69 (Suppl 5): 9- 15

Khanna S, Vieta E, Lyons B, Grossman f, Eerdekens M & Kramer M. 2005. Risperidone in the treatment of acute mania: double-blind, placebo-controlled study. *British Journal of Psychiatry* 187: 229- 234

Kramlinger KG & Post RM. 1989. The addition of Lithium to Carbamazepine. *Archives of General Psychiatry* 46: 794- 800

Kushner SF, Khan A, Lane R, Olson WH. 2006. Topiramate monotherapy in the management of acute mania: results of four double- blind placebo controlled trials. *Bipolar Disorders* 8: 15-27

Lam D, Watkins E, Hayward P, Bight J, Wright K, Kerr N & et al. 2003. A randomised controlled study of cognitive therapy of relapse prevention for bipolar affective disorder- outcome of the first year. *Archives of General Psychiatry* 60:145- 152

Macritchie K, Geddes JR, Scott J, Haslam D, de Lima M & Goodwin G. 2003. Valproate for acute mood episodes in bipolar disorder. *Cochrane Database Systematic Review* CD004052

Meehan K, Zhang F, David S, Tohen M, Janicak P, Small J & et al. 2001. A double-blind, randomised comparison of the efficacy and safety of intramuscular injections of Olanzapine, Lorazepam or placebo in treating acutely agitated patients diagnosed with bipolar mania. *Journal of Clinical Psychopharmacology* 21: 389-397

Miklowitz DJ, George EL, Richards JA, Simoneau TL, Sudhdath RL. 2003. A randomised study of family-focused psychoeducation and pharmacotherapy in the outpatient management of bipolar disorder. *Archives of general Psychiatry* 60: 904-912

Mishory A, Yaroslavsky Y, Bersudsky Y & Belmaker RH. 2000. Phenytoin as an antimanic anticonvulsant; a controlled study. *American Journal of Psychiatry* 157: 463- 465

McElroy SL, Keck PE, Stanto SP, Tugrul KC, Bennett JA & Strakowski SM. 1996. A randomised comparison of Divalproex oral loading versus Haloperidol in the initial treatment of acute psychotic mania. *Journal of Clinical Psychiatry* 57: 142-146

McElroy SL, Weisler RH, Chang W, Olausson B, Paulsson B & et al. 2010. A double-blind, placebo-controlled study of Quetiapine and Paroxetine as monotherapy in adults with bipolar depression (EMBOLDEN II study). *Journal of Clinical Psychiatry* 71: 163-174

McIntyre RS, Brecher M, Paulsson B, Huizar K & Mullen J. 2005. Quetiapine or Haloperidol as monotherapy for bipolar mania- a 12week, double-blind, randomised, parallel-group, placebo- controlled trial. *European Neuropsychopharmacology* 15: 573- 585

McIntyre RS, Konarski JZ, Jones M & Paulsson B. 2007. Quetiapine in the treatment of acute bipolar mania: Efficacy across a broad range of symptoms. *Journal of Affective Disorders* 100: suppl S5-S14

McIntyre RS, Hirschfeld R, Alphs L, Cohen M, Macek T & Panagides J. 2008. Randomised, placebo-controlled studies of Asenapine in the treatment of acute mania in bipolar I disorder. *Journal of Affective Disorders* 107 (suppl 1): 56

McIntyre RS, Cohen M, Zhao J & et al. 2009.Asenapine versus Olanzapine in acute mania: a double-blind extension study. *Bipolar Disorders* 11: 815- 826

Nemeroff CB, Evans DL, Gyulai L & et al. 2001. Double- blind, placebo-controlled comparison of Imipramine and Paroxetine in the treatment of bipolar depression. *American Journal of Psychiatry* 158: 906- 912

Nivoli AM, Murru A & Vieta E. 2010. Lithium: Still a cornerstone in the long-term treatment in bipolar disorder? *Neuropsychobiology* 62: 27- 35

Nolen W, Weisler RH, Neijber A & et al .2009. Quetiapine or Lithium versus placebo for maintenance treatment of bipolar I disorder after stabilisation on Quetiapine. Poster presented at 17th European Congress of Psychiatry; 24- 28th Jan 2009, Lisbon, Portugal; in press

Okuma T, Kishimoto A, Inoue K, Matsumoto H & Ogura A. 1973. Anti-manic and prophylactic effects of Carbamazepine on manic depressive psychosis. A preliminary report. *Folia Psychiatr Neurology* Japan 27: 283- 297

Okuma T, Inanaga K, Otsuki S, Sarai K, Takahashi R & et al. 1979. Comparison of the antimanic efficacy of Carbamazepine and Chlorpromazine: a double-blind controlled study. *Psychopharmacology* 66: 211- 217

Perlis RH, Baker RW, Zarate CA Jr, Brown EB, Schuh LM, Jamal HH & et al. 2006. Olanzapine versus Risperidone in the treatment of manic or mixed states in bipolar I disorder: a randomised, double- blind trial. *Journal of Clinical Psychiatry* 67: 1747-1753

Prien RF, Caffey EM & Klett CJ. 1972. Comparison of Lithium carbonate and Chlorpromazine in the treatment of mania. Report of the Veterans Administration and National Institute of Mental Health Collaborative Study Group. *Archives of General Psychiatry* 26: 146- 153

Post RM, Ketter TA, Uhde T & Ballenger JC. 2007. Thirty years of clinical experience with Carbamazepine in the treatment of bipolar illness: principles and practice. *CNS Drugs* 21: 47- 71

Post RM, Uhde TW, Roy-Byrne & et al. 1986. Antidepressant effects of Carbamazepine. *American Journal of Psychiatry* 43: 29- 34

Reegeer EJ, Ten HM, Rosso ML, Hakkaart- van RL, Vollebergh W & Nolen WA. 2004. Prevalence of bipolar disorder in the general population: a Reappraisal study of the Netherlands Mental Health survey and Incidence study. *Acta Psychiatrica Scandinavica* 110: 374- 382.

Rosa AR, Fountoulakis K, Siamouli M, Gonda X & Vieta E. 2011. Is anticonvulsant treatment of mania a class effect? Data from randomised clinical trials. *CNS Neurosciences & Therapeutics* 17: 167-177

Sachs GS, Grossman F, Ghaemi SN, Okmoto A & Bowden CL. 2002. Combination of mood stabiliser with Risperidone or Haloperidol for treatment of acute mania: a double-blind, placebo- controlled comparison of efficacy and safety. *American Journal of Psychiatry* 159: 1146- 1154

Sachs G, Chengappa KN, Suppes T, Mullen JA, Brecher M, Devine NA & et al. 2004. Quetiapine with Lithium or Divalproex for the treatment of bipolar mania: a randomised, double-blind, placebo- controlled study. *Bipolar Disorders* 6: 213- 233

Sachs G, Sanchez R, Marcus R, Stock E, McQuade R, Carson W & et al. 2006. Aripiprazole in the treatment of acute manic or mixed episodes in patients with bipolar I disorder: a 3-week placebo- controlled study. *Journal of Psychopharmacology* 20: 536- 546

Sanford M & Scott LJ. 2008. Intramuscular Aripiprazole: a review of its use in the management of agitation in schizophrenia and bipolar I disorder. *CNS Drugs* 22: 335- 352

Scott J, Paykel E, Morris R, Bentall R, Kinderman P, Johnson T & et al. 2006. Cognitive – behavioural therapy for severe and recurrent bipolar disorders- randomised controlled trail. *British Journal of Psychiatry* 188: 313-320

Segal J, Berk M & Brook S. 1998. Risperidone compared with both Lithium and Haloperidol in mania: a double-blind randomised controlled trial. *Clinical Neuropharmacology* 21: 176- 180

Sidor MM & McQueen GM. 2011. Antidepressants for the acute treatment of bipolar depression: a systematic review and meta-analysis. *Journal of Clinical Psychiatry* 72: 156- 167

Small JG. 1990. Anticonvulsants in affective disorders. *Psychopharmacology Bulletin* 26: 25- 36

Smith LA, Cornelius V, Warnock A, Tacchi MJ & Taylor D. 2007. Acute bipolar mania: a systematic review and meta-analysis of Co-therapy vs. Monotherapy. *Acta Psychiatrica Scandinavica* 115: 12-20

Smith LA, Cornelius V, Azorin JM, Perugi G, Vieta E, Young AH & Bowden CL. 2010. Valproate for the treatment of acute bipolar depression: systematic review and meta- analysis. *Journal of Affective Disorders* 122: 1- 9

Suppes T, Baldessarini RJ, Faedda GL & Tohen M. 1991. Risk of recurrence following discontinuation of Lithium treatment in bipolar disorder. *Archives of General Psychiatry* 48: 1082-1088

Suppes T, Webb A, Paul B, Carmody T, Kraemer H & Rush AJ. 2003. Clinical outcome in a Randomised 1-year trial of Clozapine versus treatment as usual for patients with treatment resistant illness and a history of mania. *Focus* 1: 37- 43

Swann AC, Bowden CL, Calabrese J, Dilsaver Sc & Morris DD. 2002. Pattern of response to Divalproex, Lithium, or placebo in four naturalistic subtypes of mania. *Neuropsychopharmacology* 26: 530- 536

Thase ME, Macfadden W, Weisler RH, Chang W, Paulsson B, Khan A & et al. 2006. Efficacy of Quetiapine monotherapy in bipolar I and II depression: a double-blind, placebo-controlled study (the BOLDER II study). J *Clinical Psychopharmacology* 26: 600- 609

Thomas P, Vieta E, for the SOLMANIA study group. 2008. Amisulpride plus Valproate vs. Haloperidol plus Valproate in the treatment of acute mania of bipolar I patients: a multicenter, open-label, randomised, comparative trial. *Neuropsychiatry Disorders Treatment* 4: 1- 12

Tohen M, Jacobs TG, Grundy SL, McElroy SL, Banov MC, Janicak PG & et al. 2000. Efficacy of Olanzapine in acute bipolar mania: a double- blind, placebo- controlled study. The Olanzapine HGEH Study Group. *Archives of General Psychiatry* 57: 841- 849

Tohen M, Chengappa KN, Suppes T, Zarate CA, Calabrese JR, Bowden CL & et al. 2002. Efficacy of Olanzapine in combination with Valproate or Lithium in the treatment of mania in patients partially nonresponsive to Valproate or Lithium monotherapy. *Archives of General Psychiatry* 59: 62-69

Tohen M, Goldberg JF, Gonzalez- Pinto Arrillaga AM, Azorin JM, Vieta E & et al. 2003a. A 12- week, double-blind comparison of Olanzapine vs. Haloperidol in the treatment of acute mania. *Archives of General Psychiatry* 60: 1218- 1226

Tohen M, Ketter TA, Zarate CA, Suppes T, Frye M, Altshuler L & et al. 2003b. Olanzapine versus Divalproex Sodium for the treatment of acute mania and maintenance of remission: a 47- week study. *American Journal of Psychiatry* 160: 1263-1271

Tohen M, Vieta E, Calabrese J & et al. 2003c. Efficacy of Olanzapine and Olanzapine-Fluoxetine combination in the treatment of bipolar I depression. *Archives of General Psychiatry* 60: 1079- 1088

Tohen M, Zarate CA, Hennen J & et al. 2003d. The McLean- Harvard First- Episode Mania Study: prediction of recovery and first recurrence. *American Journal of Psychiatry* 160: 2099- 2107

Tohen M, Greil W, Calabrese JR, Sachs GS, Yatham LN & et al. 2005. Olanzapine versus Lithium in the maintenance treatment of bipolar disorder: a 12- month randomised double-blind, controlled clinical trial. *American Journal of Psychiatry* 162: 1281- 1290

Tohen M, Calabrese JR, Sachs GS, Banov MD, Detke HC & et al. 2006. Randomised, placebo-controlled trial of Olanzapine as maintenance therapy in patients with bipolar I disorder responding to acute treatment with Olanzapine. *American Journal of Psychiatry* 163: 247- 256

Tohen M, Kryzhanovskaya L, Carlson G, DelBello M, Wozniak J, Kowatch R & et al. 2007. Olanzapine versus placebo in the treatment of adolescents with bipolar mania. *American Journal of Psychiatry* 164: 1547- 1556

Tohen M, Bowden CL, Smulevich AB, Bergstrom R, Quinlan T, Osuntokun O & et al. 2008. Olanzapine plus Carbamazepine alone in treating manic episodes. *British Journal of Psychiatry* 192: 135-143

Tohen M, Vieta E, Goodwin GM, Sun B, Amsterdam JD, Banov M, Shekhar A & et al. 2009. Olanzapine versus Divalproex versus placebo in the treatment of mild to moderate mania: a randomised, 12 week, double-blind study. *Journal of Clinical Psychiatry* 69: 1776- 1789

van der Loss ML, Mulder P, Hartong EG & et al for the Lamlit study group. 2009. Efficacy and safety of Lamotrigine as add-on treatment to Lithium in bipolar depression: a multi-centre, double-blind, placebo-controlled trial. *Journal of Clinical Psychiatry* 70: 223-231

van der Loss ML, Mulder P, Hartong EG & et al. 2010. Efficacy and safety of two treatment algorithms in bipolar depression consisting of a combination of Lithium, Lamotrigine or placebo and Paroxetine. *Acta Psychiatrica Scandinavica* 122: 246- 254

van der Loss ML, Mulder P, Hartong EG, Blom MB & et al. 2011. Long-term outcomes of bipolar depressed patients receiving Lamotrigine as add-on to Lithium with the possibility of the addition of Paroxetine in non-responders: a randomised, placebo-controlled trial with a novel design. *Bipolar Disorders* 13: 111- 117

Vasudev K, Goswami U, Kohli K. 2000. Carbamazepine and Valproate monotherapy: feasibility, relative safety and efficacy, and therapeutic drug monitoring in manic disorder. *Psychopharmacology (Berlin)* 150: 15-23

Vieta E. 2009. Are antidepressants useful in treating bipolar depression? *International Journal of Psychiatry in Clinical Practice* 13 (suppl 1): 15-16

Vieta E, Bourin M, Sanchez R, Marcus R, Stcok E, McQuade R & et al. 2005a. Effectiveness of Aripiprazole v. Haloperidol in acute bipolar mania: double-blind, randomised, comparative 12- week trial 4829. *British Journal of Psychiatry* 187: 235- 242

Vieta E, Ros S, Goikolea JM, Benabarre A, Popova E, Comes M & et al. 2005b. An open-label study of Amisulpride in the treatment of mania. *Journal of Clinical Psychiatry* 66: 575- 578

Vieta E, Panicali F, Goetz I, Reed C, Comes M & Tohen M. 2008. Olanzapine monotherapy and Olanzapine combination therapy in the treatment of mania: 12-week results from the European Mania in Bipolar Longitudinal Evaluation of Medication (EMBLEM) observational study. *Journal of Affective Disorders* 106: 63-72

Vieta E, Suppes T, Eggens I, Persson I, Paulsson B, Brecher M & et al. 2008b. Efficacy and safety of Quetiapine in combination with Lithium or Divalproex for maintenance of patients with bipolar I disorder. *Journal of Affective Disorders* 109: 251-263

Vieta E, Tjoen C, McQuade RD, Carson WH, Jr., Marcus RN, Sanchez R & at al. 2009a. Efficacy of adjunctive Aripiprazole to either Valproate or Lithium in bipolar mania patients partially non-responsive to Valproate/ Lithium monotherapy: A placebo-controlled study. *American Journal of Psychiatry* 165: 1316- 1325

Vieta E, Ramey TS, Keller D, English PA, Loebel AD & Miceli JJ. 2010b. Ziprasidone in the treatment of acute mania: a 12-week, placebo-controlled, Haloperidol- referenced study. *Journal of Psychopharmacology* 24: 547- 548

Vieta E, Berwaerts J, Nuamah I, Lim P, Yuen E, Palumbo J & et al. 2010a. Randomised, placebo, active- controlled study of Paliperidone extended release (ER) for acute manic and mixed episodes in bipolar I disorder. *Bipolar Disorders* 12: 230- 243

Weisler RH, Kalali AH & Ketter TA. 2004. A multicenter, randomised, double-blind, placebo- controlled trial of extended- release Carbamazepine capsules as monotherapy for bipolar disorder patients with manic or mixed episodes. *Journal of Clinical Psychiatry* 65: 478- 484

Weisler RH, Keck PE Jr, Swann AC, Cutler AJ, Ketter TA & Kalali AH. 2005. Extended-release Carbamazepine capsules as monotherapy for acute mania in bipolar disorder: a multicenter, randomised, double-blind, placebo- controlled trial. *Journal of Clinical Psychiatry* 66: 323- 330

Weissman MM, Bland RC, Canino GJ, Faravelli C, Greenwald S, Hwu HG & et al. 1996. Cross-national epidemiology of major depression and bipolar disorder. *Journal of the American Medical Association* 276: 293-299

WHO 1996 (Murray CJL & Lopez AD). The Global Burden of Disease. *Geneva, World Health Organisation, Harvard School of Public Health, World Bank*

Woods SW. 2000. The economic burden of bipolar disorder. *Journal of Clinical Psychology* 61 suppl 13: 38- 41

Yatham LN. 2005. Atypical antipsychotics for bipolar disorder. *Psychiatry Clinics of North America* 28: 325- 347

Yatham LN, Grossman F, Augustyns I, Vieta E & Ravindran A. 2003. Mood stabilisers plus Risperidone or placebo in the treatment of acute mania. International, double-blind, randomised controlled trail. *British Journal of Psychiatry* 182: 141- 147

Yatham LN, Paulsson B, Mullen J & Vagero AM. 2004. Quetiapine versus placebo in combination with Lithium or Divalproex for the treatment of bipolar mania. *Journal of Clinical Psychopharmacology* 24: 599- 606

Yildiz A, Guleryuz S, Ankerst DP, Ongur D & Renshaw PF. 2008. Protein Kinase C inhibition in the treatment of mania: a double-blind, placebo-controlled trail of Tamoxifen. *Archives of General Psychiatry* 65: 255- 263

Young LT, Joffe RT, Robb JC & et al. 2000. Double-blind comparison of addition of a second mood stabiliser versus an antidepressant to an initial mood stabiliser for treatment of patients with bipolar depression. *American Journal of Psychiatry* 157: 124- 127.

Young AH, Oren DA, Lowy A, McQuade RD, Marcus RN, Carson WH & et al. 2009. Aripiprazole monotherapy in acute mania: 12-week randomised placebo- and Haloperidol- controlled study. *British Journal of Psychiatry* 194: 40-48

Young AH, McElroy SL, Bauer M, Philips N, Chang W & et al. 2010. A double-blind, placebo-controlled study of Quetiapine and Lithium monotherapy in adults in the acute phase of bipolar depression (EMBOLDEN I study). *Journal of Clinical Psychiatry* 71: 150- 162

Zarate CA & Tohen M. 2004. Double-blind comparison of the continued use of antipsychotic treatment versus its discontinuation in remitted mania patients. *American Journal of Psychiatry* 161:169- 171

Zajecka JM, Weisler R, Sachs G, Swann AC, Wozniak P & Sommerville KW. 2002. A comparison of the efficacy, safety, and tolerability of Divalproex Sodium and Olanzapine in the treatment of bipolar disorder. *Journal of Clinical Psychiatry* 63: 1148-1155

3

Antidepressant Pharmacotherapy – Do the Benefits Outweigh the Risks?

Angela Getz, Fenglian Xu and Naweed Syed
University of Calgary, Faculty of Medicine, Department of Cell Biology and Anatomy,
Hotchkiss Brain Institute
Canada

1. Introduction

Major depressive disorder (MDD) is a debilitating and often recurrent psychiatric illness that impacts the lives of millions. Approximately 20 percent of individuals will experience at least one depressive episode during their lives, and the high rates of chronic morbidity (depressive episodes typically last for several months) and mortality (owing to suicide) attributed to this disorder constitute one of the largest global economic disease burdens (Kessler et al., 2005). Despite the considerable burden of depression, our understanding of its pathophysiology and the therapeutic mechanisms of action of antidepressant drugs remains incomplete. In fact, much of what we currently understand about the neuropathology of depression is derived from the observed effects of known antidepressants on the brain. This situation is confounded by the fact that currently available antidepressant drugs are of limited clinical efficacy – the antidepressant response typically takes several weeks to develop, and a substantial proportion of patients do not experience a significant improvement in depressive symptoms, or full clinical remission. Furthermore, because antidepressant efficacy varies significantly as a function of symptom severity, the benefit of antidepressant therapy may be limited or nonexistent in patients with mild to moderate depressive symptoms, which represent the majority of clinical cases (Fournier et al., 2010). When the inadequate efficacy profiles of antidepressant drugs are weighed against our limited understanding of depression, the therapeutic action of antidepressants, and the potential negative side effects of these drugs arising from nonspecific actions, a difficult question arises: do the benefits of antidepressant pharmacotherapy outweigh the risks?

In this chapter, we explore the development of the current theories of depression etiology, the hindrances of current antidepressant therapeutics, and how the poor understanding of the mechanism of antidepressant action contributes to a haphazard interpretation of the benefits and consequences arising from their non-specific interactions. Through the use of a simple single-synapse experimental approach, we have gained insights into the impact of non-specific antidepressant actions on neuronal function, and our findings will be discussed in this context. Finally, we will explore prospective developments in the field of depression pharmacotherapy that may hold the potential to revolutionize the way we understand and treat depression.

1.1 Identifying & understanding depression

Depression is a prevalent psychiatric condition in which the depressive affect (the immediate emotional state and a normal emotional response) becomes sustained and predominant, thus constituting a disorder of mood (a sustained emotional state). It is characterized by persistent emotional symptoms including a dysphoric mood and anhedonia (loss of interest or pleasure), low self-esteem, feelings of guilt, anguish, apathy and pessimism, and thoughts of suicide or death. Additional biological symptoms include difficulty concentrating and remembering, disturbances of sleep and appetite, loss of energy and libido, and psychomotor agitation (restlessness) or psychomotor retardation (slowing of thoughts and actions). The clinical diagnosis of depression is subjective, being based on the concurrent presence of a depressed mood, and a number of the above-mentioned biological symptoms, for a period of at least two weeks.

Because the understanding of the pathophysiology of depression is limited, reliable indicators of risk have not yet been identified. The multitude of symptom profiles that constitute a diagnosis of depression points to the heterogeneous nature of the disorder, and its probable multifactorial and polygenic etiology. Indeed, the heterogeneity of depression is evident in the markedly different occurrence of depressive symptoms, genetic predispositions, and environmental risk factors such as stressful life events, among patients that present with MDD. Depression has a strong genetic predisposition, with an estimated heritability of 40 percent (Krishnan & Nestler, 2008; Sullivan et al., 2000); and while genetic association studies have identified some MDD susceptibility genes, several of which play a role in monoaminergic neurotransmission and neuroplasticity, findings have often been inconsistent, and the role of genetic polymorphisms in the manifestation of MDD remains uncertain (López-León et al., 2008; Pezawas et al., 2008). The roles of monoamine neurotransmitters and neuroplasticity in depression will be further explored below.

The linear relationship between genetic mutations and inherited disorders, which has proven useful in understanding numerous other conditions (such as familial Alzheimer's disease or Huntington's disease), is not so evident in psychiatric disorders, where it is likely that complex interactions between genes and the environment influence neuronal networks, and ultimately behaviour. A polymorphism in the serotonin transporter (5-HTT) gene, which modulates serotonergic neurotransmission, was found to influence the occurrence of depression in response to stressful life events, providing the first direct evidence for the interplay of genes and the environment in the etiology of depression (Caspi et al., 2003). The strong contribution of both genetics and the environment to MDD provides a feasible starting point from which we can begin to understand and interpret the heterogeneity of depression, and ultimately, perhaps, even predict or prevent its onset.

1.2 Depression etiology: Insights from antidepressant drugs

Advances in understanding the etiology and developing effective therapeutics for MDD – and numerous psychiatric and neurodegenerative illnesses, for that matter – have lagged considerably behind other areas of medical research, the primary obstacle being the inherent complexity of the human brain. Research in the field of mood disorders has been hindered by both the difficulty of studying the brain directly (though modern imaging techniques have enabled considerable progress in this area), and the lack of truly representative animal models, where, while biological correlates of the disorder can be induced in animal models, the emotional and psychological characteristics that define the human condition are far from accurately paralleled.

The mechanistic understanding of both MDD and the therapeutic mode of action of antidepressants has been slow to follow the development and clinical application of antidepressant medication, particularly because the desired outcome of drug treatment is readily apparent as an elevation of mood and alleviation of depressive symptoms, whereas reversal of the causative brain abnormalities underlying MDD, such as neurochemical imbalance and/or structural alterations, are not so evident. A case in point, the primary theories of the etiology of depression have developed not from identifying the factors that underlie the neuropathology of MDD, but rather from observing the effects of antidepressant drugs on the brain and interpreting the roles of these target neuronal systems in behaviour.

1.2.1 The monoamine hypothesis

The monoaminergic theory of depression posits that the cause of depression is a functional deficit in monoaminergic neurotransmission, due to the decreased availability of monoamine neurotransmitters, of which serotonin (5-Hydroxytryptamine; 5-HT) has received considerable attention in depression. Developed from early observations that drugs fortuitously discovered to exert antidepressant effects all appeared to target monoaminergic systems, the monoamine hypothesis was the first biochemical theory of depression, and remains one of the main etiological hypotheses of the disorder (Schildkraut, 1965; Lapin et al., 1969). Serotonin in particular plays a dynamic role in the regulation of mood, cognition, attention, learning, appetite, sleep, motor function and the response to stress (Martinowich & Lu, 2008; Oberlander et al., 2009). In accordance with the monoamine hypothesis, there is an obvious parallel between the symptomatic disruption of mood and behaviour in depression, and the normal physiological role of serotonin.

The monoamine theory of MDD provides the most logical basis for understanding the therapeutic mode of action of antidepressant drugs, as nearly all available antidepressants act by potentiating the synaptic availability of monoamine neurotransmitters (López-Muñoz & Alamo, 2009), which will be further explored below. Whereas antidepressants produce a rapid biochemical effect and an almost immediate enhancement of chemical neurotransmission, there is a substantial delay in the onset of antidepressant action. Achieving clinical improvement in depressive symptoms requires several weeks of continuous antidepressant administration, highlighting two obvious limitations of both current antidepressant medications and the monoamine theory of depression: firstly, the prolonged period of therapeutic inefficacy provides a large window during which depressive symptoms remain untreated, and suicide risk is high (Licinio & Wong, 2005); and secondly, such a delay in the onset of antidepressant action indicates that the cause of depression is not simply a deficit of monoamine neurotransmitters.

1.2.2 The Neuroplasticity hypothesis

A recent neuroplasticity theory of MDD gaining acceptance and substantial evidentiary support posits that depression results from disruptions of neuronal plasticity (structural and functional alterations of the brain in response to environmental changes) at various regions of the brain (Pittenger & Duman, 2008). In depressed patients, post-mortem and neuroimaging studies have identified neuronal atrophy and aberrant activity patterns in several brain structures, most notably in the prefrontal cortex, hippocampus and amygdala (Zou et al., 2010; Drevets, 2001; Krishnan & Nestler, 2008). Remarkably, chronic stress, an environmental risk factor known to contribute to the development depression, also affects neuroplasticity in similar brain regions. These affected structures are responsible for various aspects of cognition, including executive functions (prefrontal cortex), emotional response (amygdala) and memory formation (hippocampus). Again, the normal functions of the brain regions disrupted by chronic stress and MDD parallel the symptomatology of depression, pointing to an underlying role for dysfunctional neuronal plasticity in the etiology of MDD. A powerful facet of the neuroplastic hypothesis is the ability to explain the delayed onset of antidepressant drug effects. Through a slower-acting secondary neuroplastic mechanism, long-term adaptive changes in the brain in response to antidepressants are thought to be responsible for the clinical improvement of depressive symptoms. Indeed, following chronic antidepressant treatment, the occurrence of structural and functional changes and enhanced neurogenesis that normalize neuronal networks and activity patterns correlates with the onset of the therapeutic response, and are likely to play a causal role in antidepressant action (Ressler & Mayberg, 2007; Santarelli et al., 2003; Maya Vetencourt et al., 2008). Though we lack a clear understanding of the mechanistic action of antidepressants, there is an apparent relationship between the mechanisms of neuroplasticity and MDD neuropathology, which has been illuminated by the molecular and cellular changes in the brain brought about by antidepressant action. The implication of neuroplasticity in MDD lends to the exciting possibility that the cellular and molecular mechanisms of synaptic plasticity may be effective and more direct targets for antidepressant therapeutics, providing prospective directions for investigation in a field of pharmacology that has been stagnant for decades.

1.2.3 Linking monoamines, neuroplasticity & antidepressants

The slow onset of therapeutic effects of antidepressant drugs that rapidly increase synaptic levels of monoamine neurotransmitters necessitated the development of an alternative neuromodulatory hypothesis for the mechanism of therapeutic action of antidepressant medication. However, the monoaminergic and neuroplasticity theories of depression are not mutually exclusive, as monoamines are modulatory neurotransmitters that influence neurogenesis and neuron survival, neuronal activity, synaptogenesis and synaptic plasticity by initiating molecular signalling cascades. In particular, changes in the expression levels or function of neurotrophic factors, such as brain-derived neurotrophic factor (BDNF), a growth factor that is a key regulator of synaptic plasticity and participates in a developmental feed-back loop with serotonin, has been suggested to underlie both depression neuropathology and the therapeutic antidepressant response (Martinowich & Lu, 2008). Studies demonstrating that levels of BDNF and BDNF-mediated signalling are reduced in depressed patients and increased patients receiving antidepressant medication provide a link between the expression of BDNF and the therapeutic action of antidepressants (Shimizu et al., 2003; Chen, 2001). This notion is further supported by evidence that BDNF signalling is necessary for mediating the antidepressant response in animal models (Saarelainen et al., 2003). How exactly this BDNF-mediated neuroplasticity contributes to the emotional and behavioural response in antidepressant treatment remains unidentified.

The intracellular signal transduction cascades connecting serotonin neurotransmission and BDNF expression provide a workable explanation for the ability of antidepressants that potentiate monoaminergic activity to promote neuroplasticity and an antidepressant response. All but one of the 5-HT receptor subtypes act through a G-protein coupled metabotropic mechanism, which initiates cellular responses through the activation of intracellular signalling cascades. Chronic antidepressant treatment, presumably by promoting enhanced serotonergic synaptic availability and receptor signalling, has been found to up-regulate numerous components of the cAMP signal transduction pathway, including the effector protein kinase A (PKA) and the transcription factor cAMP-response-element-binding protein (CREB) (Nestler et al., 1989; Nibuya et al., 1996; Pittenger & Duman, 2008). Notably, the cAMP-PKA-CREB cascade, which is implicated in synaptic plasticity, is downstream of a number stimulatory G-protein coupled receptors, including several serotonin receptor subtypes (Martinowich & Lu, 2008). As CREB is a key transcription factor involved in activity-dependent BDNF expression (Tao et al., 1998), the activation of CREB may be one of the mechanisms by which the antidepressant-induced elevation of monoamines acts to enhance BDNF expression and promote neuroplasticity.

1.3 Antidepressant pharmacotherapy: Limited options & limited outcomes

Nearly all currently marketed antidepressant medications act to increase the synaptic availability of monoamine neurotransmitters. This is achieved through one of two mechanisms: the prevention of degradation by inhibition of the enzyme monoamine oxidase, or the prevention of re-uptake from the synapse by inhibition of the reuptake transporter proteins. The three commonly prescribed classes of antidepressants include the Monoamine oxidase inhibitors (MAOIs), the tricyclic antidepressants (TCA), and the selective reuptake inhibitors (SRIs), including selective serotonin reuptake inhibitors (SSRIs), and serotonin-norepinephrine reuptake inhibitors (SNRIs).

MAOIs: Among the first clinically introduced antidepressants, MAOIs cause inhibition of the monoamine oxidase enzyme, which acts to degrade serotonin, norepinephrine and dopamine. In the brain, monoamine oxidase (MAO) regulates the cytoplasmic concentration of monoamine neurotransmitters, thus, the primary effect of MAOIs is to increase the cytoplasmic concentration of monoamines, thereby promoting spontaneous transmitter leakage and enhanced synaptic action. The enzyme isoform MAO-A is the primary target of MAOI-type antidepressants, and is responsible for the antidepressant effect. However, most MAOIs are not particularly selective, inhibiting both MAO-A and MAO-B isoforms, as well as several other enzymes, including those involved in drug metabolism. These non-specific interactions contribute to an extensive profile of serious adverse effects including cardiovascular complications, dietary interactions, drug interactions, and lethality in overdose.

TCAs: Another class of early antidepressants, tricyclic compounds (so named for their characteristic three-ringed chemical structure) were initially synthesized as potential antipsychotic drugs, and though found ineffective in psychosis, they did exert potent antidepressive effects. TCAs act to inhibit the reuptake of monoamines from the synapse by blocking reuptake transporters, the primary mechanism by which the length of the synaptic signal is regulated and the actions of monoamine neurotransmitters are terminated. This action enhances the synaptic availability of monoamine neurotransmitters. All of the three major classes of monoamine transporter proteins, the serotonin transporter (SERT or 5-HTT), the norepinephrine transporter (NET) and to a lesser extent the dopamine transporter (DAT), are inhibited by TCAs. As with MAOIs, the non-selective pharmacological profile of TCAs contributes to a host of unwanted effects, including inhibition of various types of neurotransmitter receptors, cardiovascular effects, sedation, drug interactions, and lethality in overdose.

SRIs: The diverse systemic side effect profiles of MAOIs and TCAs, coupled with the toxic effects in overdose that lead to the frequent use of these compounds in suicide attempts, prompted the development of new antidepressants that would be safer and more tolerable – what resulted was a diverse class of second-generation reuptake inhibitors whose clinical use rapidly overtook that of MAOIs and TCAs. Of all the available types of antidepressant drugs, selective serotonin reuptake inhibitors (SSRIs) are the most commonly prescribed. Acting in a manner analogous to TCAs, these second generation compounds block monoamine reuptake, but exhibit selectivity for blocking SERT and/or NET. While the profile of adverse drug effects of SRIs is more favourable than that of MAOIs or TCAs, these antidepressants still exhibit considerable side effects including the nonspecific inhibition of ion channels and neurotransmitter receptors, and even, surprisingly, an increased risk of suicide.

Drug Class		Examples	Conventional Mode of Action
MAOIs		Phenelzine Rasagiline Moclobemide Iproniazid	Monoamine Oxidase Inhibition (MAO-A)
TCAs		Imipramine Amitriptyline Doxepin Desipramine	Monoamine Reuptake Transporter Inhibition (SERT, NET, DAT)
SRIs	SSRI	Fluoxetine Paroxetine Citalopram Sertaline	Selective Serotonin Reuptake Inhibition (SERT)
	SNRI	Venlafaxine Duloxetine	Serotonin-Norepinephrine Reuptake Inhibition (SERT, NET)

Table 1. Classification of monoaminergic antidepressant drugs according to the conventional mechanism of action.

The advent of second-generation SRIs with a superior safety profile improved the pharmacological management of depression; however, this advance was not paralleled by an improvement in the clinical outcome of MDD pharmacotherapy. MAOIs, TCAs, and SRIs all require several weeks of continuous treatment for an improvement of depressive symptoms to appear, meanwhile the response rate is abysmally low and the relapse rate is high. Only approximately 60 percent of patients receiving antidepressants experience a meaningful improvement of depressive symptoms, with as little as one third experiencing full remission (Trivedi et al., 2006; Thase et al., 2005). A further disadvantage of the available plethora of antidepressant medications is the fact that they all essentially work through the same monoaminergic mechanism. Thus, attempting combinatorial therapy or a series of different medications in attempts to gain improvement in the clinical management of MDD faces fundamental mechanistic limitations, though this is a commonly employed but largely unproven clinical strategy (Thase, 2011). Whereas SRIs have to some extent addressed the adverse side effect profile of antidepressants, the efficacy and time course of therapeutic action are two critical aspects of antidepressant therapeutics that still must be improved.

1.4 Side effects of antidepressant pharmacotherapy: Consequences of high therapeutic doses & non-specific drug effects

Antidepressants are notoriously promiscuous substances, indiscriminately affecting a wide range of ion channels, neurotransmitter receptors, and synaptic plasticity mechanisms that ultimately results in changes in neuronal architecture and function. While these non-specific effects have been suggested to be essential for producing the antidepressant response, the fact that we do not know the mechanism of therapeutic action of antidepressants makes it difficult to separate the beneficial from the detrimental effects of these non-specific interactions.

With the reuptake blocker type of antidepressants (including TCAs and SRIs), there exists a 100-1,000 fold-magnitude of difference between the concentrations at which selective inhibition of monoamine reuptake and the therapeutic antidepressant effect occurs (Bolo et al., 2000; Torres et al., 2003; Lenkey et al., 2006). The high concentrations required for therapeutic efficacy result in a substantial loss of drug specificity. Within the therapeutic window (e.g. steady state brain concentrations in the low micromolar range), antidepressants affect a number of protein targets, inhibiting numerous types of ion channels and neurotransmitter receptors, which are critical components of neuronal electrical excitability and network activity. Documented interactions of antidepressant drugs include calcium, sodium and potassium channels, as well as serotonergic, adrenergic, dopaminergic, glutamatergic, and cholinergic receptors. The movement of ions through voltage- and ligand-gated channels underlies virtually every aspect of neuronal function – action potential generation and synaptic communication being two principle examples. Calcium (Ca^{2+}) ions in particular have a critical function as a second messengers in intracellular signalling, regulating numerous neuronal events such as the activation of Ca^{2+}-dependent proteins, the initiation of gene expression, neurite outgrowth, synapse formation, neurotransmitter release and synaptic plasticity (Feng et al., 2002; Xu et al., 2009; Hardingham et al., 1997). As the cardiovascular system similarly depends on ionic influx (i.e. Ca^{2+} for heart contraction) and neurotransmitter regulation, this opens to the possibility that the non-specific interactions of antidepressant drugs with voltage gated ion channels and neurotransmitter receptors can produce systemic dysregulation, as is seen in the cardiotoxic lethality in TCA overdose. Ultimately, the blind modulation of protein targets by antidepressant drugs contributes to systemic and neuronal side effects that may have devastating consequences.

A fundamental principle of therapeutic intervention is that the derived benefit of the therapy must outweigh the potential risks. Antidepressant medications are readily used as the first-line standard of treatment for the management of MDD, as depression constitutes a substantial personal and economic burden, and the risks associated with untreated depression are substantial (i.e. diminished quality of life, loss of productivity, comorbid diseases, suicide). In accordance with the increasing clinical prevalence of MDD, the use of antidepressant drugs has grown rapidly, being the most commonly prescribed class of medication; SSRIs in particular, with their comparatively innocuous profile of serious adverse effects, are the most widely used type of antidepressant (Olfson & Marcus, 2009). In light of the potential negative effects arising from the often overlooked non-specific interactions of antidepressant drugs, the limited benefit of antidepressants raises considerable grounds for concern. Indeed, despite their widespread use, the risk-benefit ratio of antidepressant drugs is somewhat controversial. In addition to the less-than-optimal response and remission rates resulting from antidepressant pharmacotherapy, the actual pharmacological benefit of antidepressants in the majority of patients – those below the threshold of 'very severe' depression – is largely unfounded. In a patient-level meta-analysis, Fournier et al. (2010) demonstrated that the magnitude of response to antidepressant therapy depends on the baseline depression symptom severity; such that compared to placebo, patients with mild to severe depression do not derive significant benefit from antidepressant pharmacotherapy. Furthermore, these patients with less

Target		Drug	Reference
Ion channels			
Sodium (Na⁺) channels		Fluoxetine, Amitriptyline, Desipramine, Doxepin	Pancrazio et al., 1998
	$Na_v1.3$, $Na_v1.4$, $Na_v1.7$	Duloxetine, Sertraline, Paroxetine	Wang et al., 2008; Wang et al., 2010
		Citalopram	Pacher & Kecskemeti, 2004
Potassium (K⁺) channels	HERG	Citalopram	Witchel et al., 2002
	GIRK	Citalopram, Imipramine, Amitriptyline	Kobayashi et al., 2004
	$K_V1.5$	Citalopram	Lee et al., 2010
	$K_V1.1$	Fluoxetine	Yeung et al., 1999
	$K_V3.1$	Fluoxetine	Sung et al., 2008
Calcium (Ca²⁺) channels	T, N, L- type	Fluoxetine, Citalopram	Deák et al., 2000; Witchel et al., 2002
	P/Q-type	Fluoxetine	Wang et al., 2003
Neurotransmitter Receptors			
N-Methyl-D-aspartate (NMDA)		Desipramine, Imipramine	Sernagor et al., 1989; Reynolds & Miller, 1988
Glycine		Fluoxetine	Ye et al., 2008
Nicotinic Acetylcholine (nACh)		Fluoxetine	García-Colunga et al., 1997
		Imipramine,	Rana et al., 1993
Muscarinic Acetylcholine (mACh)		Imipramine	Snyder & Yamamura, 1977
Serotonin (5-HT₃)		Fluoxetine, Phenelzine, Imipramine, Iproniazid	Fan et al., 1994

Table 2. Highlight of some of the known ion channel and neurotransmitter receptor targets of antidepressant drugs.

severe depressions represent the majority of clinical cases, and are frequently excluded from clinical trials establishing antidepressant drug efficacy, where inclusion often requires a minimum baseline symptom severity (Zimmerman et al., 2002). This apparent lack of a meaningful drug response for a large percentage of the MDD patient population tips the balance of the risk-benefit assessment of antidepressant pharmacotherapy, giving rise to the question – could antidepressant therapy be causing more harm than good?

2. Insights from a single-synapse experimental model

In addition to its function as a modulatory neurotransmitter in the adult brain, serotonin also plays a role in numerous neurodevelopmental events, including synaptogenesis and the wiring of brain circuits (Gaspar et al., 2003). As antidepressants are known to cross the placental barrier, numerous clinical and animal model studies have investigated the impact of gestational antidepressant exposure, and have identified the occurrence of severe neurodevelopmental birth defects, neuronal network mis-wiring complications, and sustained neurobehavioural effects in association with *in utero* exposure (Alwan et al., 2007; Xu et al., 2004; Homberg et al., 2009; Oberlander et al., 2009). It is, however, difficult to differentiate between the developmental effects of the maternal mental illness (in clinical studies), excessive levels of serotonin caused by the action of antidepressant drugs, and the non-specific interactions of antidepressants. Identifying the contribution of each of these factors to developmental complications is difficult to assess in the context of complex *in vivo* models. Similar neurodevelopmental events, such as neurogenesis, synaptogenesis and synaptic plasticity, occur throughout adulthood, where they are believed to underlie adaptive processes such as learning and memory. If the non-specific actions of antidepressant drugs do in fact play a role in the disruption of neuronal architecture and function in the developing brain, then the possibility also exists that the dynamic adult brain may be similarly susceptible, raising new concerns for the potential adverse effects of antidepressant drugs.

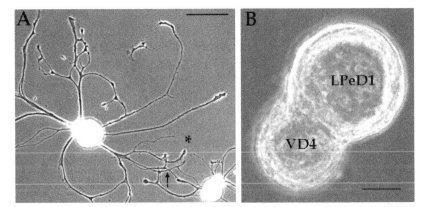

Fig. 1. The *in vitro* neuronal culture model of *Lymnaea stagnalis*. **A.** Neurons cultured in the presence of growth factors extend neurite processes and form synaptic networks with neighboring neurons (arrow). Growth cones (asterisk) actively sense and navigate the environment. Scale bar represents 50 μm. **B.** The soma-soma single synapse experimental model. When the somas (cell bodies) of neurons are juxtaposed in culture, synaptogenesis occurs without the reliance on neurite outgrowth. Scale bar represents 25 μm.

Our interest in investigating the impact of non-specific antidepressant effects on synapse formation and synaptic function was initiated by the fact that antidepressant drugs indiscriminately inhibit ion channels, and that neurotrophic signalling and synaptic plasticity mechanisms appear to be necessary for the antidepressant response. Our group employs a simple *in vitro* experimental model to explore the cellular and molecular mechanisms of synapse formation. With the invertebrate model system *Lymnaea stagnalis*, functionally defined individual neurons with known neurotransmitter phenotype can be isolated and cultured *in vitro*. In the presence of neurotrophic factors, these neurons regenerate neuronal processes, recapitulate specific synaptic connectivity and establish functional neuronal networks, resembling the developmental events seen *in vivo* (Syed et al., 1990; Ridgway et al., 1991; Feng et al., 1997). As this model enables the study of individual neurons, synapse formation and synaptic activity at the level of the single synapse, it provides us with a unique opportunity to isolate the impact of the non-specific interactions of antidepressant drugs on neuronal viability, synaptic function, and neurotrophic factor-dependent synaptogenesis.

2.1 Review of key findings from our comparative evaluation of the neuronal effects of the non-specific actions of two SSRI-type antidepressants

SSRIs represent the most widely used type of antidepressant medication, and though their action is largely regarded to be specific, or at least the most specific of available medications, there is a growing body of evidence that these compounds indiscriminately affect various aspects of neuronal function, primarily through the non-specific inhibition of ion channels and neurotransmitter receptors. For our investigation, we opted to conduct a comparative analysis of two commonly prescribed SSRI-type antidepressant drugs, fluoxetine and citalopram. Fluoxetine was the first and the most obvious choice for investigation, as it was the first clinically introduced SSRI and is furthermore the most commonly used compound in experimental settings. Within the SSRI class of antidepressants, however, fluoxetine exhibits the lowest degree of selectivity for serotonin reuptake, whereas citalopram is the most selective, and additionally is a more potent inhibitor of serotonin reuptake than fluoxetine (Hyttel, 1994). This lends to the possibility that citalopram may produce an antidepressant effect at lower therapeutic concentrations, thereby reducing the risk of non-specific inhibitory actions. These pharmacological characteristics lent to the formulation of our hypothesis that different SSRIs would exert characteristic non-specific neuronal side effects, and, because of its lesser selectivity profile, that fluoxetine would exert a more detrimental effect on synaptic physiology than citalopram. Using a combination of intracellular and patch-clamp electrophysiological recordings, calcium imaging, immunocytochemistry and various neuroimaging techniques, we have for the first time demonstrated that clinically-relevant concentrations of fluoxetine, but not citalopram (dosage range up to 5 µg/mL; Bolo et al., 2000), exhibit detrimental effects on neurite outgrowth, synapse formation, synaptic transmission and synaptic plasticity, and that the negative effects of fluoxetine on synaptic function involves a direct perturbation of both pre- and post-synaptic machinery (Xu et al., 2010; Getz et al., 2011).

2.1.1 Fluoxetine inhibits the initiation of neurite outgrowth and induces growth cone collapse and neurite retraction

The Effect: Neurite outgrowth is the initial and essential step prior to synapse formation, and is easily and routinely modelled experimentally. We therefore first sought to investigate the non-specific neuronal effects of SSRIs by examining their impact on neurite outgrowth. To this end, *Lymnaea* serotonergic or non-serotonergic neurons were cultured under control conditions (in the presence of growth media containing neurotrophic factors), or in the presence of SSRIs over a therapeutically-relevant dosage range. The neuronal ability to initiate and elongate neurite processes, spread branches and form active growth cones was monitored under these two conditions (Xu et al., 2010). We found that neurons cultured in growth media alone established extensive neurite outgrowth (massive branches with active growth cones), while neurons cultured in the presence of fluoxetine exhibited only minimal branches and shorter processes at lower doses (< 3 µg/mL), and no growth at higher concentrations (> 3 µg/mL). In neurons that had developed active growth cones, exposure to fluoxetine resulted in the collapse of growth cones within minutes, and the retraction of neurite processes within hours. These negative effects of fluoxetine were observed in *Lymnaea* neurons regardless of their neurotransmitter phenotype. We also performed a similar investigation using mammalian neurons to determine whether the inhibitory effects of fluoxetine may be attributed to the invertebrate preparation used. Fluoxetine was similarly found to inhibit neurite outgrowth and disrupt neuronal network assembly in both

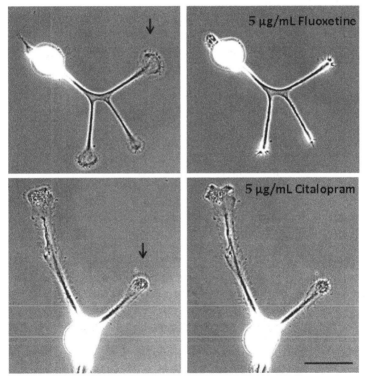

Fig. 2. Acute application of fluoxetine, but not citalopram, causes rapid growth cone collapse and neurite retraction. *Lymnaea* neurons were cultured in the presence of growth factors and allowed to develop neurite outgrowth with active growth cones (arrow). Within 30 minutes of fluoxetine exposure, all growth cones exhibited collapsed morphology, whereas citalopram application resulted in no discernable detrimental effect. Scale bar represents 50 µm

rat primary cortical neurons and neurohybridoma cells homologous to dorsal root ganglion neurons, thus validating our findings of the inhibitory effects of fluoxetine in *Lymnaea* neurons. As the negative effect of fluoxetine on neurite outgrowth and growth cone morphology was observed in neurons regardless of vertebrate or invertebrate, serotonergic or non-serotonergic phenotype, these findings suggest that fluoxetine possesses non-specific effects that are independent of its mechanistic action as an SSRI. Interestingly, exposure to citalopram did not exhibit negative effects on neurite outgrowth or growth cone morphology (Getz et al., unpublished observations), suggesting that the negative effects observed for fluoxetine may be a drug-specific property, and not a common feature of the SSRI class of antidepressants.

The Mechanism: Optimal calcium transients in growth cones have been shown to be essential for the regulation of the polymerization and depolymerisation status of cytoskeletal proteins including F-actin, and thus affect growth cone motility and behaviour (Spira et al., 2001; Welnhofer et al., 1999; Henley & Poo, 2004). In the presence of trophic factors, the growth cones of *Lymnaea* neurons exhibit small spontaneous Ca^{2+} transients, and these Ca^{2+} transients were eliminated within minutes of exposure to fluoxetine (Xu et al., 2010). Furthermore, immunocytochemical labeling identified that the fluoxetine-induced inhibition of spontaneous Ca^{2+} transients and collapse of growth cones was accompanied by a breakdown of the F-actin cytoskeleton. Thus, the perturbation of Ca^{2+} homeostasis in neuronal growth cones by the non-specific actions of fluoxetine contributes to its detrimental effect on neuronal architecture.

2.1.2 Fluoxetine, but not citalopram, inhibits synapse formation

The Effect: Because fluoxetine was found to prevent neurite outgrowth and neuronal network assembly, the use of the soma-soma synapse model, where synapse formation occurs in the absence of neuronal outgrowth, enabled us to investigate how the non-specific effects of SSRIs might affect the development of functional synapses. When paired in a soma-soma configuration, the identified *Lymnaea* neurons visceral dorsal 4 (VD4) and left pedal dorsal 1 (LPeD1) form a well characterized excitatory cholinergic synapse, in which VD4 functions presynaptically, and LPeD1 functions as the postsynaptic partner. As SSRIs distribute throughout the brain, their actions are not limited to monoaminergic neurons, thus the investigation of the non-specific effects of SSRIs on synaptogenesis and synaptic function in other neuronal systems is warranted. To determine whether SSRI exposure affects synaptogenesis between VD4 and LPeD1, these neurons were cultured in the soma-soma configuration in the presence of various concentrations of fluoxetine or citalopram. Simultaneous recordings of presynaptic action potentials (current injection-induced) and postsynaptic potentials (PSPs) were made to determine the effect of SSRI exposure on the incidence of synapse formation, by measuring the percentage of cells that exhibited a functional synapse, and the synaptic strength, by measuring the mean amplitude of PSPs in response to the presynaptic action potential. When cultured in the presence of fluoxetine, neuron pairs exhibited a dose-dependent reduction in both the incidence of synaptogenesis, and, in pairs that did form synapses, a reduction in synaptic efficacy, which was significant at higher concentrations. Interestingly, citalopram had no detrimental effect on either the incidence of synapse formation or synaptic efficacy. Again, these findings lend support to our hypothesis that different SSRIs exhibit characteristic non-specific neuronal effects, and that fluoxetine is more detrimental than citalopram.

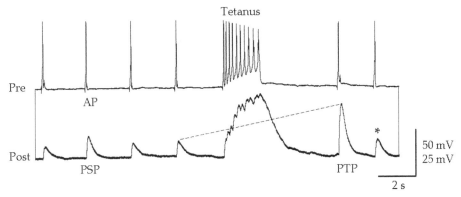

Fig. 3. The simultaneous intracellular electrophysiological recording protocol used in the soma-soma synapse model. Current injection in the presynaptic neuron (pre, VD4) results in the generation of an action potential (AP), which triggers release of neurotransmitter. The efficacy of synaptic transmission can be measured through the amplitude of the resultant excitatory post-synaptic potential (PSP) generated in the postsynaptic neuron (post, LPeD1). Triggering AP burst firing (tetanus) in the presynaptic neuron results in the induction of a use-dependent form of synaptic plasticity, pots-tetanic potentiation (PTP), measured as the ratio of PTP over PSP increase (dotted line). The efficacy of synaptic transmission rapidly returns to baseline values (asterisk), demonstrating the use-dependent characteristic of this type of synaptic plasticity.

The Mechanism: Using the *in vitro* soma-soma preparation, we have recently found that neurotrophic factor signalling, through triggering Ca^{2+} influx via voltage-gated calcium channels in the postsynaptic cell and the subsequent expression of excitatory neurotransmitter receptors, is essential for the formation of excitatory synapses (Xu et al., 2009). These trophic factor-mediated intracellular Ca^{2+} oscillations required for excitatory synapse formation were inhibited in the presence of fluoxetine, indicating that fluoxetine prevents the expression of proteins involved in synaptogenesis (Xu et al., 2010). Attesting to this, we found that the expression and synaptic localization of synaptophysin, a synaptic vesicle-associated protein and presynaptic biomarker, were significantly reduced in synapses formed in the presence of fluoxetine, but not citalopram (Getz et al., 2011). Importantly, we also demonstrated that the inhibitory effect of fluoxetine on synapse formation is reversible following prolonged drug washout, and that this recovery is dependent on protein synthesis – that is, new synapses developed following the removal of fluoxetine. Together, these data suggest that fluoxetine, through the non-specific inhibition of Ca^{2+} signalling and Ca^{2+}-dependent gene expression, affects the assembly of synaptic machinery during synapse formation, and that this contributes to a sustained, albeit reversible impairment of synaptogenesis.

2.1.3 Acute exposure to fluoxetine and citalopram affects transmission at established synapses

The Effect: Through the inhibition of ion channel and neurotransmitter receptor activity, the non-specific interactions of SSRIs also have the potential to augment the function of existing synapses. To determine whether neuronal communication at established synapses is affected by SSRI exposure, we measured the efficacy of synaptic transmission between VD4-LPeD1 soma-soma paired neurons following the acute application of various concentrations of fluoxetine or citalopram. Again, using simultaneous pre- and post-synaptic electrophysiological recordings, the mean amplitude of the PSP provided an indication of synaptic strength, which was recorded before, during and after washout of SSRIs. Following exposure to fluoxetine, the efficacy of synaptic transmission was significantly reduced at all doses examined, and this inhibition was not reversible after a brief washout period. Surprisingly, acute exposure of neuron pairs to citalopram also resulted in a reduction of synaptic transmission efficacy; however, this effect was significant only at the highest concentration evaluated. Moreover, we found that exposure to fluoxetine, and to some extent high concentrations of citalopram, often resulted in the development of presynaptic action potential clamping during burst firing (inability to sustain continuous trains of action potentials), suggesting that the intrinsic membrane properties of the neurons may be affected by both fluoxetine and citalopram exposure, for example, through the non-specific inhibition of the sodium and potassium channels that generate the action potential. Established synapses also exhibit the property of synaptic plasticity, such that synaptic communication is not fixed, but has the capacity to change in response to modulations of neuronal activity patterns. The VD4-LPeD1 synapse exhibits a well characterized use-dependent form of short term plasticity known as post-tetanic potentiation (PTP), which is initiated during periods of bursting activity in the presynaptic neuron. Taking this advantage, we investigated whether the inhibition of action potential burst firing resulting from acute SSRI exposure might also affect the occurrence of synaptic plasticity. Interestingly, whereas PTP was not affected by citalopram, exposure to fluoxetine almost completely inhibited the induction of PTP. As both SSRIs were found to affect synaptic transmission at established synapses, yet only fluoxetine affected synaptic plasticity, we postulate that the profiles of inhibitory effects on ion channels and neurotransmitter receptors are unique for these two drugs, and that these drug-specific pharmacological characteristics contribute to the differential neuronal effects seen for fluoxetine and citalopram.

The Mechanism: Synaptic machinery, the components at the synapse that mediate presynaptic neurotransmitter release and the postsynaptic response, must function collectively in order for proper synaptic transmission to occur. Presynaptically, the action potential triggers the influx of Ca^{2+} through the opening of N-type voltage-gated calcium channels, whereby Ca^{2+}-sensing proteins associated with the synaptic vesicle activate to trigger the release of neurotransmitter into the synaptic cleft. Postsynaptically, released neurotransmitters bind to either ionotropic receptors that produce depolarizing or hyperpolarizing currents in the postsynaptic cell to transfer information between neurons, or metabotropic receptors that activate signalling cascades to affect neuronal activity. Using whole-cell patch clamp recordings, we found that the Ca^{2+} current in the presynaptic VD4 neuron was significantly reduced after exposure to fluoxetine, but not citalopram, indicating that a direct inhibition of Ca^{2+} influx through voltage-gated calcium channels contributes to the fluoxetine-mediated inhibition of synaptic transmission. Furthermore, ratiometric Ca^{2+} imaging revealed that the influx of Ca^{2+} during action potential burst firing was significantly reduced by both fluoxetine and citalopram, suggesting that a loss of depolarizing driving force (i.e. through the inhibition of sodium and/or potassium channels and the development of action potential clamping) and subsequent indirect reduction in Ca^{2+} entry is most likely responsible for the citalopram-mediated reduction of synaptic transmission

(Getz et al., 2011). In *Lymnaea* neurons, the mechanism underlying the short-term plasticity of PTP has been shown to involve presynaptic Ca^{2+} entry through voltage-gated calcium channels and subsequent activation of CaMKII, a protein kinase that mediates the effects of intracellular signalling cascades (Luk et al., 2011). This mechanism illuminates how the differential effects of fluoxetine and citalopram on synaptic plasticity can be produced by their respective direct and indirect inhibition of presynaptic Ca^{2+} entry. Finally, we examined the amplitude of the receptor potential generated in the postsynaptic neuron in response to exogenously applied acetylcholine to determine whether the postsynaptic machinery was also affected by SSRI exposure. Indeed, in the presence of fluoxetine, but not citalopram, the receptor potential was significantly reduced, indicating that the inhibition of neurotransmitter receptors is another mechanism by which the non-specific actions of fluoxetine contributed to the reduction of synaptic transmission efficacy. Ultimately, we find that the negative effect of fluoxetine on synaptic function is attributable to the direct perturbation of numerous components of both pre- and post-synaptic machinery, whereas citalopram exhibits only a minor profile of adverse effects in established synapses, again providing support for the hypothesis that the distinctive auxiliary neuronal effects arise from the characteristic non-specific interactions of SSRIs.

2.1.4 The inhibitory effects of SSRIs on neuronal function: It all comes down to calcium

The occurrence of non-specific ion channel and neurotransmitter receptor inhibition by SSRIs is widely acknowledged; however, the potential impact of these effects remains largely disregarded. Taken together, our findings reveal that these non-specific interactions do in fact hold unforeseen consequences for both neurodevelopmental events and synaptic function. Nearly all of the neuronal functions impacted by fluoxetine can be either directly or indirectly attributed to calcium and its critical function as a cytosolic messenger, mediating such diverse neuronal effects as cytoskeletal dynamics, growth cone activity, gene expression, neurotransmitter release, and synaptic plasticity. As citalopram did not directly affect Ca^{2+} influx through voltage-gated calcium channels, and is additionally associated with a comparatively benign profile of adverse neuronal effects, we propose that the disruption of calcium homeostasis by fluoxetine is the primary causal factor underlying the extensive profile of detrimental neuronal effects attributed to this SSRI.

Neuronal Phenomenon	Ca^{2+}-dependent?	Fluoxetine Inhibition	Citalopram Inhibition
Neurite outgrowth	Yes	Yes	No
Growth cone dynamics	Yes	Yes	No
Synapse formation	Yes	Yes	No
Synaptic transmission	Yes	Yes	Yes
Synaptic plasticity (PTP)	Yes	Yes	No
Presynaptic I_{Ca}	Yes	Yes	No

Table 3. Summary of the differential effects fluoxetine and citalopram exhibit on neuronal architecture and function.

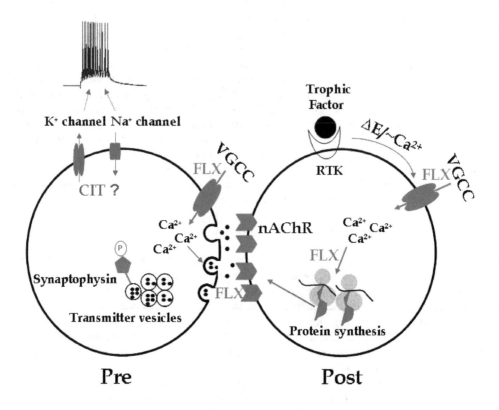

Fig. 4. The proposed mechanisms of non-specific action of SSRIs that contribute to the development of inhibitory effects on neuronal structure and function. Our data suggests that the principle mechanism underlying the fluoxetine-mediated disruption of neuronal function is the inhibition of intracellular calcium signalling. This interferes with numerous neuronal processes including neurotrophic factor signalling through receptor tyrosine kinase (RTK), synaptic protein expression (i.e. synaptophysin, the postsynaptic nACh receptor), synaptogenesis, membrane excitability, and synaptic neurotransmitter release. As citalopram did not exhibit a similar profile of detrimental effects, and did not directly inhibit intracellular calcium influx, we propose that citalopram-mediated disruption of synaptic transmission efficacy may result from the reduction of neuronal excitability, for instance, through the inhibition of the Na+ and/or K+ channels that contribute to the development of action potentials and the regulation of neuronal excitability.

While the impact of the promiscuous interactions of antidepressant medications remains largely unaccounted for, we find that one in particular – the modulation of calcium channel activity – can have devastating consequences for neuronal structure and synaptic function. Ultimately, in light of the low clinical efficacy of antidepressant medications and our limited understanding of the mechanism(s) of antidepressant action, the benefits of antidepressant pharmacotherapy, in some instances, may not outweigh the risks.

3. Conclusions: Looking to the future of antidepressant therapeutics

After more than half a century of development in the field of antidepressant pharmacotherapy, there has not been a significant improvement in the treatment paradigm or the therapeutic outcome. The last advance came in the 1990's with the introduction of the SRI class of antidepressants, which, to some extent, addressed the need for safer and more tolerable compounds, but left the issues of efficacy and time course of therapeutic action largely unresolved. Assessing the clinical safety of these compounds is complicated by the fact we do not completely understand the mechanism of therapeutic action – making it difficult to differentiate between what may be a necessary effect for therapeutic response and a detrimental effect resulting from non-specific interactions of SRIs with ion channels and neurotransmitter receptors. The limited efficacy profiles, long periods of therapeutic lag, and as we have identified, the potential for inhibitory effects on neuronal function arising from the non-specific interactions of antidepressant medications, underscores the need to develop more selective and more effective therapeutics for the treatment of MDD.

Further development in this field has been hindered by lack of certainty regarding the etiology of depression. Indeed, the complex multifactorial nature of MDD provides no obvious starting points for molecular investigation, and this situation is further confounded by the fact that much of what we currently understand about depression has been gleaned from observing the effects of antidepressant drugs, which themselves appear to act through convoluted and indirect secondary mechanisms. Though slow to gain recognition, the alternative neuroplasticity theory of depression posits that structural changes and neuroplasticity deficits are causative factors underlying MDD, and thus opens to the possibility that these pathways may be targeted directly in attempts to improve therapeutic outcome and perhaps also to reduce the unwanted non-specific effects associated with current antidepressant drugs. An exciting new therapeutic strategy that has made its way into clinical trials involves the use of the psychotropic drug ketamine, which acts as a glutamate NMDA receptor antagonist. Fascinatingly, a single dose of ketamine has been found to produce a rapid (occurring within hours) and sustained (lasting as long as two weeks) antidepressant response through the rapid activation of synaptic plasticity mechanisms (Berman et al., 2000; Li et al., 2010). However, the clinical use of ketamine is limited by its psychotrophic effects and the potential for abuse. Subunit-selective NMDA receptor antagonists that produce an antidepressant response without the development of a psychotropic reaction have more recently been developed and tested clinically, providing an alternate means to achieve the rapid acting antidepressant effects without the side effects and potential complications (Preskorn et al., 2008). As numerous antidepressant drugs have been found to antagonize NMDA receptor activity, it is possible that current antidepressant drugs may also be acting through this mechanism – just taking a roundabout and rather ineffectual way of getting there, hence the therapeutic delay and high concentration required for antidepressant response. Herein we find a striking example of the difficulty in interpreting the effects of antidepressant medications without a clear understanding of their mechanism of action, and how this impacts neuronal function.

There is an unmistakable need for a solution to the problems of the high rates of morbidity and mortality present during the extended window of therapeutic inefficacy associated with traditional antidepressants, and the cryptic consequences of their non-specific interactions. The fact that NMDA receptor antagonists produce an antidepressant response with just a single dose, and that this response is sustained beyond the period of drug metabolism and elimination, highlights the potential for this therapeutic strategy to have minimal non-specific interactions and adverse effects, providing a significant advantage over currently available antidepressant medications. Furthermore, as the onset of antidepressant action of NMDA receptor antagonists is extremely rapid, the limitation of therapeutic lag associated with traditional antidepressants is also addressed. Given the compelling evidence to date, it appears as though NMDA receptor antagonists and the mechanisms of synaptic plasticity may provide a route towards the 'magic-bullet' for depression pharmacotherapy that we have been searching for.

4. References

Alwan, S.; Reefhuis, J.; Rasmussen, S.A.; Olney, R.S. & Friedman, J.M. (2007). Use of selective serotonin-reuptake inhibitors in pregnancy and the risk of birth defects. *The New England Journal of Medicine*, Vol.356 No.26, (June 2007), pp. 2684-2692, ISSN 0028-4793

Berman, R.M.; Cappiello, A.; Anand, A.; Oren, D.A.; Heninger, G.R.; Charney, D.S. & Krystal, J.H. (2000). Antidepressant effects of ketamine in depressed patients. *Biological Psychiatry*, Vol.47, No.4, (February 2000), pp. 351-354, ISSN 0006-3223

Bolo, N.R.; Hodé, Y.; Nédélec, J.F.; Lainé, E.; Wagner, G. & Macher, J.P. (2000). Brain pharmacokinetics and tissue distribution in vivo of fluvoxamine and fluoxetine by fluorine magnetic resonance spectroscopy. *Neuropsychopharmacology*, Vol.23, No.4, (October 2000), pp. 428–438, ISSN 0893-133X

Chen, B.; Dowlatshahi, D.; Macqueen, G.M.; Wang, J.F. & Young, L.T. (2001). Increased hippocampal BDNF immunoreactivity in subjects treated with antidepressant medication. *Biological Psychiatry*, Vol.50, No.4, pp. 260-265, ISSN 0006-3223

Deák, F.; Lasztóczi, B.; Pacher, P.; Petheö, G.L.; Kecskeméti, V. & Spät, A. (2000). Inhibition of voltage-gated calcium channels by fluoxetine in rat hippocampal pyramidal cells. *Neuropharmacology*, Vol.39, No.6, (April 2000), pp. 1029–1036, ISSN 0028-3908

Drevets, W.C. (2001). Neuroimaging and neuropathological studies of depression: implications for the cognitive-emotional features of mood disorders. *Current Opinion in Neurobiol*, Vol.11, No.2, (April 2001), pp. 240-249, ISSN 0959-4388

Fan, P. (1994). Effects of antidepressants on the inward current mediated by 5-HT3 receptors in rat nodose ganglion neurons. *British Journal of Pharmacology*, Vol.112, No.3, (July 1994), pp. 741-744, ISSN 0007-1188

Feng, Z.P.; Grigoriev, N.; Munno, D.; Lukowiak, K.; MacVicar, B.A.; Goldberg, J.I. & Syed, N.I. (2002). Development of Ca2+ hotspots between Lymnaea neurons during synaptogenesis. *Journal of Physiology*, Vol.539, No.1, (February 2002), pp. 53–65, ISSN 0022-3751

Feng, Z.P.; Klumperman, J.; Lukowiak, K. & Syed, N.I. (1997). In vitro synaptogenesis between the somata of identified Lymnaea neurons requires protein synthesis but not extrinsic growth factors or substrate adhesion molecules. *The Journal of Neuroscience*, Vol.17, No.20, (October 1997), pp. 7839–7849, ISSN 0270-6476

Fournier, J.C.; DeRubeis, R.J.; Hollon, S.D.; Dimidjian, S.; Amsterdam, J.D.; Shelton, R.C. & Fawcett, J. (2010). Antidepressant drug effects and depression severity. *The Journal of the American Medical Association*, Vol.303, No.1, (January 2010), pp. 47-53, ISSN 0098-7484

García-Colunga, J.; Awad, J.N. & Miledi, R. (1997). Blockage of muscle and neuronal nicotinic acetylcholine receptors by fluoxetine (Prozac). *Proceedings of the National Academy of Sciences of the United States of America*, Vol.94, No.5, (March 1997), pp.2041-2044, ISSN 0027-8424

Gaspar, P.; Cases, O. & Maroteaux, L. (2003). The developmental role of serotonin: news from mouse molecular genetics. *Nature Reviews. Neuroscience*, Vol.4, No.12, (December 2003), pp. 1002-1012, ISSN 1471-003X

Getz, A.; Xu, F.; Zaidi, W. & Syed, N.I. (2011). The antidepressant fluoxetine but not citalopram suppresses synapse formation and synaptic transmission between Lymnaea neurons by perturbing presynaptic and postsynaptic machinery. *European Journal of Neuroscience*, Vol.34, No.2, (July 2011), pp. 221-234, ISSN 0953-816X

Hardingham, G.E.; Chawla, S.; Johnson, C.M. & Bading, H. (1997). Distinct functions of nuclear and cytoplasmic calcium in the control of gene expression. *Nature* Vol.385, No.6613, (January 1997), pp. 260-265, ISSN 0028-0836

Henley, J. & Poo, M.M. (2004). Guiding neuronal growth cones using Ca2+ signals. *Trends inCell Biology*, Vol.14, No.6, (June 2004), pp. 320-330, ISSN 0962-8924

Homberg, J.R.; Schubert, D. & Gaspar, P. (2009). New perspectives on the neurodevelopmental effects of SSRIs. *Trends in Pharmacological Science*, Vol.31, No.2, (February 2009), pp. 60-65, ISSN 0165-6147

Hyttel, J. (1994). Pharmacological characterization of selective serotonin reuptake inhibitors (SSRIs). *International Clinical Psychopharmacology*, Vol.9, No.1, (March 1994), pp. 19–26, ISSN 0268-1315

Kessler, R.C.; Berglund, P.; Demler, O.; Jun, R.; Merikangas, K.R. & Walters, E.E. (2005). Lifetime prevalence and age-of-onset distributions of DSM-IV disorders in the national comorbidity survey replication. *Archives of General Psychiatry*, Vol.62, No.6, (June 2005), pp. 593-602, ISSN 0003-990X

Kobayashi, T.; Washiyama, K. & Ikeda, K. (2004). Inhibition of G protein-activated inwardly rectifying K+ channels by various antidepressant drugs. *Neuropsychopharmacology*, Vol.29, No.10, (October 2004), pp. 1841-1851, ISSN 0893-133X

Krishnan, V. & Nestler, E.J. (2008). The molecular neurobiology of depression. *Nature*, Vol.455, No.7215, (October 2008), pp. 894-902, ISSN0028-0836

Lapin, J.P. & Oxenkrug, G.F. (1969). Intensification of the central serotonergic processes as a possible determinal of the thymoleptic effect. *Lancet*, Vol.1, No.7586, (January 1969), pp. 132-136, ISSN 0140-6736

Lee, H.M.; Hahn, S.J. & Choi, B.H. (2010). Open channel block of Kv1.5 currents by citalopram. *Acta Pharmacologica Sinica*, Vol.31, No.4, (April 2010), pp. 429-435, ISSN 1671-4083

Lenkey, N.; Karoly, R.; Kiss, J.P.; Szasz, B.K.; Vizi, E.S. & Mike, A. (2006). The mechanism of activity-dependent sodium channel inhibition by the antidepressants fluoxetine and desipramine. *Molecular Pharmacology*, Vol.70, No.6, (December 2006), pp. 2052-2063, ISSN 0026-895X

Li, N.; Lee, B.; Liu, R.-J.; Banasr, M.; Dwyer, J.M.; Iwata, M.; Li, X.-Y.; Aghajanian, G. & Duman, R.S. (2010). mTOR-dependent synapse formation underlies the rapid antidepressant effects of NMDA antagonists. *Science*, Vol.329, No.5994, (August 2010), pp. 959-964, ISSN 0036-8075

Licinio, J. & Wong, M.-L. (2005). Depression, antidepressants and suicidality: a critical appraisal. *Nature Reviews. Drug Discovery*, Vol.4, No.2, (February 2005), pp. 165-171, ISSN 1474-1776

López-León, S.; Janssens, A.C.; González-Zuloeta Ladd, A.M.; Del-Favero, J.; Claes, S.J.; Oostra, B.A. & van Duijn, C.M. (2008). Meta-analyses of genetic studies on major depressive disorder. *Molecular Psychiatry*, Vol.13, No.8, (August 2008), pp. 772–785, ISSN 1359-4184

Luk, C.C.; Naruo, H.; Prince, D.; Hassan, A.; Doran, S.A.; Goldberg, J.I. & Syed, N.I. (2011). A novel form of presynaptic CaMKII-dependent short-term potentiation between Lymnaea neurons. *European Journal of Neuroscience*, Vol.34, No.4, (August 2011), pp. 848-856, ISSN 0953-816X

Olfson, M. & Marcus, S.C. (2009). National patterns in antidepressant medication treatment. *Archives of General Psychiatry*, Vol.66, No.8, (August 2009), pp. 848-856, ISSN 0003-990X

Martinowich, K. & Lu, B. (2008). Interaction between BDNF and serotonin: role in mood disorders. *Neuropsychopharmacology* Vol.33, No.1, (January 2008), pp. 73-83, ISSN 0893-133X

Maya Vetencourt, J.F.; Sale, A.; Viegi, A.; Baroncelli, L.; De Pasquale, R.; O'Leary, O.F.; Castrén, E. & Maffei, L. (2008). The antidepressant fluoxetine restores plasticity in the adult visual cortex. *Science*, Vol.320, No.5874, (April 2008), pp. 385–388, ISSN 0036-8075

Nestler, E.J.; Terwilliger, R.Z. & Duman, R.S. (1989). Chronic antidepressant administration alters the subcellular distribution of cyclic AMP-dependent protein kinase in rat frontal cortex. *Journal of Neurochemistry*, Vol.53, No.5, (Novemer 1989), pp. 1644–1647, ISSN 0022-3042

Nibuya, M.; Nestler, E.J. & Duman, R.S. (1996). Chronic antidepressant administration increases the expression of cAMP response element binding protein (CREB) in rat hippocampus. *The Journal of Neuroscience*, Vol.16, No.7, (April 1996), pp. 2365–2372, ISSN 0270-6474

Oberlander, T.F.; Gingrich, J.A. & Ansorge, M.S. (2009). Sustained neurobehavioral effects of exposure to SSRI antidepressants during development: molecular to clinical evidence. *Clinical Pharmacology & Therapeutics*, Vol.86, No.6, (December 2009), pp. 672-677, ISSN 0009-9236

Pacher, P. & Kecskemeti, V. (2004). Cardiovascular side effects of new antidepressants and antipsychotics: new drugs, old concerns? *Current Pharmaceutical Design*, Vol.10, No.20, (August 2004), pp. 2463-2475, ISSN 1381-6128

Pancrazio, J.J.; Kamatchi, G.L.; Roscoe, A.K. & Lynch, C. III. (1998). Inhibition of neuronal Na+ channels by antidepressant drugs. *The Journal of Pharmacology and Experimental Therapeutics*, Vol. 284, No.1, (January 1998), pp. 208-214, ISSN 0022-3565

Pezawas, L.; Meyer-Lindenberg, A.; Goldman, A.L.; Verchinski, B.A.; Chen, G.; Kolachana, B.S.; Egan, M.F.; Mattay, V.S.; Hariri, A.R. & Weinberger, D.R. (2008). Evidence of biologic epistasis between BDNF and SLC6A4 and implications for depression. *Molecular Psychiatry*, Vol.13, No.7, (July 2008), pp. 709-716, ISSN 1359-4184

Pittenger, C. & Duman, R.S. (2008). Stress, depression, and neuroplasticity: a convergence of mechanisms. *Neuropsychopharmacology*, Vol.33, No.1, (Jan 2008), pp. 88-109, ISSN 0893-133X

Preskorn, S.H.; Baker, B.; Kolluri, S.; Menniti, F.S.; Krams, M. & Landen, J.W. (2008). An innovative design to establish proof of concept of the antidepressant effects of the NR2B subunit selective N-methyl-D-aspartate antagonist, CP-101,606, in patients with treatment-refractory major depressive disorder. *Journal of Clinical Psychopharmacology*, Vol.28, No.6, (December 2008), pp. 631-637, ISSN 0271-0749

Rana, B.; McMorn, S.O.; Reeve, H.L.; Wyatt, C.N.; Vaughan, P.F. & Peers, C. (1993). Inhibition of neuronal nicotinic acetylcholine receptors by imipramine and desipramine. *European Journal of Pharmacology*, Vol.250, No.2, (December 1993), pp. 247-251, ISSN 0014-2999

Ressler, K.J. & Mayberg, H.S. (2007). Targeting abnormal neural circuits in mood and anxiety disorders: from the laboratory to the clinic. *Nature Neuroscience*, Vol.10, No.9, (September 2007), pp. 1116-1124, ISSN 1097-6256

Reynolds, I.J. & Miller, R.J. (1988). Tricyclic antidepressants block N-methyl-D-aspartate receptors: similarities to the action of zinc. *British Journal of Pharmacology*, Vol.95, No.1, (September 1988), pp. 95-102, ISSN 0007-1188

Ridgway, R.L.; Syed, N.I.; Lukowiak, K. & Bulloch, A.G. (1991). Nerve growth factor (NGF) induces sprouting of specific neurons of the snail Lymnaea stagnalis. *Journal of Neurobiology*, Vol.22, No.4, (June 1991), pp. 377-390, ISSN 0022-3034

Saarelainen, T.; Hendolin, P.; Lucas, G.; Koponen, E.; Sairanen, M., MacDonald, E.; Agerman, K.; Haapasalo, A.; Nawa, H.; Aloyz, R.; Ernfors, P. & Castrén, E. (2003). Activation of the TrkB neurotrophin receptor is induced by antidepressant drugs and is required for antidepressant-induced behavioural effects. *The Journal of Neuroscience*, Vol.23, No.1, (January 2003), pp. 349-357, ISSN 0270-6474

Santarelli, L.; Saxe, M.; Gross, C.; Surget, A.; Battaglia, F.; Dulawa, S.; Weisstaub, N.; Lee, J.; Duman, R.; Arancio, O.; Belzung, C. & Hen, R. (2003). Requirement of hippocampal neurogenesis for the behavioural effects of antidepressants. *Science*, Vol.301, No.5634, (August 2003), pp. 805-809, ISSN 0036-8075

Schildkraut, J.J. (1965). The catecholamine hypothesis of affective disorders: a review of supporting evidence. *The American Journal of Psychiatry*, Vol.122, No.5, (November 1965), pp. 509-522, ISSN 0002-953X

Sernagor, E.; Kuhn, D., Vyklicky, L. Jr. & Mayer, M.L. (1989). Open channel block of NMDA receptor responses evoked by tricyclic antidepressants. *Neuron*, Vol. 2, No.3, (March 1989), pp. 1221-1227, ISSN 0896-6273

Shimizu, E.; Hashimoto, K.; Okamura, N.; Koike, K.; Komatsu, N.; Kumakiri ,C.; Nakazato, M.; Watanabe, H.; Shinoda, N., Okada, S. & Iyo, M. (2003). Alterations of serum levels of brain-derived neurotrophic factor (BDNF) in depressed patients with or without antidepressants. *Biological Psychiatry*, Vol.54, No.1, (July 2003), pp. 70-75, ISSN 0006-3223

Snyder, S.H. & Yamamura, H.I. (1977). Antidepressants and the muscarinic acetylcholine receptor. *Archives of General Psychiatry*, Vol.34, No.2, (February 1977), pp. 236-239, ISSN 0003-990X

Spira, M.E.; Oren, R.; Dormann, A.; Ilouz, N. & Lev, S. (2001). Calcium, protease activation, and cytoskeleton remodelling underlie growth cone formation and neuronal regeneration. *Cellular and Molecular Neurobiology*, Vol.21, No.6, (December 2001), pp. 591-604, ISSN 0272-4340

Sullivan, P.F.; Neale, M.C. & Kendler, K.S. (2000). Genetic epidemiology of major depression: review and meta-analysis. *The American Journal of Psychiatry*, Vol.157, No.10, (October 2000), pp. 1552–1562, ISSN 0002-953X

Sung, M.J.; Ahn, H.S.; Hahn, S.J. & Sung, H.C. (2008). Open channel block of Kv3.1 currents by fluoxetine. *Journal of Pharmacological Sciences*, Vol.106, No.1, (January 2008), pp. 38-45, ISSN 1347-8613

Syed, N.I.; Bulloch, A.G. & Lukowiak, K. (1990). In vitro reconstruction of the respiratory central pattern generator of the mollusc Lymnaea. *Science*, Vol.250, No.4978, (October 1990), pp. 282-285, ISSN 0036-8075

Tao, X.; Finkbeiner, S.; Arnold, D.B.; Shaywitz, A.J. & Greenberg, M.E. (1998). Ca2+ influx regulates BDNF transcription by a CREB family transcription factor-dependent mechanism. *Neuron*, Vol.20, No.4, (April 1998), pp.709-726, ISSN 0896-6273

Thase, M.E. (2011). Antidepressant combinations: widely used, but far from empirically validated. *Canadian Journal of Psychiatry*, Vol.56, No.6, (June 2011), pp. 317-323, ISSN 0706-7437

Thase, M.E.; Haight, B.R.; Richard, N.; Rockett, C.B.; Mitton, M.; Modell, J.G.; VanMeter, S.; Harriett, A.E. & Wang, Y. (2005). Remission rates following antidepressant therapy with bupropion or selective serotonin reuptake inhibitors: a meta-analysis of original data from 7 randomized controlled trials. *The Journal of Clinical Psychiatry*, Vol.66, No.8, (August 2005), pp. 974–981, ISSN 0160-6689

Torres, G.E.; Gainetdinov, R.R. & Caron, M.G. (2003). Plasma membrane monoamine transporters: structure, regulation and function. *Nature Reviews. Neuroscience*, Vol.4, No.1, (January 2003), pp. 13-25, ISSN 1471-003X

Trivedi, M.H.; Rush, A.J.; Wisniewski, S.R.; Nierenberg, A.A.; Warden, D.; Ritz, L.; Norquist, G.; Howland, R.H.; McGrath, P.J.; Shores-Wilson, K.; Biggs, M.M.; Balasubramani, G.K.; Fava, M. & STAR*D Study Team. (2006). Evaluation of outcomes with citalopram for depression using measurement-based care in STAR*D: implications for clinical practice. *The American Journal of Psychiatry*, Vol.163, No.1, (January 2006), pp. 28–40, ISSN 0002-953X

Wang, G.K.; Mitchell, J. & Wang, S.Y. (2008). Block of persistent late Na+ currents by antidepressant sertraline and paroxetine. *The Journal of Membrane Biology*, Vol.222, No.2, (March 2008), pp. 79-90, ISSN 0022-2631

Wang, S.J.; Su, C.F. & Kuo, Y.H. (2003). Fluoxetine depresses glutamate exocytosis in the rat cerebrocortical nerve terminals (synaptosomes) via inhibition of P/Q-type Ca2+ channels. *Synapse*, Vol.48, No.4, (June 2003), pp. 170-177, ISSN 0887-4476

Wang, S.-Y.; Calderon, J. & Kuo Wang, G. (2010). Block of neuronal Na+ channels by antidepressant duloxetine in a state-dependent manner. *Anesthesiology*, Vol.113, No.3, (September 2010), pp. 655-665, ISSN 0003-3022

Welnhofer, E.A.; Zhao, L. & Cohan C.S. (1999). Calcium influx alters actin bundle dynamics and retrograde flow in Helisoma growth cones. *The Journal of Neuroscience*, Vol.19, No.18, (September 1999), pp. 7971-7982, ISSN 0270-6474

Witchel, H.J.; Pabbathi, V.K.; Hofmann, G.; Paul, A.A. & Hancox, J.C. (2002). Inhibitory actions of the selective serotonin re-uptake inhibitor citalopram on HERG and ventricular L-type calcium currents. *FEBS Letters*, Vol.512, No.1-3, (February 2002), pp. 59-66, ISSN 0014-5793

Xu, Y.; Sari, Y. & Zhou, F.C. (2004). Selective serotonin reuptake inhibitor disrupts organization of thalamocortical somatosensory barrels during development. *Developmental Brain Research*, Vol.150, No.2, (June 2004), pp. 151-161, ISSN 0165-3806

Xu, F.; Hennessy, D.A.; Lee, T.K. & Syed, N.I. (2009) Trophic factor-induced intracellular calcium oscillations are required for the expression of postsynaptic acetylcholine receptors during synapse formation between Lymnaea neurons. *The Journal of Neuroscience*, Vol.29, No.7, (February 2009), pp. 2167–2176, ISSN 0270-6474

Xu, F.; Luk, C.; Richard, M.P.; Zaidi, W.; Farkas, S.; Getz, A.; Lee, A.; van Minnen, J. & Syed, N.I. (2010). Antidepressant fluoxetine suppresses neuronal growth from both vertebrate and invertebrate neurons and perturbs synapse formation between Lymnaea neurons. *European Journal of Neuroscience*, Vol. 31, No.6, (March 2010), pp. 994-1005, ISSN 0953-816X

Ye, Z.Y.; Lu, Y.G.; Sun, H.; Cheng, X.P.; Xu, T.L. & Zhou, J.N. (2008). Fluoxetine inhibition of glycine receptor activity in rat hippocampal neurons. *Brain Research*, Vol.1239, (November 2008), pp. 77-84, ISSN 0006-8993

Yeung, S.Y.; Millar, J.A. & Mathie, A. (1999). Inhibition of neuronal KV potassium currents by the antidepressant drug, fluoxetine. *British Journal of Pharmacology*, Vol.128, No.7, (December 1999), pp. 1609-1615, ISSN 0007-1188

Zimmerman, M.; Posternak, M.A. & Chelminski, I. (2002). Symptom severity and exclusion from antidepressant efficacy trials. *Journal of Clinical Psychopharmacology*, Vol.22, No.6, (December 2002), pp. 610-614, ISSN 0271-0749

Zou, K.; Deng, W.; Li, T.; Zhang, B.; Jiang, L.; Huang, C.; Sun, X. & Sun, X. (2010). Changes of brain morphometry in first-episode, drug-naïve, non-late-life adult patients withmajor depression: an optimized voxel-based morphometry study. *Biological Psychiatry*, Vol.67, No.2, (January 2010), pp. 186-188, ISSN 0006-3223

4

Cognitive-Behavioural Therapy Combined with Antidepressants for Major Depressive Disorder

Narong Maneeton

Department of Psychiatry, Faculty of Medicine, Chiang Mai University
Thailand

1. Introduction

Major depressive disorder (MDD) is a common psychiatric illness. Its 1-year prevalence rates varied in the different regions, for instance 5.1% in Australia, 6.7% in New Zealand, 5.8% in Netherlands, 7.1% in Hungary, 6.2 in Italy, 15-23 % in Republic region of Udmurtia (rural area), 3.5%-10.3% in USA and 4.1%-4.6% in Canada (Handerson et al., 2000; Oakley-Browne et al., 1989; Pakriev et al., 1998; Bijl et al., 1998; Szadoczky et al., 1998; Faravelli et al., 1990; Bourdon et al., 1992; Offord et al., 1996; Bland et al., 1988). However, its prevalence in Taiwan is in a lower range of 0.6%-1.1% (Hwu et al., 1989). According to a meta-analysis of 11 clinical studies, the mean average of its 1-year prevalence rate is 4.1% (95%CI, 2.4% to 6.2%), and its sex-specific 1-year prevalence rates for men and women are 4.9% (95%CI, 3.3% to 7.1%) and 10.0% (95%CI, 6.4% to 14.6%) respectively (Waraich et al., 2004). The lifetime prevalence for MDD patients is 12.6% in New Zealand, 15.4% in Netherlands, 15.1% in Hungary, 13.1% in Italy, 15.7%-22.8% in Switzerland, 9.0% in Germany, 5.9%-17.1% in USA and 8.6%-29.6% in Canada (Oakley-Browne et al., 1989; Bijl et al., 1998; Szadoczky et al., 1998, Carta et al., 1995; Wacker et al.1992; Wittchen et al., 1992 ; Kessler et al., 1994; Bourdon et al., 1992; Murphy et al., 2000; Fournier et al. 1997; Bland et al., 1988). For Asian countries, the prevalence is 1.9% in Hon Kong, 3.4% in Korea and 0.88%-1.7% in Taiwan (Chen et al., 1993; Lee et al., 1987; Hwu et al., 1989). Its prevalence in Puerto Rico is 4.6% (Canino et al., 1987). A meta-analyis of data obtained from several countries revealed that its lifetime prevalence is approximate 3.8% (95%CI, 2.4% to 23.1%) for men and 7.5% (95%CI, 4.5% to 11.3%) for women (Waraich P, 2004).

Depression is associated with various chronic medical conditions, including cardiovascular disease, hypertension, diabetes, arthritis and back pain. Recent evidence suggested that it is a primary risk factor for coronary heart disease (CHD), including myocardial infarction (MI) and cardiac death (Lett et al., 2004; Rugulies, 2002). In the contrary, patients with myocardial infarction (MI) and cardiac death also have an increased risk of depression. Depression is also associated with hypertension (Patten, 2001; DiMatteo et al., 2002). Despite of the heterogeneity of results, depression was found to be a risk of poor adherence to antihypertensive medications (Eze-Nliam et al., 2010).

Diabetic patients also have a high risk for depression. A systemic review has found that diabetes doubles the odds of comorbid depression (Anderson et al., 2001) and increases the risk for depression for 24% (Nouwen et al., 2010). In the contrary, depression also increases the risk of diabetes development. In addition, depression has been associated with hyperglycemia, diabetic complications, functional disability and mortality among diabetic patients (Rustad et al., 2011).

The relationship of arthritis and depression has been well documented. A recent study has shown a strong association of depression and functional severity of rheumatoid arthritis (RA) and its related diseases (Godha et al., 2010). Another study also suggested that depression is highly correlated with the disease activity of rheumatoid arthritis (RA), especially the number of swollen joints and joint functional class (Khongsaengdao et al., 2000).

Depression is a major burden for individuals, communities and health services throughout the world. The study of global burden of diseases in the year 2000 indicates that depression is an important causes of disease burden accounting for 4.4% of total disability adjusted life years (DALYs) in the year 2000, which is almost 12% of all total years lived with disability worldwide (Üstün et al., 2004). Effective pharmacological and psychosocial interventions to resolve depressive symptoms promptly could be reduce this burden.

Pharmacotherapy, psychotherapy and their combinations are effective treatment for MDD. Tricyclic antidepressants (TCAs), selective serotonin reuptake inhibitors (SSRIs), serotonin-norepinephrine reuptake inhibitors (SNRIs) are examples of medications approved for the treatment of MDD. Examples of effective psychotherapy techniques are cognitive therapy (CT), cognitive behavioural therapy (CBT), interpersonal therapy (IT) and mindfulness-based cognitive therapy (MBCT). Although most patients respond to these interventions, a considerable proportion of them may not respond or only partially respond to them. Combined psychotherapy and pharmacotherapy is therefore a choice for the latter group of patients.

The aim of this chapter is to summarize the efficacy and safety of CBT combined with antidepressants. However, the efficacy and safety of antidepressants alone and CBT alone are also addressed.

2. Cognitive behavioral therapy

2.1 Cognitive model of depression

The cognitive model of depression is supported by several research findings. The cognitive theory addressed in several studies comprises of three components: cognitive triad in depression, negatively biased cognitive processing of stimuli and identifiable dysfunctional beliefs (Beck, 2005).

The components of cognitive triad include the patterns of depressed patients interpreting experiences, viewing themselves and viewing future in a negative way. The first triad is the negative interpretation of experience. Persistently, depressed patients tend to interpret the interaction between themselves and environment as representation of defeat, deprivation and disparagement. They perceive that their lives are plentiful of burdens, obstacle and traumatic events. The second triad is the negative evaluation of the self. Patients view themselves as deficiency, inadequacy and worthlessness. They tend to regard themselves as having a physical, mental or moral defect. They usually reject themselves because of those unpleasant defects. The last triad is the negative expectation of future. Depressed patients assume that the current difficulties and suffering will last forever. Their lives have endless obstacles, frustration and deprivation. These cognitive distortions are cause of depression (Beck, 1967).

There are some of common maintenance processes in the depressed patients. The vicious cycle linking a depressed mood with cognitive bias, and negative appraisal causes the negative view of self, then maintaining the depressive symptoms. The negative appraisals and depressive symptoms could reduce depressed patients' activities usually providing the pleasure and sense of achievement for them, and thus the decreased activities continue the depression. The symptoms of depression and negative appraisal may decrease the ability to cope and deal with their difficulties. They may feel hopelessness and continue to be depressed (Wrestbrook et al. 2007).

2.2 Cognitive behavioral therapy for depression
CBT is a collaborative, short-term, structured, focused approach psychotherapeutic intervention. The aims of CBT are to help the patients to understand the relationship of cognitions, emotions or affect, behaviours and physiology influenced by external stimuli. In addition, it would educate the patients on two-way relationship between cognition and behaviour in which cognitive processes can influence behavioural patterns, and behavioural changes can influence cognition (Wright, 2006).

For the treatment of depression, CBT allows to use several techniques. In the early phase of treatment, the behavioural technique such as exercise or activity scheduling is used to reduce the depressive symptoms. For instance, high level physical exercise appears to be effective in reducing the depressive symptoms, and behavioural activities could prevent the reduction of activity in depressed patients. Then, the early cognitive technique is used to distract the patients from their negative automatic thoughts (NATs) and/or to change the attitude toward them. Some depressive symptoms may be relieved or reduced. The last, main cognitive behavioural technique is applied. In this phase, the patients learn to identify the NATs and alternative thoughts, self monitoring, thought records or behavioural experiment to disconfirm their NATs and to prove alternative hypothesis. In addition, the therapist also teaches the depressed patient to use the problem solving skills to reduce the depressive symptoms and risk of suicide (Wrestbrook et al. 2007).

Besides the treatment of depression, CBT is widely used for several mental health conditions, e.g. anxiety disorders, personality disorders, eating disorders and substance use disorders (Beltman et al., 2010; Hofmann & Smits, 2008; Linehan et al., 1991; Fairburn et al., 1995; Magill et al., 2009). CBT adjunct with medications is also beneficial for schizophrenia and bipolar disorder (Turkington et al., 2004; da Costa et al., 2010).

3. Treatment for major depressive disorder

3.1 Short-term treatment (acute phase) (6-12 weeks)
In this phase, the patient experiences severe symptoms of depression. The goal is to relieve those symptoms. Most patients turn to be a remission at the end of this phase.

3.1.1 Antidepressants
There have been several randomized-controlled trials and meta-analyses comparing the efficacy and tolerability of antidepressants among MDD patients. While the efficacy of most antidepressants is relatively comparable, their tolerability appears to be varied based on their mechanisms of action.

3.1.1.1 Tricyclic antidepressants
3.1.1.1.1 Tricyclic antidepressants vs. Placebo

Several systemic reviews demonstrated the efficacy of tricyclic antidepressants (TCAs) for MDD. In a meta-analysis of 32 placebo-controlled trials with 4314 patients, Storosum et al.

(2001), compared the short-term efficacy of TCAs with placebo. Their results suggested that TCAs are effective in the short-term treatment of MDD. Another meta-analysis of Furukawa et al. (2003, 2002) including 35 studies (2013 participants) compared low-dose TCAs (75-100 mg/day) withplacebo for the treatment of depression. The findings suggested that low dose TCAs is superior to placebo in term of response rates while the tolerability of those TCAs is not significantly different from placebo.

Although several lines of evidence support that TCAs is effective for adult depression, their efficacy for depression in children and adolescents is still controversial. A meta-analysis of Hazell et al. (1995) reviewed 12 randomised controlled trials comparing the efficacy of tricyclic antidepressants with placebo in depressed children and adolescents. The review showed that TCAs might not be effective for the treatment of depression in this age group. Another meta-analysis of TCAs for depressive disorders in children and adolescents including nine randomized, placebo-controlled trials supports the earlier findings (Maneeton et al., 2000).

3.1.1.1.2 Tricyclic antidepressants vs. selective serotonin reuptake inhibitors

Several systemic reviews compared TCAs with SSRIs in the treatment of MDD. A meta-analysis of efficacy and tolerability in hospitalized depressed patients suggested that some TCAs, in particular amitriptyline, may be superior to SSRIs. A dual action of both 5-HT and noradrenaline reuptake inhibitors of those TCAs may be a possible explanation for the superiority. However, the meta-analysis found that SSRIs had a modest advantage in terms of tolerability (Anderson 1998, 2000).

In the contrary, a few systemic reviews found no superiority of TCAs over SSRIs. A meta-analysis of 11 studies including 2,951 participants comparing SSRIs with TCAs in the treatment of depression showed that their efficacy were comparable but the TCA patients dropped out more frequently. Another meta-analysis of 181 randomized clinical trials (47% were inpatients, and 53% were outpatients), compared amitriptyline with SSRIs (Barbui et al., 2004). Amitriptyline therapy was not superior to SSRIs in both outpatients and inpatients.

A meta-analysis of Arroll et al. (2005) reviewed ten studies of TCAs and SSRIs as comparison to placebo for treatment of depression in primary care. One half of those studies were at low methodological quality, and nearly all studies were short-term trials (six to eight weeks). The review showed that TCAs and SSRIs are more effective than placebo. In addition, the efficacy of low-dose and high-dose TCAs is comparable.

TCAs may be less tolerable than SSRIs. A meta-analysis of Anderson et al. (2000) reviewed 62 randomized controlled trials including 6,029 patients with MDD comparing SSRIs with TCAs in term of treatment discontinuation. Most study durations of included trials were between four and eight weeks. The analysis showed that the discontinuation rate due to side effect but that not due to treatment failure was more in the TCA-treated patients. Another meta-analysis of randomized, controlled trials also revealed that the overall discontinuation rates of tricyclic/heterocyclic antidepressants were greater than those of SSRIs (Hotopf, et al., 1997). Another meta-analysis of Montgomery (2001) examined the efficacy and tolerability of paroxetine (n = 1924) and tricyclic antidepressants (TCAs; n = 1693) in the treatment of major depression, it included studies from 39 randomized, double-blind, parallel-group studies. The durations of all included studies were six weeks or less. The findings indicated that paroxetine and TCAs have comparable efficacy, but paroxetine is more tolerable. In addition, a meta-analysis of Montgomery et al. (1994) examined 42 published randomized controlled studies also shows a lower discontinuation rate due to side effects as compared with TCAs.

From those reviews, most TCAs and SSRIs are effective in the treatment of MDD. The superiority of amitriptyline to SSRIs is still controversial. As compared with SSRIs, the adverse effects of TCAs are more common and severe. Low dose TCAs should be considered in depressed patients intolerable to the moderate and high doses.

Numerous systemic reviews are conducted to summarize the efficacy and tolerability of SSRIs in treating elderly patients with depression. A meta-analysis of Dunbar (1995) including ten studies carried out in elderly depressed patients demonstrated that paroxetine is as effective as other agents (amitriptyline, clomipramine, doxepin, mianserin). However, the adverse effects of paroxetine might be less frequent and less. These findings suggested that paroxetine might be an alternative first-line treatment to elderly depressed patients.

3.1.1.1.2 Tricyclic antidepressants vs. serotonin norepinephrine reuptake inhibitors

Only few systemic reviews compared TCAs with serotonin norepinephrine reuptake inhibitors (SNRIs). A meta-analysis of van den Broek et al. (2009) compared venlafaxine and TCAs (imipramine, clomipramine, amitriptyline, nortriptyline and desipramine). The average doses of venlafaxine and TCAs were 103.5 and 106.1 mg/day respectively. This review did not find any significant difference of efficacy and tolerability between groups.

3.1.1.2 Selective serotonin reuptake inhibitors

Several systemic reviews have indicated that SSRIs are effective for MDD. In meta-analysis of Bech & Cialdella (1992), citalopram was more effective and more tolerable than placebo. Its dose of 20 mg/day may be enough for patients with mild depression or first depressive episode. However, 40 mg/day may be needed for those with severe or recurrent depression (Montgomery et al., 1994). Another meta-analysis of Tignol et al. (1992) reviewed 178 patients treated with paroxetine and 66 patients treated with placebo and suggested that paroxetine is superior to placebo in the treatment of melancholic depression.

Very few systemic reviews examined efficacy, safety and tolerability of SSRIs in depressed children and adolescents. A systemic review of published and unpublished randomised controlled trials comparing the efficacy and adverse events of SSRIs with placebo suggested that only fluoxetine therapy is effective. However the adverse events and risk of suicidal ideation and behaviour were increased the SSRIs-treated group (Hetrick et al., 2007). The meta-analyses of Whittington et al. (2004) and Usala et al. (2008) also supported the previous review.

From several reviews, SSRIs is effective and acceptable in the treatment of MDD. However, in children and adolescents, fluoxetine may be the only one effective in this population. Since SSRIs have adverse effects and may increase the suicide risk, the use of them in this age group should carefully balance between the risk and its benefits.

3.1.1.3 Serotonin norepinephrine reuptake inhibitors

3.1.1.3.1 Serotonin norepinephrine reuptake inhibitors vs. Placebo

Several systemic reviews have summarized the efficacy and acceptability of serotonin norepinephrine reuptake inhibitors (SNRIs) as comparison with placebo. A meta-analysis of six comparable double-blind placebo-controlled studies comparing venlafaxine with placebo indicated that it is effective for depression regardless of age, gender, presence of melancholia, and severity or duration of depression (Entsuah et al., 1995). In addition, another meta-analysis also showed that venlafaxine is superior to placebo in reducing symptoms of anxiety in depressed patients (Rudolph et al., 1998).

Desvenlafaxine is another SNRI that is effective, safe and well tolerated for patients with MDD. A pooled study of two studies showed that, after eight weeks of treatment, it is superior to placebo in the treatment of MDD. Its adverse effects are comparable to placebo (Lieberman et al., 2008). Another review of nine studies also demonstrated its short-term efficacy for MDD (Thase et al., 2009). Another meta-analysis of eight clinical trials suggested that desvenlafaxine could improve the functioning and well-being among MDD patients (Soares et al., 2009).

Several reviews have suggested that duloxetine at the doses of 40-60 mg/day is safe and effective in acute phase treatment of MDD (Mallinckrodt et al., 2006). A meta-analysis of Mallinckrodt et al. (2005) reviewed eight double-blind, placebo-controlled clinical trials for up to nine weeks of treatment indicated that duloxetine was superior to placebo in the treatment of depressive disorder both melancholic and non-melancholic types. Another review of two 9-week trials, also demonstrated that duloxetine, as comparison to placebo, has a greater response rate at week two and a greater remission rate at week 5 (Hirschfeld et al., 2005). In addition, the significant difference of efficacy between male and female is not found (Kornstein et al., 2006).

In comparison to venlafaxine, duloxetine may be less effective in the treatment of MDD. There is a systemic review of eight trials, including 1754 patients for efficacy and 791 patients for discontinuation/safety, to compare the efficacy and safety of extended-release (XR) venlafaxine and duloxetine in treating MDD (Vis et al., 2005). The results showed that remission and response rates of venlafaxine were significantly greater than those of placebo and duloxetine. However the adverse events of both drugs are comparable. Another meta-regression analysis also indicated that duloxetine appears to be less effective than venlafaxine in acute phase treatment of adult patients with MDD (Eckert & Lançon, 2006).

From previous reviews, SNRIs are effective for MDD, with comparable tolerability to placebo. However, venlafaxine may be more effective than duloxetine. Venlafaxine, therefore, may be beneficial in patients with severe depressive symptoms.

3.1.1.3.2 Serotonin norepinephrine reuptake inhibitors vs. Selective serotonin reuptake inhibitors

Some reviews compared the efficacy between venlafaxine and SSRIs. Remission rate of MDD during venlafaxine treatment appear to be superior to SSRIs and placebo. A meta-analysis of Thase et al. (2001) compared the remission rate in MDD of venlafaxine with SSRIs/placebo. The study showed that remission rate for venlafaxine is 45 %, while SSRIs and placebo are 35% and 25% respectively. The difference between venlafaxine and SSRIs appear to be significantly different at week 2 while the difference between SSRIs and placebo is significantly different at week 4. Another meta-analysis of eight double-blind, active-controlled, randomized clinical trials also demonstrated that the remission rate of venlafaxine in the treatment of MDD is higher than that of SSRIs (remission rate at week 8: venlafaxine, 40%-55% vs. SSRI, 31%-37%). The recent systemic review of remission between venlafaxine and SSRIs also supports those of findings (Nemeroff et al., 2008).

Another systemic review of 32 double-blind, randomized, controlled trials compared venlafaxine with other antidepressants in the treatment of depression. Its findings indicated that venlafaxine was superior to SSRIs (Smith et al., 2002). Another meta-analysis of five six-week, double-blind, randomized studies including 1,454 outpatients with major depression from comparing the efficacy of venlafaxine with fluoxetine showed that venlafaxine was not only superior to but also had a more rapid onset of action than fluoxetine (Davidson et al., 2002). The rapid onset of remission for venlafaxine treatment over SSRIs does not differ in age or gender (Entsuah et al., 2001). A recent systemic review comparing venlafaxine and TCAs or SSRIs in MDD also supports the previous reviews (Bauer et al., 2009). The findings showed that venlafaxine might be more effective than SSRIs, and at least as effective as TCAs, for the treatment of MDD and treatment-resistant depression.

Not all systematic reviews support the greater efficacy of venlafaxine over SSRIs. A meta-analysis of 17 trials summarized the remission, response and discontinuation rates between venlafaxine and SSRIs. The results demonstrated that a remission rate of venlafaxine is not superior to SSRIs, while response rate is only small significant over SSRIs (Weinmann et al., 2008).

Although venlafaxine may provide a highly effective antidepressant property, it tends to be associated with high blood pressure. A meta-analysis of venlafaxine affecting blood pressure summarized the results of controlled clinical trials including 3744 patients with major depression. The findings indicated that venlafaxine had a dose-dependent effect on supine diastolic blood pressure (Thase, 1998). Venalfaxine, therefore, may be avoided in depressed patients with hypertension.

There are a few systemic reviews comparing the efficacy of duloxetine and SSRIs in the treatment of MDD. In a meta-analysis, duloxetine showed its comparable efficacy in the treatment of MDD patients as compared with SSRIs. However, its remission rates among patients with moderate to severe depression appears to be higher (Thase et al., 2007).

Milnacipran is another SNRI effective for MDD. A meta-analysis of Puech et al. (1997) reviewed controlled trials comparing milnacipran with imipramine or SSRIs in MDD patients. The study findings showed that milnacipran was as effective as imipramine and might be superior to SSRIs. Milnacipran is as tolerable as SSIRS but more tolerable than TCAs in terms of general and cardiovascular side effects. Another meta-analysis of six studies including 1,082 outpatients with MDD compared the response rates between milnacipran and SSRIs (Papakostas & Fava 2007). The findings suggested that, for the treatment of MDD, milnacipran is as effective as SSRIs.

From those reviews, SNRIs may be as effective as TCAs in the treatment of MDD. Their tolerability and safety are comparable to SSRIs. Venlafaxine and milnacipran may be superior to SSRIs in the treatment of MDD. However venlafaxine is associated with high blood pressure.

3.1.1.4 Monoamine oxidase inhibitors

Monoamine oxidase inhibitors (MAOIs) are a class of antidepressants. They appear particularly effective for atypical depression. There is a meta-analysis of eight studies comparing MAOIs with other antidepressants or placebo in the treatment of atypical depression. Most clinical trials were conducted on reversible MAOIs. The findings showed that MAOIs might be superior to TCA in the treating of MDD with atypical features (Henkel et al., 2006).

Moclobemide, a reversible Inhibitor of MAO-A, have shown its efficacy in treating MDD in many trials. A meta-analysis, as compared with other antidepressants, moclobemide, imipramine, and clomipramine therapies may lead to a higher response rate in patients with depression (Angst et al., 1993). Another meta-analysis of 12 trials including 1,207 outpatients with MDD also showed that efficacy of moclobimide is comparable to that of SSRIs

(Papakostas & Fava, 2006). However SSRIs therapy might have greater rates of nausea, headaches, and treatment-emergent anxiety than that of moclobemide.

From those reviews, MAOIs are effective for atypical depression. The evidences suggest that only moclobimide is as effective as TCAs and SSRIs for the treatment of MDD.

3.1.1.5 Other antidepressants

3.1.1.5.1 Escitalopram

Escitalopram is effective in the treatment of MDD. A previous meta-analysis showed that, after six weeks of treatment, escitalopram was superior to placebo and comparable to TCAs. However escitalopram had fewer adverse events than those of TCAs (Bech & Cialdella, 1992). A systemic review of four studies carried out in primary care settings also demonstrated that remission and response rates of escitalopram were superior to placebo and citalopram, but not venlafaxine-XR. However, its side effects are comparable with other antidepressants (Einarson, 2004). Another meta-analysis of ten clinical trials involving 2,687 patients also supported the previous review results. The findings showed that escitalopram might be superior to SSRIs and comparable to venlafaxine in the treatment of patients with MDD (Kennedy et al., 2006).The results of a recently meta-analysis in eight-week treatment trials of MDD indicated that escitalopram (10-20 mg/day) is superior to and more tolerable than duloxetine (60 mg/day) (Lam et al., 2008). Another systemic review involving clinical trials of escitalopram versus SNRIs (two trials with duloxetine and two with venlafaxine extended release) in outpatients (18-85 years of age) with moderate-to-severe MDD summarized that, over the eight week treatment period, escitalopram was as effective as but more tolerable than SNRIs (venlafaxine XR and duloxetine) (Kornstein et al., 2009). In addition, two meta-analyses showed that the efficacy and tolerability of escitalopram was superior to SSRIs and SNRIs (Kennedy et al., 2009; Lam et al., 2010). Escitalopram may also have a more rapid onset of action than other antidepressants (Kasper et al., 2006).The minimal effective dose for depression is 20 mg/day. However patients with severe or recurrent depression tend to respond to its higher dose (40 mg/day), and less severe depression may respond to its minimal effective dose (20 mg/day) (Montgomery et al., 1994). However, recent meta-analysis findings indicated that the effective doses of escitalopram may be lower than those in previous reviews. The recent review showed that the optimal dose of escitalopram in the treatment of moderate DSM-IV MDD is 10 mg/day, while the effective dose of escitalopram in patients with moderate to severe depression is 20 mg/day.

According to several review findings, escitalopram is effective for MDD. Its efficacy may be greater than that of SSRIs. With a more tolerable profile, it appears to be superior TCAs and SNRIs. The dose range for moderate depression is 10-20 mg/day and for moderate to severe depression is 20-40 mg/day.

3.1.1.5.2 Mirtazapine

A number of systemic reviews have summarized the efficacy and safety of mirtazpine for MDD. A meta-analysis of four clinical studies comparing mirtazapine with amitriptyline and placebo suggested that mirtazapine was as effective as amitriptyline in the treatment of MDD. However, mirtazapine was better tolerated than amitriptyline with respect to adverse events, particularly anticholinergic and cardiac side effects (Stahl et al., 1997). Another meta-analysis including 405 patients demonstrated that mirtazapine and amitriptyline were equally effective for severely depressed patients (Kasper et al., 1997). A systemic review of eight studies also showed that mirtazapine might be superior to placebo and comparable to amitriptyline for patients with MDD predominant with anxiety/agitation or anxiety/somatisation symptoms (Fawcett & Barkin, 1998). In comparison to SSRIs, a systemic review of ten clinical trials including 1,904 outpatients with MDD showed that mirtazapine and SSRIs were equally effective, but mirtazapine had a preferable side effect profile (Papakostas, et al., 2008). In addition, a meta-analysis of 14 studies involving 1,108 patients with MDD, mirtrazapine appears to have lesser sexual dysfunction than SSRIs (Chen et al., 2008). A meta-analysis of remission rates and time to remission of 15 six-week, clinical trials of mirtazapine and SSRIs showed a higher remission rates in mirtazapine-treated patients after 1, 2, 3, 4 and 6 weeks of treatment. Mirtazapine may have a more rapid onset of action than SSRIs (Thase et al., 2010).

With regard to those reviews, mirtazapine is as effective as amitriptyline and may be superior to SSRIs in the treatment of MDD. The side effect profile of mirtazapine appears to be different from those of amitriptyline and SSRIs.

3.1.1.5.3 Bupropion

Several systemic reviews supported the efficacy, safety and tolerability of bupropion. In a pooled study of clinical studies in MDD patients, at week 8 or end point, bupropion and SSRIs were equally effective and tolerable (Thase et al., 2005). In another meta-analysis of summarized that bupropion XL had a better sexual tolerability than that of escitalopram with similar antidepressant efficacy (Clayton et al., 2006). A systemic review of six clinical trials in MDD patients indicated that bupropion had a greater resolution of sleepiness and fatigue than SSRIs treatment (Papakostas et al., 2006).

From those reviews, bupropion is an effective and tolerable antidepressant. Patients treated with bupropion appear to have less sexual dysfunction than those with SSRIs. It is also beneficial for sleepy and fatigue patients.

3.1.1.5.4 Trazodone

A meta-analysis summarized the efficacy, safety and tolerability of trazodone. Trazodone was compared with imipramine in six treatment studies of depression. The findings suggested that both active drugs were equally efficacious (Patten, 1992). A meta-analysis of nine studies including 988 patients showed that trazodone might be comparable to nefazodone and SSRIs (Papakostas & Fava, 2007). From two review, trazodone seems to be equi-effective and –tolerable as other antidepressants in the treatment of depression.

3.1.1.5.5 Agomelatine

Agomelatine, melatonergic agonist (MT1 and MT2 receptors) and 5-HT2C antagonist, is indicated for the treatment of adult MDD. Most clinical trial results supported it efficacy in general depressed patients. A meta-analysis of three clinical studies also suggested that 25-50 mg/day of agomelatine was also effective for severe depression.

3.1.2 Cognitive-behavioural therapy

CBT is effective for MDD. A meta-analysis of four short-term, randomized trials comparing antidepressants and CBT in severely depressed outpatients showed that CBT was as effective as antidepressants (DeRubeis et al., 1999). In comparison to psychodynamic psychotherapy, included studies with at least 13 therapy sessions and a at least 20 patients per group. The review findings suggested that short-term psychodynamic psychotherapy and CBT or behavioural therapy have similar remission or improvement judged by the patients (Leichsenring, 2001). Another meta-analysis of Beltman (2010) including 29 studies found the effectiveness of CBT for the reduction of depressive symptoms in depressed patients with a diversity of somatic diseases.

In addition, a meta-analysis comparing found that CBT, behavioral therapy, and psychodynamic therapy seem to be superior to pharmacological treatment in elderly depressed patients. However, those nondrug and antidepressant therapies are comparable in treatment those depressed patients (Gerson et al., 1999). There is a systemic review of 57 controlled trials to assess the effects of psychotherapy and other behavioral interventions in depressed older patients. About 19% of the participants discontinued their treatment, with the higher discontinuation rates in group therapies and in longer therapies. The reviews summarized that CBT and reminiscence seemed to be effective and acceptable for older patients with depression. Seven to twelve sessions appear to optimize effectiveness and minimize dropout rates (Pinquart et al., 2007).

Several reviews have shown the efficacy of CBT in patients with depression. Its efficacy for the treatment of depression is comparable to that of antidepressants and other psychotherapy such as short-term psychodynamic psychotherapy. CBT may be beneficial or an alternative treatment for children, adolescents and elderly patients intolerable to antidepressants.

Several reviews have shown that CBT is effective for depression in children and adolescents. A meta-analysis of six randomized trials compared the efficacy of CBT with inactive interventions in depressed patients aged between 8 and 19 years. Most included trials are based on relatively mild cases of depression and moderate quality. The review suggested that CBT may be beneficial for the treatment of depressive disorder with moderate severity in children and adolescents but not recommended for severe depression (Harrington et al., 1998). Another meta-analysis also demonstrated that CBT appears to be effective for depressed adolescents (Lewinsohn & Clarke, 1999; Klein et al., 2007). Since there is a limitation for antidepressant use in children and adolescents, CBT may be an alternative and effective treatment of those patients with MDD.

Although some clinical studies and reviews showed the efficacy of CBT in treating depressed patients, an overestimation of its efficacy from each study may not be overlooked. In a meta-analysis of Cuijpers et al. (2010) examined the effect sizes of 117 studies with 175 comparisons between psychotherapy and control conditions demonstrated that the benefits of psychotherapy for adult depression appeared to be overestimated considerably due to publication bias.

3.1.3 Cognitive-behavioural therapy combined with antidepressants

Although antidepressant or CBT therapy alone shows its efficacy for MDD, significant proportion patients, particular those with severe or recurrent MDD, do not or partially respond to either monotherapy. Combined treatment is, therefore, a choice to raise the response and remission rates. Although many types of combined therapy for MDD are available, psychotherapy, particularly CBT, combined with antidepressants is effective and possibly less adverse effects than other combinations, e.g., combination of two antidepressants. The effectiveness of CBT combined with antidepressant is widely reported. A systemic review of 18 studies including 1,838 subjects receiving psychological treatment alone or combined treatment consisting of the same psychological treatment plus an antidepressant. The review showed that combined treatment is more effective than psychological treatment alone (Cuijpers et al., 2009). However the advantage of combination appears to be less when an antidepressant is added to CBT (Cuijpers et al., 2009). The clinical study of Thompson et al. (2001) compared the efficacy of desipramine-alone, CBT-alone and their combination for elderly outpatients with depression. The findings indicated that the combined therapy might be effective for severely depressed patients.

The MDD patients who do not respond to an adequate dose and duration of antidepressant treatment are indicated for combined therapy. Many studies show that psychotherapy combined with antidepressants is effective for these patients. In the STAR*D study, the MDD patients who had received inadequate benefits from a initial antidepressant medication were assigned to treat with other strategies. The findings showed that CBT augmentation to citalopram is as effective as pharmacologic augmentation, although, the latter augmentation had more rapid remission than the CBT augmentation (Thase et al., 2007). Regarding the evidence from other ethnic groups, an open study also demonstrated the adding CBT to fluoxetine in Thai patients with MDD who did not respond to four weeks treatment of fluoxetine has significantly more efficacy than previous fluoxetine treatment alone (Maneeton et al., 2010).

4. Long-term treatment (continuation and maintenance phase)

After the successful treatment of MDD in the acute phase, the discontinuation of antidepressant therapy usually leads to a relapse or recurrent. Long-term treatment is, therefore, desperately needed for most patients. The ultimate goal of treatment phase is to sustain the remission period and prevent a new episode of MDD.

4.1 Antidepressants

Many reviews supported the antidepressant continuation for the prevention of early relapse for a period of 9-12 months after remission. Maintenance therapy of antidepressants is effective for preventing the recurrence of depressive episodes (Paykel, 2001). A systemic review of 31 studies including 4,410 participants demonstrated that antidepressant continuation treatment could reduce the relapse rate as comparison with placebo (41% for placebo vs. 18% for antidepressants) (Geddes, et al., 2003). Another meta-analysis of four comparative and 23 placebo-controlled trials reviewed the efficacy and effectiveness of second-generation antidepressants for preventing MDD relapse and recurrence during continuation and maintenance phases of treatment. Duloxetine and paroxetine, fluoxetine and sertraline, fluvoxamine and sertraline, and trazodone and venlafaxine were comparable for the relapse prevention of a depressive episode. A meta-analysis of those second-generation antidepressants indicated the overall benefits of continuation- and maintenance-phase treatment for patients with MDD (Hansen et al., 2008). In addition, a meta-analysis of 30 studies involving 4,890 participants also summarized that antidepressants could reduce a relapse risk in the maintenance phase, regardless of clinical and pharmacologic factors. However, the larger number of depressive episodes may suggest a relative resistance against the prophylactic treatment from antidepressant (Kaymaz et al., 2008).

A meta-analysis of Kok et al. (2011) reviewed eight studies of continuation and maintenance treatment in the elderly with 925 participating patients. The results showed that continuing treatment with antidepressants appeared to be efficacious as compared with placebo. The efficacy and tolerability during long-term treatment of both TCAs and SSRIs are comparable.

From those reviews, antidepressants appear to be effective in prevention relapse and recurrence of a depressive episode in MDD patients. However, the prophylactic effects of antidepressants in patients with many depressive episodes may not be as effective as those with a single episode.

4.2 Cognitive behavioral therapy

The review of Paykel (2001) showed that CBT appeared to be effective in preventing relapse from unipolar depression, particularly in patients with residual symptoms. A systemic review of 28 trials involving 1,880 adult patients suggested that acute treatment of CBT might be more effective than pharmacotherapy in reducing a relapse or recurrence of depressive episode. To compare with other active continuation treatments, continuation treatment with CBT in those responding to acute antidepressant therapy can reduce the relapse and recurrence at the end of continuation treatment and follow-up (Vittengl et al., 2007).

Several evidences also show the advantage of long-term treatment with CBT for depression. The clinical study of Fava et al. (1996) determined whether CBT of residual symptoms of depression can prevent further relapses. Forty MDD patients with successfully antidepressant therapy were randomly assigned to either CBT or standard clinical management. Antidepressant medications in both groups were gradually tapered. The result showed that CBT was effective for the reduction of relapse in the depressed patients.

As an intervention during the continuation and maintenance phase, CBT is beneficial for prevention of depressive episodes.

4.3 Cognitive-behavioural therapy combined with antidepressants

There is some evidence on the long-term benefits of psychotherapy combined with antidepressants. This combined therapy is particular effective in preventing a relapse of depressive episode. Although short-term antidepressant treatment is effective for MDD patients, some of them still behave and believe as if they depressed, and some still have low self-esteem or interpersonal difficulties. These residual symptoms, therefore, may be addressed with CBT. A 6-month, randomized controlled trial (RCT) compared the efficacy of continuation treatment with fluoxetine plus CBT or fluoxetine alone in 56 patients (ages 11-18 years) with MDD who have responded to acute pharmacotherapy. The findings indicated that fluoxetine plus CBT might be able to reduce the risk of relapse as compared with fluoxetine alone (Kennard et al., 2008). In an open trial, 19 patients who failed to respond to at least two trials of antidepressants with adequate doses and durations were treated with CBT augmentation. The remaining 16 patients improved significantly, and 12 patients were considered to be in remission (Fava et al., 1997).

In contrast, there is a 6-month, continuation treatment study in patients with MDD who were remitted from an 8-week, open-label, fixed dose, acute treatment of fluoxetine. The study compared the continuation treatment of fluoxetine only and fluoxetine plus CBT. The findings showed no significant differences in the respects of relapse rates and 17 HAM-D scores (Petersen et al., 2004).

5. Further research

Several lines of evidence suggest that antidepressants, CBT and their combination are effective for the treatment and prevention of depressive episodes. Most studies involved the treatment in acute phase and the rests were in the continuation and maintenance phases. Although several reviews and clinical studies in acute phase treatment of MDD have been done, most of them involve only either antidepressant or CBT monotherapy. In addition, only few clinical studies and systematic reviews of MDD treatments in continuation and maintenance phases, particularly the cognitive-behavioural therapy combined with antidepressants, have been carried out. Further RCTs and systemic reviews with well-designed methodology, large sample sizes and consistent outcomes may be helpful in clarifying the benefits of this combination therapy in both acute and long-term treatments of MDD.

6. Conclusion

In the acute phase of MDD, combination of CBT and antidepressants appears to be more efficacious than antidepressant or CBT monotherapy, particularly in severely depressed patients. However this is a lack of evidence of this combination in depressed children and adolescents.

For long-term treatment of MDD, antidepressant medications, CBT and its combination appear to be effective in preventing a depressive episode in both continuation and maintenance phase. Since there were only limited studies of this, we could not conclude that this combination is superior to antidepressant or CBT monotherapy in these phases. More well-designed studies are, therefore, necessary to determine the superiority of this combination over antidepressant and CBT monotherapy.

7. Acknowledgment

I would like to thank Professor Manit Srisurapanont MD., Department of Psychiatry, Faculty of Medicine, Chiang Mai University, Thailand, who reviewed and edited this chapter.

8. References

Anderson, I. (2000). Selective serotonin reuptake inhibitors versus tricyclic antidepressants: A meta-analysis of efficacy and tolerability. *Journal of affective disorders*, Vol. 58, No.1, pp: 19-36

Anderson, R.J., Freedland, K.E., Clouse, R.E. & Lustman P.J. (2001). The prevalence of comorbid depression in adults with diabetes: a meta-analysis. *Diabetes Care.*, Vol. 24, No.6, pp: 1069-1078

Angst, J., Scheidegger, P. & Stabl, M. (1993). Efficacy of moclobemide in different patient groups. Results of new subscales of the hamilton depression rating scale. *Clinical neuropharmacology*, Vol. 16 (Supplement 2), pp: S55-62

Arroll, B., Macgillivray, S., Ogston, S., Reid, I., Sullivan, F., Williams, B. & Crombie, I. (2005). Efficacy and tolerability of tricyclic antidepressants and SSRIs compared with placebo for treatment of depression in primary care: A meta-analysis *Annals of family medicine*, Vol. 3, No. 5, pp: 449-456

Barbui, C., Guaiana, G. & Hotopf, M. (2004). Amitriptyline for inpatients and SSRIs for outpatients with depression? Systematic review and meta-regression analysis. *Pharmacopsychiatry*, Vol. 37, No. 3, pp: 93-97

Bauer, M., Tharmanathan, P., Volz, H.P., Moeller, H.J. & Freemantle, N. (2009). The effect of
    venlafaxine compared with other antidepressants and placebo in the treatment of
    major depression: a meta-analysis. *European archives of psychiatry and clinical
    neuroscience*. Vol. 259, No. 3, pp:172-185

Bech, P. & Cialdella, P. (1992). Citalopram in depression--meta-analysis of intended and
    unintended effects. *International clinical psychopharmacology*, Vol. 6 (Supplement 5),
    pp: 45-54

Beck, A.T. (1967). *Depression: Clinical, experimental and theoretical aspects*, Harper & Row, New
    York

Beck, A.T. (2005). The current state of cognitive therapy: a 40-year retrospective. *Archives of
    General Psychiatry*, Vol. 62, pp: 953–959

Beltman, M., Voshaar, R. & Speckens, A. (2010). Cognitive-behavioural therapy for
    depression in people with a somatic disease: Meta-analysis of randomized
    controlled trials. *The British journal of psychiatry*, Vol. 197, No. 1, pp: 11-19

Bijl ,R., Ravelli, A. & van Zessen, G. (1998). Prevalence of psychiatric disorder in the general
    population: results of the Netherlands Mental Health Survey and Incidence Study
    (NEMESIS). *Social psychiatry and psychiatric epidemiology*, Vol. 33, pp: 587–595

Bland, R.C., Newman, S.C. & Orn, H. (1988). Period prevalence of psychiatric disorders in
    Edmonton. *Acta psychiatrica Scandinavica. Supplementum*, Vol. 77, pp: 33–42

Bourdon, K.H., Rae, D.S., Locke, B.Z., Narrow, W.E. & Regier, D.A. (1992). Estimating the
    prevalence of mental disorders in US adults from the Epidemiologic Catchment
    Area Survey. *Public Health Reports*, Vol. 107, No. 6, pp: 663–668

Canino, G.J., Bird, H.R., Shrout, P.E., Rubio-Stipec, M., Bravo, M., Martinez, R. & others.
    (1987). The prevalence of specific psychiatric disorders in Puerto Rico. *Archives of
    general psychiatry*, Vol. 44, pp: 727–735

Carta, M.G., Carpiniello, B., Kovess, V., Porcedda, R., Zedda, A. & Rudas, N. (1995) Lifetime
    prevalence of major depression and dysthymia: results of a community survey in
    Sardinia. *European neuropsychopharmacology*, Vol. 5 (Supplement), pp: 103–107

Chen C.N., Wong, J., Lee, N., Chan-Ho, M.W., Lau, J.T. & Fung, M. (1993). The Shatin
    Community Mental Health Survey in Hong Kong. *Archives of general psychiatry*,
    Vol. 50, No. 2, pp: 125–133

Chen, Z., Wang, H. & Jin, W. (2008). Selective serotonin reuptake inhibitor is more likely to
    induce sexual dysfunction than mirtazapine in treating depression. *National journal
    of andrology*, Vol.14, No.10, pp: 896-899

Clayton, A., Croft, H., Horrigan, J., Wightman, D., Krishen, A., Richard, N. & Modell, J.
    (2006). Bupropion extended release compared with escitalopram: Effects on sexual
    functioning and antidepressant efficacy in 2 randomized, double-blind, placebo-
    controlled studies. *The Journal of clinical psychiatry*, Vol. 67, No. 5, pp: 736-746

Cuijpers, P., Van Straten, A., Warmerdam, L. & Andersson, G. (2009). Psychotherapy versus
    the combination of psychotherapy and pharmacotherapy in the treatment of
    depression: A meta-analysis. *Depression and anxiety*, Vol. 26, No. 3, pp: 279-288

Cuijpers, P., van Straten, A., Warmerdam, L., Andersson, G. (2009). Psychotherapy versus
    the combination of psychotherapy and pharmacotherapy in the treatment of
    depression: a meta-analysis. *Depression and Anxiety*, Vol. 26, No. 3, pp: 279-288

da Costa, R., Rangé, B., Malagris, L., Sardinha, A., De Carvalho, M. & Ae, N. (2010) Cognitive-behavioral therapy for bipolar disorder. *Expert Review of Neurotherapeutics*, Vol.10, No. 7, pp: 1089-1099

Davidson, J., Meoni, P., Haudiquet, V., Cantillon, M. & Hackett, D. (2002). Achieving remission with venlafaxine and fluoxetine in major depression: Its relationship to anxiety symptoms. *Depression and anxiety*, Vol.16, No. 1, pp: 4-13

DeRubeis, R., Gelfand, L., Tang, T. & Simons, A. (1999). Medications versus cognitive behavior therapy for severely depressed outpatients: Mega-analysis of four randomized comparisons. *The American journal of psychiatry*, Vol.156, No.7, pp: 1007-1013

DiMatteo, M.R., Lepper, H.S. & Croghan, T.W. (2000). Depression is a risk factor for noncompliance with medical treatment: meta-analysis of the effects of anxiety and depression on patient adherence. *Archives of internal medicine*, Vol. 160, No.14, pp: 2101–2107

Dunbar, G. (1995). Paroxetine in the elderly: A comparative meta-analysis against standard antidepressant pharmacotherapy. *Pharmacology*, Vol. 51, No. 3, pp: 137-144

Eckert, L. & Lançon, C. (2006). Duloxetine compared with fluoxetine and venlafaxine: Use of meta-regression analysis for indirect comparisons. *BMC psychiatry*, Vol. 6, No. 30

Einarson, T. (2004) Evidence based review of escitalopram in treating major depressive disorder in primary care. *International clinical psychopharmacology*, Vol. 19, No. 5, pp: 305-310

Entsuah, A., Rudolph, R. & Chitra, R. (1995). Effectiveness of venlafaxine treatment in a broad spectrum of depressed patients: A meta-analysis. *Psychopharmacology bulletin*, Vol. 31, No. 4, pp: 759-66

Entsuah, A., Huang, H. & Thase, M. (2001). Response and remission rates in different subpopulations with major depressive disorder administered venlafaxine, selective serotonin reuptake inhibitors, or placebo. *The Journal of clinical psychiatry*, Vol. 62, No. 11, pp: 869-877

Eze-Nliam, C.M., Thombs, B.D., Lima, B.B., Smith, C.G. & Ziegelstein, R.C. (2010). The association of depression with adherence to antihypertensive medications: a systematic review. *Journal of hypertension*, Vol. 28, No. 9, pp: 1785-1795

Fairburn, C.G., Norman, P.A., Welch, S.L., O'Connor, M.E., Doll, H.A. & Peveler, R.C. (1995). A prospective study of outcome in bulimia nervosa and the long-term effects of three psychological treatments. *Archives of general psychiatry*, Vol. 52, No.4, pp: 304–312

Faravelli, C., Degl'Innocenti, B.G., Aiazzi, L., Incerpi, G. & Pallanti, S. (1990). Epidemiology of mood disorders: a community survey in Florence. *Journal of affective disorders*, Vol. 20, No.2, pp: 135–141

Fava, G., Grandi, S., Zielezny, M., Rafanelli, C. & Canestrari, R. (1996). Four-year outcome for cognitive behavioral treatment of residual symptoms in major depression. *The American journal of psychiatry*, Vol. 153, No. 7, pp: 945-947

Fava, G,A., Savron, G., Grandi, S., & Rafanelli, C. (1997). Cognitive-behavioral management of drug-resistant major depressive disorder. *The Journal of clinical psychiatry*. Vol. 58, No. 6. pp: 278-282

Fawcett, J. & Barkin, R. (1998). A meta-analysis of eight randomized, double-blind, controlled clinical trials of mirtazapine for the treatment of patients with major depression and symptoms of anxiety. *The Journal of clinical psychiatry*, Vol. 59, No. 3, pp: 123-127

Fournier, L., Lesage, A.D., Toupin, J. & Cyr, M. (1997). Telephone surveys as an alternative for estimating prevalence of mental disorders and service utilization: a Montreal catchment area study. *Canadian journal of psychiatry*, Vol. 42, No. 7, pp: 737-743

Furukawa, T., Mcguire, H. & Barbui, C. (2002). Meta-analysis of effects and side effects of low dosage tricyclic antidepressants in depression: Systematic review. *BMJ*, Vol. 325, No. 7371, pp: 991

Furukawa, T., Mcguire, H. & Barbui, C. (2003). Low dosage tricyclic antidepressants for depression. *Cochrane database of systematic reviews*, No. 3 (CD003197)

Geddes, J.R., Carney, S.M., Davies, C., Furukawa, T.A., Kupfer, D.J., Frank, E. & Goodwin, G.M. (2003). Relapse prevention with antidepressant drug treatment in depressive disorders: a systematic review. *Lancet*, Vol. 361, No. 9358, pp: 653-661

Gerson, S., Belin, T., Kaufman, A., Mintz, J. & Jarvik, L. (1999). Pharmacological and psychological treatments for depressed older patients: A meta-analysis and overview of recent findings. *Harvard review of psychiatry*, Vol. 7, No. 1, pp: 1-28

Godha, D., Shi, L. & Mavronicolas, H. (2010). Association between tendency towards depression and severity of rheumatoid arthritis from a national representative sample: the Medical Expenditure Panel Survey. *Current medical research and opinion*, Vol. 26, No.7, pp: 1685-1690

Hansen, R., Gaynes, B., Thieda, P., Gartlehner, G., Deveaugh-Geiss., A, Krebs, E. & Lohr, K. (2008). Meta-analysis of major depressive disorder relapse and recurrence with second-generation antidepressants. *Psychiatric services*, Vol. 59, No. 10, pp: 1121-1130

Harrington, R., Whittaker, J. S., P & Campbell, F. (1998). Systematic review of efficacy of cognitive behaviour therapies in childhood and adolescent depressive disorde. *BMJ*, Vol. 316, No.7144, pp: 1559-1563

Hazell, P., O'Connell, D., Heathcote, D., Robertson, J. & Henry, D. (1995). Efficacy of tricyclic drugs in treating child and adolescent depression: a meta-analysis. *BMJ*. Vol. 310, No.6984, pp: 897-901

Henderson, S., Andrews, G. & Hall, W. (2000). Australia's mental health: overview of the general population survey. *The Australian and New Zealand journal of psychiatry*, Vol. 34, No.2, pp: 197–205

Henkel, V., Mergl, R., Allgaier, A., Kohnen, R., Möller, H. & Hegerl, U. (2006). Treatment of depression with atypical features: A meta-analytic approach. *Psychiatry research*, Vol.141, No. 1, pp: 89-101

Hetrick, S., Merry, S., McKenzie, J., Sindahl, P. & Proctor, M. (2007). Selective serotonin reuptake inhibitors (SSRIs) for depressive disorders in children and adolescents. *Cochrane database of systematic reviews*, No. 3 (CD004851)

Hirschfeld, R., Mallinckrodt, C., Lee, T. & Detke, M. (2005). Time course of depression-symptom improvement during treatment with duloxetine. *Depression and anxiety*, Vol. 21, No. 4, pp: 170-177

Hofmann, S.G., & Smits, J.A. (2008). Cognitive-behavioral therapy for adult anxiety. *The Journal of clinical psychiatry*, Vol. 69, No. 4, pp: 621-632.

Hotopf, M., Hardy, R. & Lewis, G. (1997). Discontinuation rates of SSRIs and tricyclic antidepressants: a meta-analysis and investigation of heterogeneity. *The British journal of psychiatry*, Vol. 170, pp: 120-127

Hwu, H.G., Yeh, E.K. & Chang, L.Y. (1989). Prevalence of psychiatric disorders in Taiwan defined by the Chinese Diagnostic Interview Schedule. *Acta psychiatrica Scandinavica*, Vol. 79, No.2, pp: 136–147

Kasper, S., Zivkov, M., Roes, K. & Pols, A. (1997). Pharmacological treatment of severely depressed patients: A meta-analysis comparing efficacy of mirtazapine and amitriptyline. *European neuropsychopharmacology*, Vol. 7, No. 2, pp: 115-124

Kasper, S., Spadone, C., Verpillat, P. & Angst, J. (2006). Onset of action of escitalopram compared with other antidepressants: Results of a pooled analysis. *International clinical psychopharmacology*, Vol. 21, No. 2, pp: 105-110

Kaymaz, N., van Os, J., Loonen, A.J. & Nolen, W.A. (2008). Evidence that patients with single versus recurrent depressive episodes are differentially sensitive to treatment discontinuation: a meta-analysis of placebo-controlled randomized trials. *The Journal of clinical psychiatry*, Vol. 69, No. 9, pp: 1423-1436

Kennard, B.D., Emslie, G.J., Mayes, T.L., Nightingale-Teresi, J., Nakonezny, P.A., Hughes JL, Jones, JM., Tao, R., Stewart, SM. & Jarrett, RB. (2008). Cognitive-behavioral therapy to prevent relapse in pediatric responders to pharmacotherapy for major depressive disorder. *Journal of the American Academy of Child and Adolescent Psychiatry*, Vol. 47, No. 12, pp: 1395-1404

Kennedy, S., Andersen, H. & Lam, R. (2006). Efficacy of escitalopram in the treatment of major depressive disorder compared with conventional selective serotonin reuptake inhibitors and venlafaxine XR: A meta-analysis. *Journal of psychiatry & neuroscience*, Vol. 31, No. 2, pp: 122-131

Kennedy, S., Andersen, H. & Thase, M. (2009) Escitalopram in the treatment of major depressive disorder: A meta-analysis. *Current medical research and opinion*, Vol. 25, No. 1, pp: 161-175

Kessler. R.C., McGonagle, K.A., Zhao, S., Nelson, C.B., Hughes, M., Eshleman, S., Wittchen, H.U. & Kendler, K.S. (1994). Lifetime and 12-month prevalence of DSM-III-R psychiatric disorders in the United States. Results from the National Comorbidity Survey. *Archives of general psychiatry*, Vol. 51, No. 1, pp: 8-19

Khongsaengdao, B., Louthrenoo, W. & Srisurapanont, M. (2000). Depression in Thai patients with rheumatoid arthritis. *Journal of the Medical Association of Thailand*, Vol. 83, No.7, pp: 743-747

Klein, J., Jacobs, R. & Reinecke, M. (2007). Cognitive-behavioral therapy for adolescent depression: A meta-analytic investigation of changes in effect-size estimates. *Journal of the American Academy of Child and Adolescent Psychiatry,* Vol. 46, No. 11, pp: 1403-1413

Kok, R.M., Heeren, T.J. & Nolen, W.A. (2011). Continuing treatment of depression in the elderly: a systematic review and meta-analysis of double-blinded randomized controlled trials with antidepressants. *The American journal of geriatric psychiatry*, Vol. 19, No. 3, pp: 249-255

Kornstein, S., Wohlreich, M., Mallinckrodt, C., Watkin, J. & Stewart, D. (2006). Duloxetine efficacy for major depressive disorder in male vs. Female patients: Data from 7 randomized, double-blind, placebo-controlled trials. *The Journal of clinical psychiatry*, Vol. 67, No. 5, pp: 761-770

Kornstein, S., Li, D., Mao, Y., Larsson, S., Andersen, H. & Papakostas, G. (2009). Escitalopram versus SSRI antidepressants in the acute treatment of major depressive disorder: Integrative analysis of four double-blind, randomized clinical trials. *CNS spectrums*, Vol. 14, No. 6, pp: 326-333

Lam, R., Andersen, H. & Wade, A. (2008) Escitalopram and duloxetine in the treatment of major depressive disorder: A pooled analysis of two trials. *International clinical psychopharmacology*, Vol. 23, No. 4, pp: 181-187

Lam, R., Lönn, S. & Despiégel, N. (2010). Escitalopram versus serotonin noradrenaline reuptake inhibitors as second step treatment for patients with major depressive disorder: A pooled analysis. *International clinical psychopharmacology*, Vol. 25, No. 4, pp: 199-203

Lee, C.K., Kwak, Y.S., Rhee, H., Kim, Y.S., Han, J.H., Choi, J.O. & Lee Y.H. (1987). The nationwide epidemiological study of mental disorders in Korea. *Journal of Korean medical science*, Vol. 2, No.1, pp: 19-34

Leichsenring, F. (2001). Comparative effects of short-term psychodynamic psychotherapy and cognitive-behavioral therapy in depression: A meta-analytic approach. *Clinical psychology review*, Vol. 21, No. 3, pp: 401-419

Lett, H., Blumenthal, J., Babyak, M., Sherwood, A., Strauman, T. & Robins, C. (2004). Depression as a risk factor for coronary artery disease: evidence, mechanisms, and treatment. *Psychosomatic medicine*, Vol. 66, No.3, pp: 305-315

Lewinsohn, P. & Clarke, G. (1999). Psychosocial treatments for adolescent depression. *Clinical psychology review*, Vol. 19, No. 3, pp: 329-342

Lieberman, D., Montgomery, S., Tourian, K., Brisard, C., Rosas, G., Padmanabhan, K., Germain, J. & Pitrosky, B. (2008). A pooled analysis of two placebo-controlled trials of desvenlafaxine in major depressive disorde. *International clinical psychopharmacology*, Vol. 23, No. 4, pp: 188-197

Linehan, M.M., Armstrong, H.E., Suarez, A., Allmon, D. & Heard, H.L. (1991). Cognitive-behavioral treatment of chronically parasuicidal borderline patients. *Archives of general psychiatry*, Vol. 48, No. 12, pp: 1060-1064

Magill, M. & Ray, L. (2009). Cognitive-behavioral treatment with adult alcohol and illicit drug users: A meta-analysis of randomized controlled trials. *Journal of studies on alcohol and drugs*, Vol. 70, No. 4, pp: 516-527

Mallinckrodt, C., Watkin, J., Liu, C., Wohlreich, M. & Raskin, J. (2005). Duloxetine in the treatment of major depressive disorder: A comparison of efficacy in patients with and without melancholic features. *BMC psychiatry*, Vol. 5, pp: 1

Mallinckrodt, C., Prakash, A., Andorn, A., Watkin, J. & Wohlreich, M. (2006). Duloxetine for the treatment of major depressive disorder: A closer look at efficacy and safety data across the approved dose range. *Journal of psychiatric research*, Vol. 40, No. 4, pp: 337-348

Maneeton, N., & Srisurapanont, M. (2000).Tricyclic antidepressants for depressive disorders in children and adolescents: a meta-analysis of randomized-controlled trials. *Journal of the Medical Association of Thailand*, Vol. 83, No. 11, pp: 1367-1374

Maneeton, N., Thongkam, A. & Maneeton, B. (2010). Cognitive-behavioral therapy added to fluoxetine in major depressive disorder after 4 weeks of fluoxetine-treatment: 16-

week open label study. *Journal of the Medical Association of Thailand*, Vol. 93, No. 3, pp: 337-342

Montgomery, S., Henry, J., Mcdonald, G., Dinan, T., Lader, M., Hindmarch, I., Clare, A. & Nutt, D. (1994). Selective serotonin reuptake inhibitors: Meta-analysis of discontinuation rates. *International clinical psychopharmacology*, Vol. 9, No. 1, pp: 47-53

Montgomery, S., Pedersen, V., Tanghøj, P., Rasmussen, C. & Rioux, P. (1994). The optimal dosing regimen for citalopram--a meta-analysis of nine placebo-controlled studies. *International clinical psychopharmacology*, Vol. 9 (Supplement 1), pp: 35-40

Montgomery, S. (2001). A meta-analysis of the efficacy and tolerability of paroxetine versus tricyclic antidepressants in the treatment of major depression. *International clinical psychopharmacology*, Vol. 16, No. 3, pp: 169-178

Murphy, J.M., Monson, R.R., Laird, N.M., Sobol, A.M. & Leighton, A.H. (2000). A comparison of diagnostic interviews for depression in the Stirling County Study. Challenges for psychiatric epidemiology. *Archives of general psychiatry*, Vol. 57, No.3, pp: 230-236

Nemeroff, C., Entsuah, R., Benattia, I., Demitrack, M., Sloan, D. & Thase, M. (2008). Comprehensive analysis of remission (COMPARE) with venlafaxine versus SSRIs. *Biological psychiatry*, Vol. 63, No. 4, pp: 424-434

Nouwen, A., Winkley, K., Twisk, J., Lloyd, C.E., Peyrot, M., Ismail, K., Pouwer, F. & European Depression in Diabetes (EDID) Research Consortium. (2010). Type 2 diabetes mellitus as a risk factor for the onset of depression: a systematic review and meta-analysis. *Diabetologia*. Vol. 53, No. 12, pp: 2480-2486

Oakley-Browne, M.A., Joyce, P.R., Wells, E., Bushnell, J.A. & Hornblow, A.R. (1989). Christchurch Psychiatric Epidemiology Study: Part II. Six-month and other period prevalences of specific psychiatric disorders. *The Australian and New Zealand journal of psychiatry*, Vol. 23, No.3, pp: 327-340

Offord, D.R., Boyle, M.H., Campbell, D., Goering, P., Lin, E., Wong, M. & Racine, Y.A. (1996). One-year prevalence of psychiatric disorder in Ontarians 15 to 64 years of age. *Canadian journal of psychiatry*, Vol. 41, No.9, pp: 559-563

Pakriev, S., Vasar, V., Aluoja, A., Saarma, M. & Shlik, J. (1998). Prevalence of mood disorders in the rural population of Udmurtia. *Acta psychiatrica Scandinavica*, Vol. 97, No. 3, pp: 169-174

Papakostas, G. & Fava, M. (2006). A metaanalysis of clinical trials comparing moclobemide with selective serotonin reuptake inhibitors for the treatment of major depressive disorder. *Canadian journal of psychiatry*, Vol. 51, No. 12, pp: 783-790

Papakostas, G., Nutt, D., Hallett, L., Tucker, V., Krishen, A. & Fava, M. (2006). Resolution of sleepiness and fatigue in major depressive disorder: A comparison of bupropion and the selective serotonin reuptake inhibitors *Biological psychiatry*, Vol. 60, No. 12, pp: 1350-1355

Papakostas, G. & Fava, M. (2007). A meta-analysis of clinical trials comparing milnacipran, a serotonin--norepinephrine reuptake inhibitor, with a selective serotonin reuptake inhibitor for the treatment of major depressive disorder. *European neuropsychopharmacology*, Vol. 17, No. 1, pp: 32-36

Papakostas, G. & Fava, M. (2007). A meta-analysis of clinical trials comparing the serotonin (5HT)-2 receptor antagonists trazodone and nefazodone with selective serotonin reuptake inhibitors for the treatment of major depressive disorder. *European,* Vol. 22, No. 7, pp: 444-447

Papakostas, G., Homberger, C. & Fava, M. (2008). A meta-analysis of clinical trials comparing mirtazapine with selective serotonin reuptake inhibitors for the treatment of major depressive disorder. *Journal of psychopharmacology,* Vol. 22, No. 8, pp: 843-848

Patten, S.B. (1992). The comparative efficacy of trazodone and imipramine in the treatment of depression. *CMAJ,* Vol.146, No. 7, pp: 1177-1182

Patten, S.B. (2001). Long-term medical conditions and major depression in a Canadian population study at wave 1 and 2. *Journal of affective disorders,* Vol. 63, No. 1-3, pp: 35-41

Paykel, E. (2001). Continuation and maintenance therapy in depression. *British medical bulletin,* Vol. 57, pp: 145-159

Petersen, T., Harley, R., Papakostas, G., Montoya, H., Fava, M. & Alpert, J. (2004). Continuation cognitive-behavioural therapy maintains attributional style improvement in depressed patients responding acutely to fluoxetine. *Psychological medicine,* Vol. 34, No. 3, pp: 555-561

Pinquart, M., Duberstein, P. & Lyness, J. (2007). Effects of psychotherapy and other behavioral interventions on clinically depressed older adults: A meta-analysis. *Aging & mental health,* Vol. 11, No. 6, pp: 645-657

Puech, A., Montgomery, S., Prost, J., Solles, A. & Briley, M. (1997). Milnacipran, a new serotonin and noradrenaline reuptake inhibitor: An overview of its antidepressant activity and clinical tolerability. *International clinical psychopharmacology,* Vol. 12, No. 2, pp: 99-108

Rudolph, R., Entsuah, R. & Chitra, R. (1998). A meta-analysis of the effects of venlafaxine on anxiety associated with depression. *Journal of clinical psychopharmacology,* Vol. 18, No. 2, pp: 136-144

Rugulies, R. (2002). Depression as a predictor for coronary heart disease. A review and meta-analysis. American journal of preventive medicine, Vol. 23, No.1, pp: 51-61

Rustad, J.K., Musselman, D.L. & Nemeroff, C.B. (2011).The relationship of depression and diabetes: Pathophysiological and treatment implications. *Psychoneuroendocrinology,* (April)

Smith, D., Dempster, C., Glanville, J., Freemantle, N. & Anderson, I. (2002). Efficacy and tolerability of venlafaxine compared with selective serotonin reuptake inhibitors and other antidepressants: A meta-analysis. *The British journal of psychiatry,* Vol.180, pp: 396-404

Soares, C., Kornstein, S., Thase, M., Jiang, Q. & Guico-Pabia, C. (2009) Assessing the efficacy of desvenlafaxine for improving functioning and well-being outcome measures in patients with major depressive disorder: A pooled analysis of 9 double-blind, placebo-controlled, 8-week clinical trials. *The Journal of clinical psychiatry,* Vol. 70, No. 10, pp: 1365-1371

Stahl, S., Zivkov, M., Reimitz, P., Panagides, J. & Hoff, W. (1997). Meta-analysis of randomized, double-blind, placebo-controlled, efficacy and safety studies of mirtazapine versus amitriptyline in major depression. *Acta psychiatrica Scandinavica. Supplementum,* vol. 391, pp: 22-30

Szadoczky, E., Papp, Z., Vitrai, J., Rihmer, Z. & Furedi, J. (1998). The prevalence of major depressive and bipolar disorders in Hungary. Results from a national epidemiologic survey. *Journal of affective disorders*, Vol. 50, No. 2-3, pp: 153–162

Thase, M. (1998). Effects of venlafaxine on blood pressure: A meta-analysis of original data from 3744 depressed patients. *The Journal of clinical psychiatry*, Vol. 59, No. 10, pp: 502-508

Thase, M., Entsuah, A. & Rudolph, R. (2001) Remission rates during treatment with venlafaxine or selective serotonin reuptake inhibitors. *The British journal of psychiatry*, Vol. 178, pp: 234-241

Thase, M., Haight, B., Richard, N., Rockett, C., Mitton, M., Modell, J., Vanmeter, S., Harriett, A. & Wang, Y. (2005). Remission rates following antidepressant therapy with bupropion or selective serotonin reuptake inhibitors: A meta-analysis of original data from 7 randomized controlled trials. *The Journal of clinical psychiatry*, Vol. 66, No. 8, pp: 974-981

Thase, M,E., Friedman, E,S., Biggs, M,M., Wisniewski, S,R., Trivedi, M,H., Luther, J,F., Fava, M., Nierenberg, A,A., McGrath, P,J., Warden, D., Niederehe, G., Hollon, S,D & Rush, A,J. (2007). Cognitive therapy versus medication in augmentation and switch strategies as second-step treatments: a STAR*D report. *The American journal of psychiatry*, Vol. 164, No. 5, pp: 739-752

Thase, M., Pritchett, Y., Ossanna, M., Swindle, R., Xu, J. & Detke, M. (2007). Efficacy of duloxetine and selective serotonin reuptake inhibitors: Comparisons as assessed by remission rates in patients with major depressive disorder. *Journal of clinical psychopharmacology*, Vol. 27, No. 6, pp: 672-676

Thase, M., Kornstein, S., Germain, J., Jiang, Q., Guico-Pabia, C. & Ninan, P. (2009). An integrated analysis of the efficacy of desvenlafaxine compared with placebo in patients with major depressive disorder. *CNS spectrums*, Vol.14, No. 3, pp: 144-154

Thase, M., Nierenberg, A., Vrijland, P., Van Oers, H., Schutte, A. & Simmons, J. (2010). Remission with mirtazapine and selective serotonin reuptake inhibitors: A meta-analysis of individual patient data from 15 controlled trials of acute phase treatment of major depression. *International clinical psychopharmacology*, Vol. 25, No. 4, pp: 189-198

Thompson, L., Coon, D., Gallagher-Thompson, D., Sommer, B. & Koin, D. (2001). Comparison of desipramine and cognitive/behavioral therapy in the treatment of elderly outpatients with mild-to-moderate depression. *The American journal of geriatric psychiatry*, Vol. 9, No. 3, pp: 225-240

Tignol, J., Stoker, M. & Dunbar, G. (1992). Paroxetine in the treatment of melancholia and severe depression. *International clinical psychopharmacology*, Vol. 7, No. 2, pp: 91-94

Turkington, D., Dudley, R., Warman, D. & Beck, A.T. (2004). Cognitive-behavior therapy for schizophrenia: a review. *Journal of psychiatric practice*, Vol. 10, No. 1, pp: 5–16

Usala, T., Clavenna, A., Zuddas, A. & Bonati, M. (2008). Randomised controlled trials of selective serotonin reuptake inhibitors in treating depression in children and adolescents: a systematic review and meta-analysis. *European neuropsycho-pharmacology.* Vol. 18, No. 1, pp:62-73

Ustün, T.B., Ayuso-Mateos, J.L., Chatterji, S., Mathers, C. & Murray, C.J. (2004). Global burden of depressive disorders in the year 2000. *The British journal of psychiatry*, Vol.184, pp: 386-392

Van Den Broek, W., Mulder, P., Van Os, E., Birkenhäger, T., Pluijms, E. & Bruijn, J. (2009). Efficacy of venlafaxine compared with tricyclic antidepressants in depressive disorder: A meta-analysis. *Journal of psychopharmacology*, Vol. 23, No. 6, pp: 708-713

Vis, P., Van Baardewijk, M. & Einarson, T. (2005), Duloxetine and venlafaxine-xr in the treatment of major depressive disorder: A meta-analysis of randomized clinical trials. *The Annals of pharmacotherapy*, Vol. 39, No. 11, pp: 1798-1807

Vittengl, J., Clark, L., Dunn, T. & Jarrett, R. (2007). Reducing relapse and recurrence in unipolar depression: A comparative meta-analysis of cognitive-behavioral therapy's effects. *Journal of consulting and clinical psychology*, Vol. 75, No. 3, pp: 475-488

Wacker, H.R., Mullejans, R., Klein, K.H. & Battegay, R. (1992). Identification of cases of anxiety disorders and affective disorders in the community according to ICD-10 and DSM-III-R by using the Composite International Diagnostic Interview (CIDI). *International journal of methods in psychiatric research*, Vol. 2, pp: 91–100

Waraich, P., Goldner, E.M., Somers, J.M. & Hsu, L. (2004). Prevalence and incidence studies of mood disorders: A systemic review of the literature. *Canadian journal of psychiatry*, Vol. 49, No.2, pp: 124-138

Weinmann, S., Becker, T. & Koesters, M. (2008). Re-evaluation of the efficacy and tolerability of venlafaxine vs. SSRIs: Meta-analysis. *Psychopharmacology bulletin*, Vol. 196, No. 4, pp: 511-520

Whittington, C.J., Kendall, T., Fonagy, P., Cottrell, D., Cotgrove, A. & Boddington, E. (2004). Selective serotonin reuptake inhibitors in childhood depression: systematic review of published versus unpublished data. *Lancet.* Vol. 363, No. 9418, pp:1341-1345

Wittchen, H.U., Essau, C.A., von Zerssen, D,, Krieg, J.C. & Zaudig, M. (1992). Lifetime and six-month prevalence of mental disorders in the Munich Follow-up Study. *European archives of psychiatry and clinical neuroscience*, Vol. 241, No.4, pp: 247–258

Wrestbrook, D., Kennnerley, H. & Kirk J. (2007). *An introduction to cognitive behavioral therapy: Skill and applications* (1st edition), Sage Publication Ltd, London, ISBN: 978-1-4129-0839-9

Wright, J. (2006). Cognitive behavior therapy: Basic principles and recent advances. *The journal of lifelong learning in psychiatry*, Vol. 2, No. 2, pp; 173-178

Part 2

Implications

5

Responding to the Challenge of Mental Health Recovery Policy

Lindsay G. Oades
University of Wollongong
Australia

1. Introduction

The movement towards recovery-oriented mental health service provision has emerged from growing consumer interest to define recovery in terms of personal experience, rather than symptom reduction. In many Western nations, this developing interest has helped to shape governmental health policy (Slade, Amering, & Oades, 2008). Slade, Amering and Oades (2008) state that policy in mental health recovery has become widespread in the English speaking world. They make a distinction between clinical recovery and the more consumer defined view of personal recovery, arguing that the term 'recovery' has become increasingly visible in mental health services, referring to personal recovery. Rather than the traditional medical meaning of cure as the remission of symptoms, the term "recovery" is being used to describe the personal and transformational process of consumers living with mental illness (Andresen, Oades & Caputi, 2003). The guiding principle for mental health policy in many predominantly English-speaking countries is mental health recovery, particularly now personal recovery: Australia (Australian Health Ministers, 2003), Canada (Piat & Sabetti, 2009), England (Department of Health, 2001), Ireland (Mental Health Commission, 2005), New Zealand (Mental Health Commission, 1998) and the United States (New Freedom Commission on Mental Health, 2005). This policy consensus has now become professional rhetoric. Using England as just one example, the principles of recovery have been adopted by clinical psychology (British Psychological Society Division of Clinical Psychology, 2000), mental health nursing (Department of Health, 2006), occupational therapy (College of Occupational Therapists, 2006) and psychiatry (Care Services Improvement Partnership, Royal College of Psychiatrists, & Social Care Institute for Excellence, 2007).

Slade, Amering and Oades (2008) use the term "rhetorical consensus" to refer to the consensus about the policy, which conceals the complexity and confusion around the term recovery. Since this article, further developments regarding mental health recovery have been impacting in European and Asian countries. Despite this increasing interest at the policy level, much of professional training remains symptom focussed, and many organisations continue on similar models.

To respond to the challenge of recovery policy it is important to have a clear definition of the phenomenon. It can then be measured. Services can then be developed based on the concept. Whilst this seems rudimentary- strong empirical work in this regard remains in its infancy. This chapter provides a descriptive overview of definitions of mental health recovery, and recovery oriented service provision. The first section of the chapter will define mental health recovery, including links to the science of wellbeing. Advances in measuring mental health recovery will be described. At an organisational level, mental health service providers (e.g. clinical mental health services, community organisations) have typically been symptom focused and have not celebrated the potential of consumers with mental disorders. The final section of the chapter will examine the development of recovery oriented service provision.

2. What is mental health recovery?

One of the most commonly cited definitions of personal recovery is as "*a deeply personal, unique process of changing one's attitudes, values, feelings, goals, skills and roles. It is a way of living a satisfying, hopeful, and contributing life even with limitations caused by the illness. Recovery involves the development of new meaning and purpose in one's life as one grows beyond the catastrophic effects of mental illness*" (Anthony, 1993). Slade, Amering and Oades (2008) assert that notwithstanding the significant increase in the use of the term 'recovery' in English speaking mental health systems, there is still a need for greater conceptual clarity. These authors refer to "clinical recovery" as a sustained remission of symptoms- which is consistent with the definition traditionally used in mental health services. They contrast this with "personal recovery" which emerged from patients who have lived with long-term illness emphasizes the individually defined and lived experience. Andresen, Oades and Caputi (2003) provide a definition consistent with personal recovery, known as psychological recovery, as the establishment of a fulfilling, meaningful life and a positive sense of identity founded on hopefulness and self-determination. This involves moving towards a preferred identity and a life of meaning - a framework where growth is possible - and challenging fatalistic diagnoses such as schizophrenia, whose prognoses suggest little room for the possibility of clinical healing or a meaningful life (Andresen et al, 2003).

Slade et al (2008) report a previous consensus statement involving ten principles and descriptions of personal recovery as follows: (1) *Self-direction* - Consumers lead, control, exercise choice over, and determine their own path of recovery; (2) *Individualised and Person-Centred* - There are multiple pathways to recovery based on the individual's unique needs, preferences, and experiences; (3) *Empowerment* - Consumers have the authority to exercise choices and make decisions that impact on their lives and educated and supported in so doing; (4) *Holistic* - Recovery encompasses the varied aspects of an individual's life including mind, body, spirit, and community; (5) *Nonlinea*r - Recovery is not a step-by-step process but one based on continual growth with occasional setbacks; (6) *Strengths-Based* - Recovery focuses on valuing and building on the strengths, resilience, coping abilities, inherent worth, and capabilities of the individual; (7) *Peer Support* - The invaluable role of mutual support, in which consumers encourage one another in recovery is recognised and promoted; (8) *Respect* - Community, system, and societal acceptance and appreciation of consumers - including the protection of consumer rights and the elimination of discrimination and stigma - are crucial in achieving recovery; (9) *Responsibility* - Consumers have responsibility for their own self-care and journeys of recovery; and (10) *Hope* - Recovery provides the essential and motivating message that people can and do overcome the barriers and obstacles that confront them.

Definitions of recovery have not remained static, and Resnick and Rosenheck (2006) highlighted the parallel themes and potential synergies between aspects of positive psychology, particularly strengths and their relationship to personal recovery. Other parallels include the emphasis on exploring phenomena other than illness. That is, recovery ideas that conceptualise the person's process of growth without using illness as the core framework. Positive psychology likewise does not use a negative starting point. Slade et al., (2008) report that an increased focus on recovery is being advocated as the guiding principle for mental health policy in many English-speaking countries, including Australia, England, Ireland and the United States of America. However, this momentum has not been matched by a clear conceptual framework or an agreed set of practices (Davidson, O'Connell, Tondora, Styron, & Kangas, 2006). Oades, Andresen and Caputi (2011) examine the numerous parallels between positive psychological constructs including strengths, resilience, hope, meaning and wellbeing. They argue that positive psychology as a science of optimal human functioning may provide an "empirical bridge" between the lived experience of mental health consumers, and an empirical science that is consistent with a philosophy of growth and autonomy. These authors use psychological recovery to refer to five processes of hope, meaning, identity, finding personal meaning and taking responsibility of health and wellbeing. They report a five stage model of psychological recovery, in which people living with mental illness move from moratorium, to awareness, preparation, rebuilding to a final dynamic stage of growth. This stage model to be described further below, is part of a broader endeavour to enable the tighter definition and measurement of psychological recovery, to further assist the development and evaluation of recovery oriented service provision. Measurement issues of recovery are now explored.

3. How is mental health recovery measured?

There remains no universally-accepted criterion for operationalising the concept of recovery. As recovery is represented by consumers as a unique, personal journey, there has been a reticence to define it as an outcome, however, some recovery measures have been developed. Campbell-Orde et al. (2005) compiled the Compendium of Recovery Measures, which includes measures of individual recovery and measures of recovery-promoting environments. Measures of individual recovery may be categorised into two domains: those that focus on psychological processes of the person, and those that assess satisfaction with various life domains and treatment. Measures of the intrapersonal process of psychological recovery include hope and optimism, self-determination, resilience, positive identity and finding meaning and purpose in life. Examples of measures that could be considered to fit this definition include: the Recovery Assessment Scale (RAS; Corrigan et al.,1999), the Mental Health Recovery Measure (MHRM; Young and Ensing, 1999) the Stages of Recovery Instrument (STORI) and the Self Identified Stages of Recovery (SISR) (Andresen, Oades, Caputi, 2011). Moreover, whilst there is some resistance to the idea, there exists a substantial literature, based on qualitative research, describing recovery as taking place in stages or phases. Davidson and Strauss (1992), for example, identified four aspects of recovery of the sense of self in severe mental illness. These were "(1) discovering the possibility of possessing a more active sense of self, (2) taking stock of strengths and weaknesses and assessing possibilities for change, (3) Putting into action some aspects of the self and integrating the results as reflecting one's actual capabilities and (4) using an enhanced sense of self to provide some refuge to provide a resource against the effects of the illness and [such things as stigma]" (Davidson and Strauss, 1992, p. 134).

Whilst Davidson and Strauss state that these four aspects do not necessarily occur in a linear fashion, but are related and overlapping, there is a logical order to the four aspects. Similarly three emotional stages of recovery were described by Baxter and Diehl (1998): (1) Recuperation, a stage of dependence following crisis; (2) Rebuilding, a time of building independence, and (3) Awakening, a time of building interdependence. Three phases were also posited by Young and Ensing (1999) in a model encompassing six aspects and numerous processes of recovery. The three phases of recovery were described as: Phase I, Overcoming "stuckness"; Phase II, Regaining what was lost and moving forward; and Phase III, Improving quality of Life (Young and Ensing, 1999). Spaniol et al. (2002) identified four phases of recovery in the literature: (1) Overwhelmed by the disability; (2) Struggling with the disability; (3) Living with the disability, and (4) Living beyond the disability. Spaniol et al. were able to place research participants in each of the first three phases, but not in the fourth phase. Tooth et al. (1997) and Lapsley et al. (2002) also found references to stages of recovery in large qualitative studies in Australia and New Zealand respectively.

Andresen, Oades and Caputi, (2003; 2011) combined much of this work, and examined consumer narratives to develop the construct of psychological recovery and a five stage model of psychological recovery. They state that there are four psychological processes reported by people living with enduring mental illness: (1) managing hope (2) meaning and purpose (3) establishing or re-establishing a preferred identity (4) taking responsibility for health and wellbeing. These authors then report five stages across which these processes fluctuate (1) moratorium, where there is much confusion and life is effectively on hold, (2) awareness, in which the person gets an awareness that life could be different (3) preparation, in which the person starts to prepare to make changes to his or her life (4) rebuilding, in which the person commences making changes and finally (5), the growth stage in which the person experiences and meaningful life and preferred identity and continues to strive and grow, despite potentially still having mental health symptoms. There are several measurement tools associated with this model including the Stages of Recovery Instrument (STORI), and Self Identified Stage of Recovery (SISR). The former has been translated into four languages. This model is closely related to the Collaborative Recovery Model (Oades et al, 2005) which is one attempt to assist the development of recovery oriented service provison. This endeavour to operationalise mental health recovery policy is now considered.

4. How do we develop recovery-oriented service provision?

The phrases *recovery-oriented practice* and *recovery-oriented service provision* usually refer to practices and services that are informed by the principles underpinning personal recovery. This is part of the challenge of responding to mental health recovery policy. As has been argued, there is no established criterion on what exactly personal recovery is, and hence how to measure it, and the corollary of that is that there is debate about what constitutes recovery-oriented service provision. Moreover, there is confusion, and conflation of what is the personal lived experience of a personal with mental illness (i.e. personal or psychological recovery) and the services that may be oriented to supporting this process (i.e. recovery-oriented service provision).

Davidson, Tondora, Staeheli Lawless, O'Connell and Rowe (2009) describe ten principles of recovery-oriented community based care to assist with developing some clarity about recovery- oriented care. (1) Care is oriented to promoting recovery (2) Care is strengths-based (3) Care is community- focussed (4) Care is person-driven (5) Care allows for reciprocity in relationships (6) Care is culturally responsive (7) Care is grounded in the person's life-context (8) Care addresses the socioeconomic context of the person's life (9) Care is relationally mediated; and (10) care optimises natural supports.

Like most organisational change, there is often resistance experienced. In this regard Davidson, O'Connell, Tondora, Styron, and Kangas (2006) had previously outlined the top ten concerns about recovery encountered. In increasing importance these are as follows: (10) Recovery is old news, (9) Recovery-oriented care adds to the burden of mental health practitioners who already are stretched thin by demands that exceed their resources, (8) "recovery" means the person is cured, (7) recovery in mental health is an irresponsible fad that sets people up for failure, (6) recovery happens for very few people with serious mental illness, (5) recovery only happens after, and as a result of, active treatment and cultivation of insight, (4) recovery can only be implemented with additional resources, through the introduction of new services, (3) recovery-oriented services are neither reimbursable nor evidence-based, (2) recovery approaches devalue the role of professional intervention, and (1) recovery increases provider exposure to risk and liability.

Davidson, Tondora, Staeheli Lawless, OConnell, and Rowe (2009) further describe the concept of a recovery guide. A recovery guide is similar to the concept of the recovery coaching, described by Oades et al (2009) in reference to the Collaborative Recovery Model. The Collaborative Recovery Model, a modularised model that guides systemic interventions, is proposed to facilitate the challenge of implementing recovery oriented service provision, and as discussed, is informed by positive psychology and positive organisational scholarship which provide a useful base upon which to build service reform and human growth. Oades, Crowe and Nguyen (2009) report that the CRM was originally developed as a model to assist practitioners to use evidence based skills with consumers in a manner consistent with the recovery movement (Deane et al, 2006). The model includes assumptions and practices that champion human growth, hope (Salgado et al, 2010), meaning and self-determination - issues that have not been the mainstay in the history of psychiatric practice.

Table 1 illustrates the two guiding principles and four components of the model, detailing the knowledge, skills and competencies required of practitioners.

Guiding Principle #1: Recovery as an individual process

As shown in Table 1, the first principle emphasises the personal subjective ownership of the recovery process, including hopefulness and personal meaning. It covers issues related to personal identity, particularly the need to move beyond the illness and towards one's best possible self. Finally it encourages individuals to take responsibility for their own wellbeing (Andresen, Oades & Caputi, 2003).

There are significant conceptual overlaps between Keyes' (2002) notion of flourishing and the idea of personal recovery as a journey that involves moving beyond illness, that is, living a meaningful life despite experiencing symptoms of illness. Within CRM, the *focus of recovery* concept is used to clarify the intervention or approach that is being utilised. For example, is the focus of a practitioner's team or unit mainly to remove or avoid symptoms, or is it to promote wellbeing? These are not fixed foci, and may change dependent on the illness.

Module	Knowledge Domains	Protocol, Skills and Attitudes	Competency
Recovery as an individual process (Guiding Principle 1)	Psychological recovery as a staged individual process involving: (i) hope (ii) meaning (ii) identity (iv) responsibility The "system of recovery" concept The "focus of recovery" concept	Protocol: Self Identified Stage of Recovery: Attitude: A "growth mindset" - hopefulness towards consumers' ability to set, pursue and attain personally valued life goals	Employs the principle, in all interactions and across all protocols, that psychological recovery from mental illness is an individualised process
Collaboration and autonomy support (Guiding Principle 2)	Working alliance Power and empowerment Relationship rupture Autonomy support Barriers to collaboration Working with relationship dynamics	Skill: Develop and maintain a working alliance Attitude: Positive towards genuine collaboration	Employs the principle, in all interactions and across all protocols, of maximum collaboration and support of consumer autonomy
Change enhancement (Component 1)	Stage of psychological recovery Decisional balance Motivational readiness and resistance Psychological needs Importance and confidence Fixed versus growth mindset	Protocol: Motivational interviewing, particularly decisional balance Skill: Use decisional balance techniques appropriate to assist consumer to clarify ambivalence regarding change Attitude: To take partial responsibility for role in interactional aspects of motivation	Enhances consumer change by skilful use of motivational enhancement that is appropriate to the stage of recovery of the consumer
Collaborative strengths and values (Component 2)	Values clarification Values use Strengths identification Strengths use	Protocol: "Camera" values and strengths clarification method Skill: Assist a consumer to elicit personal values and strengths and assess how well they have been implemented recently	Assists consumers to clarify values and strengths and use them in the here and now

Module	Knowledge Domains	Protocol, Skills and Attitudes	Competency
		Attitude: To value reflective exercises notwithstanding current difficulties or symptoms	
Collaborative life visioning and goal striving (Component 3)	Personal life vision Valued directions Goal identification, setting and striving Meaning/manageability trade-off Autonomous goals Approach and avoidance Goals Proximal and distal goals	Protocol: "Compass" vision and goal striving method Skill: Elicit meaningful vision and manageable goals Attitude: To be persistent in the face of obstacles	Persists flexibly and collaboratively with the components within the Compass to assist recovery by way of the development of an integrated meaningful life vision, valued directions, and manageable goals, which provide a broader purpose for actions.
Collaborative action planning and monitoring (Component 4)	Health behaviour change Action planning Homework Self-efficacy Monitoring Self-management	Protocol: "MAP" action planning method Skill: To assist with the development of comprehensive action plans Attitude: To value "small actions" between the meetings of staff and consumers (between session activity)	Systematically and collaboratively assigns actions, and monitors progress toward action completion and goals, to enhance self-efficacy of consumer

Table 1. Training and Coaching Competencies for Collaborative Recovery Model

Guiding Principle #2: Collaboration and autonomy support

This principle emphasises important aspects of the working alliance in assisting human growth. Autonomy support as outlined in Ryan, Huta and Deci's (2008) self-determination theory, underscores the importance of autonomy to wellbeing. This is particularly salient in mental health contexts due to the history of paternalism and control that has pervaded so many aspects of the systems and patient care (Andresen, Oades & Caputi, 2003).

There is substantial evidence regarding the association of the strength of the working alliance between the mental health worker and the person being supported in recovery and the degree of engagement and recovery outcomes (Martin, Garske & Davis, 2000). However, maintaining a strong working alliance often requires the mental health worker to: manage interpersonal strains or alliance ruptures, reflect on his/her own reactions to the dynamics of the working relationship (e.g. increased frustration, desire to fix things or rescue the person, etc), and maintain professional boundaries whilst striving to remain present with the person they are supporting. This is important as it encourages the worker to track and adjust her/his approach as required (e.g. rebuild trust, establish safety, confront, explore feelings, etc), particularly in light of the sometimes subtle changes that can occur in the relationship. As CRM is growth and future focused, it is conceptualised as a strengths-based coaching model, in which the relationships are coaching relationships rather than counseling relationships (Oades, Crowe, Nguyen, 2009)..

CRM Component #1: Change enhancement

This component recognises that many people (including consumers, carers and practitioners) within the context of enduring mental illnesses such as schizophrenia tend not to believe that positive change is possible. Change enhancement draws on skills from motivational interviewing, and directly challenges fixed mindsets (Dweck, 2006), regarding the potential for change. This component of the model also highlights the importance of intrinsic motivation and the personal meanings underpinning human change. It aims to shift both attitudes and beliefs about the potential for change.

Component #2: Collaborative Strengths and Values

The clarification and use of personal strengths and values is central to the model, and is the most popular component for consumers and practitioners alike. Whilst Rapp's (1998) strengths model is well known to mental health practitioners in a case management context, the CRM predominantly draws from contemporary research on character strengths, values and committed action (e.g. Petersen & Seligman, 2004; Hayes, 2004).

Component #3: Collaborative life visioning and goal striving

This third component assumes that despite adversity, a person is still capable of developing a vision for life. The vision involves articulating their best possible self and striving towards approach goals that are consistent with their personal values and while using their strengths. Clarke et al (2006) describe the goal technology that has been used to operationalise the goal component of CRM. The Collaborative Goal Technology (CGT) uses a range of evidence-based practices in goal setting (e.g. goals being specific and time limited) to assist mental health practitioners and consumers to collaboratively develop goals. In a subsequent study, Clarke, Crowe et al., (2009) found that practitioners trained in CRM, which included the CGT, were more likely to apply these evidence-based principles. Additionally, Clarke and colleagues (Clarke, Oades et al, 2009) in another investigation of CRM found that the goal attainment of people with enduring mental illness mediated the relationship between the distress caused by their symptoms and their perception of personal recovery. This finding suggests that goals are central to the recovery process and is consistent with the growth philosophy of the recovery movement. Positive psychology research continues to deepen our understanding of effective goal striving and its relationship to wellbeing (Brandtstadter, 2006).

Component #4: Collaborative action planning and monitoring

The fourth and final component of CRM is informed by research on the role of homework in cognitive-behavioural therapies (Kazantzis, Deane & Ronan, 2000). The term "action planning" is used in CRM because it does not carry the somewhat negative connotations of the word homework, which often stem from unhappy school experiences. Meta-analyses have found that therapy outcomes are significantly better for those who receive and complete homework assignments (Kazantzis, Whittington & Dattilio, 2010). Although this research has mostly focused on the treatment of depression and anxiety, there is increasing evidence of its importance in treating persistent and recurring mental illnesses such as schizophrenia (Deane, Glaser, Oades & Kazantzis, 2005; Kelly & Deane, 2009). Working on agreed actions between meetings is thus an essential ingredient of CRM.

The Collaborative Recovery Model as a Coaching Model

The CRM has been conceptualised as a strength-based person-centred coaching model (Oades, Crowe & Nguyen, 2009). The Life Journey Enhancement Tools (LifeJET) (Oades & Crowe, 2008) have been designed to operationalise key components of the CRM delivered in a coaching style, where the relationship is more person-centred and focused on personal goals (rather than clinician-centred and focused on clinical goals). Based on the root metaphor of a journey (of recovery), the protocols are called the Camera, Compass and MAP (see Figures 2 to 4), and are designed to stimulate future-oriented and hope-inducing activities. The Camera, Compass and MAP are modularized tools. Thus while it is preferable for them to be used in sequence they can be used alone.

The Camera is used to help the individuals to identify valued life domains and strengths, examine the extent to which these have recently been pursued, and to focus their attention on areas of potential change.

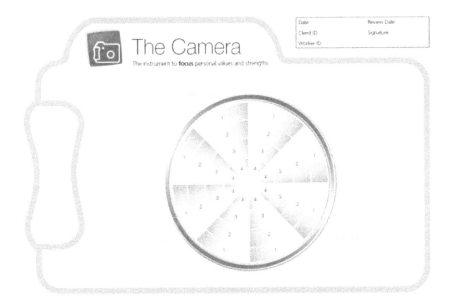

Fig. 1. The Camera values and strengths use coaching tool

The Compass evolved from the previously mentioned goal technology (Clarke et al, 2006). It is used to assist people to link their values with their goals, to quantify relative goal importance and to identify different levels of potential attainment. The Compass enables ratings of successful goal pursuit as a function of importance and attainment. Goal attainment weighted by perceived importance can be calculated as a numeric index if desired.

Last, the MAP (an abbreviation for My Action Plan) is an action-planning tool used to assist with homework setting for goal attainment tasks.

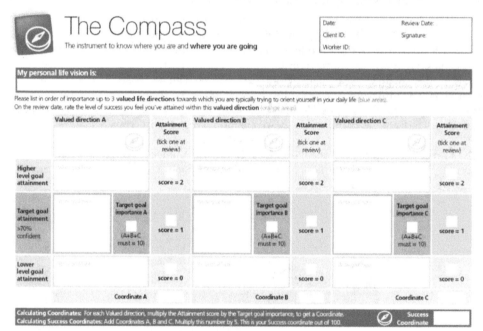

Fig. 2. The Compass valued direction and goal striving coaching tool

The Collaborative Recovery Model as a Systemic Intervention

Unlike many discrete and individual positive psychological interventions (Magyar-Moe, 2009) the Collaborative Recovery Model (CRM) (Oades et al, 2005), is a broad systemic framework guiding a range of interventions with consumers, carers, staff and organisational systems. The systemic nature of the interventions is imperative given the ingrained culture and history of psychiatric service provision. As Park and Petersen (2003) assert, positive institutions enable people to use their positive traits such as strengths and values, which in turn yields positive experiences and positive emotions. In mental health services, organisations require change to enable staff and consumers to utilise strengths, to enable the possibility of the benefits of positive emotions. Without such comprehensive change, recovery oriented services are unlikely to succeed. The CRM has been developed to assist with recovery-oriented service provision for people with enduring mental illness, and is informed by the principles, evidence and practices of positive psychology and positive organisational scholarship (Cameron, Dutton & Quinn, 2003).

The MAP

My Action Plan: The instrument to plan **what to do next**

Valued Direction
(from Compass)

Target goal
(from Compass)

Action name:

Action Description: What specific action is required to achieve the target level goal?

Date Set:

How often

When

Where

Social support

Resources
Who can give me
practical help?
With what?

Information
Who can give me
information when needed?
What information?

Emotional
Who can
listen to and
support me?

Monitoring actions

How will I monitor actions?

Barriers

What are my barriers?

Solutions

What are some solutions or backup plans?

Confidence
(circle level of confidence)

Not at all confident   0 10 20 30 40 50 60 70 80 90 100   Very confident

Specific action listed above. Repeat if not over 70% confident.

Review date:

Review outcome:

Make as soon as possible

Date:	Client ID:	Worker ID:	Review Date:	Signature

Fig. 3. The MAP action planning coaching tool

The relationship between mental health workers and the individual's wider support system is central to the recovery process. From a Collaborative Recovery perspective this system includes four parts nested in a broader community. The four interlinked parts are self of consumer, family carers, staff members and organisations (e.g., treatment services) in the community.

Currently, there is research and practice being conducted using the LifeJET tools and CRM principles in all four parts of the mental health system. The extent to which that community encourages social inclusion and non-stigmatising attitudes can greatly support an individual's recovery (e.g., Quinn & Knifton, 2005). Similarly, mental health organisations that are attempting to deliver recovery-oriented treatment may also need to make wider "systems" changes to do so successfully.

The CRM is deliberately being developed as a systemic intervention rather than one restricted to solely focusing on individual interventions with clients. The guiding principles, components and LifeJET protocol may be used for the self-development of individuals (self-coaching), used as part of a practitioner-client coaching relationship (practitioner coaching), used for carer recovery (carer coaching) and used at the organisational level, which may include practitioners coaching other practitioners (coaching) towards personal and professional development. This comprehensive systems intervention is seen as necessary to bring about the systemic and cultural transformation needed to generate recovery oriented service provision.

5. Conclusion

Mental health recovery policy, based on definitions of personal recovery from people living with mental illness, has become mainstream in most English speaking nations, and is growing in popularity across Europe and Asia. The challenge remains however as to gaining (a) more consensus about the concept referring to varied consumer experience (b) improved ways to measure the concept and (c) improve ways and organisaitonal support to develop services based around the concept, with the need for individual tailoring. This transformation is more profound than the development of "new interventions to treat mental illness". Rather it refers to a major reconsideration of the endeavour itself, a review of what is possible, and a major transformation of the mental health workforce. The Collaborative Recovery Model (CRM) is one example of an attempt towards this endeavour.

6. References

Andresen, R., Caputi, P., & Oades, L. G. (2010). Do clinical outcome measures assess consumer-defined recovery? *Psychiatry Research*, 177, 309-317.

Andresen, R., Oades, L. G., & Caputi, P. (2003). The experience of recovery from schizophrenia: Towards an empirically validated stage model. *Australian and New Zealand Journal of Psychiatry*, 37, 586-594.

Andresen, R, Oades, L. G. Caputi, P. (2011). Psychological Recovery: Beyond Mental Illness. Chichester: Wiley Blackwell.

Anthony W.A. (1993). Recovery from mental illness: the guiding vision of the mental health system in the 1990s. Innovations and Research 2, 17-24.

Anthony, W. A., Cohen, M., Farkas, M., & Cohen, B. F. (2000). Clinical care update: The chronically mentally ill. Case management-more than a response to a dysfunctional system. *Community Mental Health Journal, 36,* 97-105.

Australian Health Ministers (2003). *National Mental Health Plan* 2003-2008. Australian Government: Canberra.

Baumeister, R.R., & Vohs, K.D. (2002). *The pursuit of meaningfulness in life.* In C.R. Snyder & S.J. Lopez (eds)., Handbook of Positive Psychology, pp, 459-471.

Baxter E.A. & Diehl S. (1998). Emotional stages: Consumers and family members recovering from the trauma of mental illness. *Psychiatric Rehabilitation Journal,* 21:349–355.

Brandtstadter, J. (2006). Adaptive resources in later life: Tenacious goal pursuit and flexible goal

British Psychological Society Division of Clinical Psychology (2000). *Recent Advances in Understanding Mental Illness and Psychotic Experiences.* British Psychological Society: Leicester.

Cameron, K., Dutton, J. E., and Quinn, R. E. (eds.). (2003). *Positive Organizational Scholarship: Foundations of a New Discipline.* San Francisco: Berrett-Koehler Publishers.

Campbell-Orde, T., Chamberlin, J., Carpenter, J., et al *(2005) Measuring the Promise: A Compendium of Recovery Measures,* Vol. *II.* Human Services Research Institute Evaluation Center.

Care Services Improvement Partnership, Royal College of Psychiatrists & Social Care Institute for Excellence (2007). *A Common Purpose: Recovery in Future Mental Health Services.* CSIP: Leeds.

Carver, C., & Scheier, M. (1990). Origins and function of positive and negative affect: A control process review. *Psychological Review, 97,* 19-35.

Clarke, S. P., Crowe, T. P., Oades, L. G., & Deane, F. P. (2009). Do goal setting interventions improve the quality of goals in mental health services? *Psychiatric Rehabilitation Journal, 32(4),* 292-299.

Clarke, S. P., Oades, L.G., Crowe, T. P., & Deane, F. P. (2006). Collaborative Goal Technology: Theory and Practice. *Psychiatric Rehabilitation Journal, 30,* 129 -136.

Clarke, S., Oades, L., Crowe, T., Caputi, P. & Deane, F. P. (2009). The role of symptom distress and goal attainment in assisting the psychological recovery in consumers with enduring mental illness. *Journal of Mental Health, 18,* 389-397.

Clarke, S., Oades, L.G, Crowe, T.P. (accepted 19.7.2011). Recovery in mental health: a movement towards wellbeing and meaning in contrast with an avoidance of symptoms. *Psychiatric Rehabilitation Journal.*

College of Occupational Therapists (2006). *Recovering Ordinary Lives: The Strategy for Occupational Therapy in Mental Health Services 2007-2017.* College of Occupational Therapists: London.

Corrigan, P. W., Giffort, D., Rashid, F., Leary, M., & Okeke, I. (1999). Recovery as a psychological construct. *Community Mental Health Journal, 35,* 231-239.

Crowe, T. P., Deane, F.P., Oades, L.G., Caputi, P. & Morland, K.G. (2006). Effectiveness of a collaborative recovery training program in Australia in promoting positive views about recovery. *Psychiatric Services, 57 (10),* 1497-1500.

Davidson, L., O'Connell, M., Tondora, J., Styron, T. & Kangas, K. (2006). The Top 10 concerns about recovery encountered in mental health system transformation. *Psychiatric Services*, 57, 640-645.

Davidson L, Strauss JS. (1992). Sense of self in recovery from severe mental illness. *British Journal of Medical Psychology*, 65:131-145.

Davidson, L., Tondora, J., Staeheli Lawless, M., OConnell, M., & Rowe, M. (2009). A practical guide to recovery-oriented practice. New York: Oxford University Press.

Deane, F. P., Crowe, T., King, R., Kavanagh, D., & Oades, L. G. (2006). Challenges in implementing evidence-based practice into mental health services. *Australian Health Review*, 30, 305-309.

Deane, F.P., Glaser, N.M. Oades, L.G. & Kazantzis, N. (2005). Psychologists' use of homework assignments with clients who have schizophrenia. *Clinical Psychologist*, 9 (1), 24-30.

Department of Health (2006). *From Values to Action: The Chief Nursing Officer's Review of Mental Health Nursing*. HMSO: London.

Department of Health (2001). *The Journey to Recovery – The Government's Vision for Mental Health Care*. Department of Health: London

Dweck, C.S. (2006). Mindset : The new psychology of success. New York : Random House.

Elliot, A. J. & Friedman, R. (2007). *Approach-avoidance: A central characteristic of personal goals*. In B. R. Little, K. Salmela-Aro, & S. D. Phillips (Eds.), Personal project pursuit: Goals, actions, and human flourishing (pp. 97-118). Mahwah, New Jersey: Lawrence Erlbaum Associates, Publishers.

Elliot, A. J., Sheldon, K. M. & Church, M. A (1997). Avoidance personal goals and subjective well-being. *Personality and Social Psychology Bulletin*, 23, 915-927. doi: 10.1177/0146167297239001

Frederickson, B.L. (2001). The role of positive emotions in positive psychology: The broaden and build theory. *American Psychologist*, 56, 218-226.

Green, L.S., Oades, L.G. Grant, A.M. (2006). Cognitive-Behavioural, Solution-Focused Life Coaching: Enhancing Goal Striving, Well-Being and Hope. *Journal of Positive Psychology*, 1(3), 142-149.

Hadikin, R., (2004). Effective coaching in healthcare. London: Elsevier Science.

Hayes, S.C. (2004). Acceptance and commitment therapy, relational frame theory, and the third wave of behavioural and cognitive therapies. *Behaviour Therapy*, 35(4), 639-665.

Kazantzis, N., & Deane, F. P. & Ronan, K. (2000). Homework assignments in cognitive and behavioral therapy: A meta-analysis. *Clinical Psychology: Science & Practice*, 7, 189-202.

Kazantzis, N., Whittington, C., Dittilio, F. (2010). Meta-Analysis of Homework Effects in Cognitive and Behavioral Therapy: A Replication and Extension. *Clinical Psychology: Science and Practice*, 17, 2, 144-156.

Kelly, P., J. & Deane, F. P. (2009). Does homework improve outcomes for individuals diagnosed with severe mental illness? *Australian and New Zealand Journal of Psychiatry*, 43, 968-975.

Keyes , C.L.M. (2002). The Mental health continuum: From languishing to flourishing in life. *Journal of Health and Social Behavior*, 43, 207-222.

King, L. A. (1998). Personal goals and personal agency: Linking everyday goals to future images of the self. In M. Kofta, G. Weary & G. Sedek (Eds.), *Personal control in action: Cognitive and motivational mechanisms* (pp.109-128). New York, NY: Plenum Press.

Lapsley H., Nikora L.W. & Black R. (2002). *Kia Mauri Tau! Narratives of Recovery from Disabling Mental Health Problems*. Mental Health Commission: Wellington.

Linley, P.A. & Harrington, S. (2006). Strengths coaching: A potential-guided approach to coaching psychology. *International Coaching Psychology Review*, 1(1), 37-46.

Magyar,-Moe, J.L. (2009). *Therapist's guide to positive psychological interventions*. New York: Elsevier.

Malachowski. C.K. (2009). Optimizing System and Patient Recovery. Rediscover and Recovery: The Shared Journey Project. *International Journal of Psychosocial Rehabilitation*, 13(2), 49-64.

Marshall, S., Oades, L., & Crowe, T. (2009). Mental health consumers' perceptions of receiving recovery-focused services. *Journal of Evaluation in Clinical Practice, 15*, 654-659.

Marshall, S., Oades, L., Crowe, T., Deane, F. P., & Kavanagh, D. (2007). A review of consumer involvement in evaluations of case management: Consistency with a recovery paradigm. *Psychiatric Services, 58*, 396-401.

Martin DJ, Gaske JP, Davis MK. (2000). Relation of the therapeutic alliance with outcome and other variables: a meta-analytic review. *Journal of Consulting and Clinical Psychology*, 68: 438–450.

Maslow, A. H. (1987). *Motivation and personality* (3rd ed.). New York, NY: Harper and Row, Publishers.

Mental Health Commission (1998). *Blueprint for Mental HealthServices in New Zealand*. Mental Health Commission: Wellington.

Mental Health Commission (2005). *A Vision for a Recovery Model in Irish Mental Health Services*. Mental Health Commission: Dublin.

National Association of State Mental Health Program Directors (2006). *Morbidity and mortality in people with serious mental illness*. Medical Directors Council.

New Freedom Commission on Mental Health (2005). *Achieving the Promise: Transforming Mental Health Care in America*. U.S.Department of Health and Human Services: Rockville, MD.

Oades L.G., Andresen R., Crowe T.P., Malins G., Marshall S., and Turner A. (2008). *A Handbook to Flourish: A Recovery-Based Self-Development Program*. Illawarra Institute for Mental Health, University of Wollongong, NSW, Australia.

Oades, L., Crowe, T., Deane, F., Kavanagh, D., Lambert, W. G., & Lloyd, C. (2005). Collaborative recovery: An integrative model for working with individuals who experience chronic and recurring mental illness. *Australasian Psychiatry, 13*, 279-284.

Oades, L.G. & Crowe, T.P. (2008). *Life Journey Enhancement Tools (Life JET)*. ISBN. 978-1-74128-156-9. Illawarra Institute for Mental Health, University of Wollongong.

Oades, L.G., Crowe, T.P. & Nguyen, M. (2009). Leadership coaching transforming mental health systems from the inside out: The Collaborative Recovery Model as person-centred strengths based coaching psychology. *International Coaching Psychology Review*, 4(1), 25-36.

Park, N. and Peterson, C.M. (2003). *Virtues and organizations.* In Cameron, K.S., Dutton, J.E., and Quinn, R.E. (Eds.) Positive Organizational Scholarship: Foundations of a New Discipline. San Francisco: Berrett-Koehler.

Petersen, C. & Seligman, M.E.P. (2004). *Character strengths and virtues: A handbook and classification.* New York: Oxford University Press.

Piat, M., & Sabetti, J. (2009). The Development of a Recovery-Oriented Mental Health System in Canada: What the Experience of Commonwealth Countries Tells Us. Canadian Journal of Community Mental Health. 28 (2), 17-33.

Quinn, N., & Knifton, L. (2005). Promoting recovery and addressing stigma: Mental health awareness through community development in a low-income area. *International Journal of Mental Health Promotion, 7,* 37-44.

Rapp, C.A. (1998). *The Strengths Model: Case management with people suffering from severe and persistent mental illness.* New York: Oxford University Press.

Resnick, S.G. & Rosenheck, R.A. (2006). Recovery and positive psychology: Parallel themes and potential synergies. *Psychiatric Services, 57*(1), 120-122.

Ryan, R.M., Huta, V., & Deci, E.L. (2008). Living well: A self determination theory perspective on eudaimonia. *Journal of Happiness Studies, 9,* 139-170.

Salgado, D, Deane, F.P., Crowe, T.P. & Oades, L.G. (2010). Hope and Improvements in Mental Health Service Providers' Recovery Attitudes Following Training. *Journal of Mental Health, 19,* 243-248.

Seligman, M. E. P., & Csikszentmihalyi, M. (2000). Positive psychology: An introduction. *American Psychologist, 55,* 5-14.

Sheldon, K.M., Kasser, T., Simth, K., & Share, T. (2002). Personal goals and psychological growth: Testing an intervention to enhance goal attainment and personality integration. *Journal of Personality, 70*(1), 5-31.

Slade, M. (2009). *Personal recovery and mental illness. A guide for mental health professionals.* Cambridge: Cambridge University Press.

Slade, M. (2010). Mental illness and well-being: The central importance of positive psychology and recovery approaches. *BMC Health Services Research,* 10, 26, http://www.biomedcentral.com/1472-6963/10/26

Slade, M., Amering, M. & Oades, L.G. (2008). Recovery: an international perspective. *Epidemiologia e Psichiatria Sociale, 17*(2), 128-137.

Smith-Merry, J., Freeman, R., & Sturdy, S. (2011). Implementing recovery: an analysis of the key technologies in Scotland. *International Journal of Mental Health Systems* 2011, 5:11

Spaniol L, Wewiorski N, Gagne C, Anthony W.A. (2002). The process of recovery from schizophrenia. *International Review of Psychiatry,* 14:327–336.

Tooth BA, Kalyanansundaram V, Glover H. (1997). *Recovery from schizophrenia: A consumer perspective. Final Report to Health and Human Services Research and Development Grants Program* (RADGAC) Canberra: Department of Health and Aged Care.

Uppal, S., Oades, L.G., Crowe, T.P. & Deane. F.P. (2010). Barriers to transfer of collaborative recovery training into clinical practice. *Journal of Evaluation in Clinical Practice.16,* 451-455.

Young SL, Ensing DS. (1999). Exploring recovery from the perspective of people with psychiatric disabilities. *Psychiatric Rehabilitation Journal,* 22:219–231.

6

Primary Mental Healthcare and Integrated Services

Marie-Josée Fleury and Guy Grenier
McGill University, Douglas Hospital Research Centre, Quebec, Canada

1. Introduction

Mental disorder, which ranges in prevalence from 4.3 to 26.4% a year worldwide, is a critical healthcare issue (Demyttenaere et al., 2004). It is a leading cause of morbidity. Its cost and impact on productivity and on individual and family quality of life are substantial. It is associated with greater stigmatization of individuals, family burden, and a range of risk factors (for example, poverty, social isolation, criminal behavior, tobacco use, suicide attempts). Along with addiction, it is a major cause of work absenteeism and accounts for more lost work days in Canada than physical ailments (Kirby, 2006). Given the longstanding impact of mental disorder, the World Health Organization (WHO, 1978; 2001; 2008), emulated by countries such as Australia, New Zealand, the United Kingdom, and Canada (Smith, 2009), has advocated primary care reinforcement as a leading priority in mental healthcare. Primary care is defined as "the provision of first contact, person-focused, ongoing care over time that meets the health-related needs of individuals, referring only those too uncommon to maintain competence, and coordinated care when individuals receive services at other levels of care" (Starfield, 2008, p. 5). Usually, mental disorders that are considered to be managed in primary care are well-defined disorders, for which there are effective pharmacological and psychological treatments (Bower, 2002).

Robust primary care systems are deemed to achieve better organizational and patient outcomes (Starfield et al., 2005). Compared to specialized care, they are considered to be more accessible, less stigmatizing, and more comprehensive since they manage physical problems along with mental disorder (Rothman & Wagner, 2003). Studies report that most patients with chronic conditions prefer receiving services in primary care if the quality of services is perceived as good (Upshur & Weinreb, 2008). According to Heymans (2005), primary healthcare should handle 90% of health problems. As the main entry and service point for primary healthcare (Bambling et al., 2007), general practitioners constitute the cornerstone of the system. Every year, an estimated 75 to 80% of the general population consult a general practitioner (Nabalamba & Millar, 2007), with up to a third of these visits for a mental disorder (Rockman et al., 2004). General practitioners see more patients with mental disorders than psychiatrists do. In Canada, about 10% of the population seek mental healthcare yearly: 45% of these patients consult a general practitioners; and 25%, other healthcare practitioners (Lesage et al., 2006).

General practitioners' ability to detect, diagnose, and treat patients with mental disorder adequately, however, is often considered unsatisfactory (Walters et al., 2008; Upshur and

Weinreb, 2008). A comparison of research interview results reveals that 30 to 70% of mental disorders in general practitioners' patients go undetected (Walters et al., 2008). However, according to longitudinal studies, after three years, only 14% of patients with depression or anxiety remained unrecognized. The literature underscores the importance of early intervention in the onset of mental disorder for better prognosis (Reavley & Jorm, 2010). Unfortunately, the time to initial treatment contact following the onset of symptoms is generally quite long. It is estimated to range from 6 to 8 years for mood disorders and from 9 to 23 years for anxiety disorders (Wang et al., 2005a). However, compared to specialized care, it is pointed out that detection and diagnosis in primary care are more complex, concurrent disorders of physical and substance abuse being highly associated with mental disorder, and patients present with discrete illnesses and early symptoms that they themselves do not necessarily recognize (Walters et al., 2008). In addition, as general practitioner consultations last in general only few minutes, detection and diagnosis are more difficult to perform, compared to specialized care (Tyrer, 2009).

As regards treatment when mental disorder is diagnosed, Wang and colleagues (2007), comparing 10 high-income countries involved in the WHO Mental Health Survey Initiative, have provided estimates of minimum adequacy standards ranging from 18 to 42% among patients receiving treatment for anxiety, mood, and substance disorders. For depression, Mykletun and colleagues (2010) evaluated that less than 30% of patients receive proper treatment. In the province of Quebec in Canada, a recent study estimated that 54% of patients diagnosed with major depression and covered by the public drug insurance plan stop taking their medication before six months, in spite of best-treatment guidelines (*Conseil du médicament*, 2011) that recommend taking them at least for eight months. Moreover, only 31% of these patients consult their general practitioners at least eight times, wherever guidelines prescribed a minimum of ten visits (*Conseil du médicament*, 2011). In a similar study in the Netherlands (Seekles et al., 2009), about 30% of patients stopped using antidepressant medication within the first month of treatment, while 40% reached the recommended therapeutic dosage of the antidepressant drug.

In addition, a number of studies have revealed instances of fragmentation and duplication of services or major gaps in the range of mental healthcare systems, resulting in inefficient provision of care, and in preventable emergency-room visits or hospitalizations (Bachrach, 1996; Provan & Milward, 1995). The lack of integration between primary and specialized care, and of interdisciplinary collaboration has also received repeated mention in the literature (Fleury, 2006). Globally, the primary healthcare system has "often been viewed as poor care for poor people" (Desjardins, 2011, p. 10). Therefore, to help general practitioners manage patients with mental disorders more effectively, great efforts have been made, particularly in the past decade, to develop models of integrated care and best practices in the field of primary mental healthcare services.

On the basis of an international literature review of primary mental healthcare and two research projects focusing on general practitioner management of patients with mental disorder in Quebec, this chapter examines patient profiles in primary mental healthcare, determinants of service utilization of these patients, and primary mental healthcare reforms with a spotlight on best practices. The research projects are designed to describe the clinical and collaborative role of general practitioners in mental healthcare, uncover enabling and hindering factors associated with the management of patients with mental disorder, and cast light on general practitioners' strategies and recommendations to improve patient management. The Quebec/Canada public mental healthcare system offers an interesting setting for exploration of these topics. It has undergone significant transformation over the years in efforts to reinforce primary mental healthcare and integrated care; however, the quality of Canada's primary healthcare system and ease of accessibility rank poorly compared to international best practices (Katz et al., 2009). As a result, improvement is needed. As increasing attention worldwide is devoted to the development of optimal integrated models of primary care, this chapter makes a contribution to the discussion surrounding service planning in the field of mental healthcare. It also considers the most effective components and strategies for enhancing care collaboration and integration. While it focuses on research in a specific context (Quebec/Canada), this chapter is of wide-ranging interest and relevance since primary mental healthcare in most industrialized countries (including the United Kingdom, Australia, Ireland, and the United States) share similar reform objectives and organizational and practice features (Gask et al., 2008).

2. Methods

2.1 Study population and data collection

This chapter is based on a major literature review on primary mental healthcare, including both epidemiological and organizational research initiatives. General practitioner data from Quebec presented in this chapter were sourced from two studies. The first study (conducted using a cross-sectional design) targeted all general practitioners from nine Quebec local healthcare networks in five administrative healthcare regions (Quebec features 18 regions and 95 local networks), corresponding to 20% of the general practitioner population in the province. Quebec is the second most populated province in Canada, with about 7.9 million inhabitants (23% of the Canadian population). The province is home to 7,199 equivalent full-time general practitioners (1 GP per 1,041 inhabitants) (Savard & Rodrigue, 2007). In Quebec, local healthcare networks constitute the core of the healthcare system, where providers combine primary and specialized care services to ensure a comprehensive care spectrum (Fleury, 2006). The local healthcare networks selected for this study represent urban, semi-urban, and rural areas; some of these networks include university-affiliated psychiatric facilities. They encompass diversified work settings for general practitioners: solo private clinics; group private clinics; walk-in clinics; community care centers; family medicine groups; network clinics; and hospital centers (acute, psychiatric, or long-term). Family medicine groups correspond to a primary care setting where patients are registered with general practitioners (n= 8 to 10 equivalent full time), and where nurses work closely with general practitioners; nurses are responsible for patient screening, follow-up, and referral. Network clinics (n= 10 or more general practitioners equivalent full time) are similar, but patients are not registered with general practitioners and nurses act mainly as liaison agents, coordinating services between organizations. In community care centers, interdisciplinary teams are onsite.

To select the study sample, a list of all general practitioners in the nine local healthcare networks was provided by the Quebec Federation of General Practitioners (FMOQ), which represents all Quebec general practitioners. Every general practitioner in these local healthcare networks (n=1,415) was asked to participate in the study. The survey was mailed from September 2005 to February 2007. The Quebec public register for all general practitioner medical acts (*Régie de l'assurance maladie du Québec* (RAMQ) database, 2006) was also analyzed to compare the study's sample with the general practitioner population of Quebec as a whole wherever possible for the purpose of data validation (for example, gender, age, types of territories, diagnoses). More information on the instruments and study methods employed are provided in other publications (Fleury et al., 2008; 2009; Ouadahi et al., 2009).

The second study arose from the first. Out of the general practitioners who participated in the initial research initiative, 60 physicians (12 per region) where selected for qualitative investigation in efforts to enhance understanding of mental disorder management. Recruitment took place from April 2009 to March 2010. A 27-item questionnaire and interview guide were used. Both instruments were tested on three general practitioners not included in the final sample. The questionnaire, a shorter version of the survey used in the previous research project, covered four dimensions: (1) general practitioners' socio-demographic profile and practice location; (2) continuing medical education; (3) clinical practice features and profile of patients with mental disorder; and (4) comfort level in managing patients with mental disorder. It included categorical or continuous items, with some 5 or 10-point Likert Scale questions. It was self-administered and required 10 minutes to complete. Development of the interview guide was based on a literature review of primary care and the previous research project. The guide included three sections, relating to general practitioners': (1) clinical practice; (2) relationships with mental healthcare networks, evaluation of availability of mental healthcare resources in their territory, and views on healthcare reform; and (3) needs for support and collaboration and ideal practice models for treating mental disorder. Seventy-minute interviews were conducted (25% face-to-face and 75% by phone), recorded, and transcribed (with respondents' anonymity respected throughout). All participants from both studies signed a consent form approved by the research ethics board at the Douglas University Institute of Mental Health.

2.2 Data analysis

Quantitative and qualitative analyses were carried out. Quantitative investigation involved descriptive and inferential statistics, computed with SPSS Statistics 17.0. Analyses are well described in other publications (Fleury et al., 2008; 2009; 2010a). As for qualitative data (the second study), transcripts were read by the research team and subsequently coded using NVivo 8. The codes were derived from the primary-care literature on themes in the interview guide. Transcript analysis generated new codes. The researchers ensured coding accuracy and refined the interpretation of results. Data analysis also involved the reduction and synthesis of information. Reports integrating quantitative and qualitative data were produced to summarize pertinent results, which were read and discussed by all researchers. In addition, a second-step analysis was performed using data associated with general practitioners' main practice settings (where general practitioners spent most of their work hours), for example, solo private clinics, community care centers, and so on. Data-grouping permitted comparison of general practitioner collaborative practices with respect to their main settings. Wherever pertinent, data analysis also compared general practitioners' collaboration strategy for patients diagnosed with common mental disorder (for example, anxiety, depression) and patients with serious disorders (schizophrenia, bipolar disorder) with or without concomitant disorders (for example, physical problems, substance abuse).

3. Contextual background

3.1 Profiles of patients with mental disorders

The concept of mental health is usually considered in terms of an ecological model that includes, beyond the illness, individuals' adjustment within their communities, the state of their well-being, and their self-fulfillment (empowerment). This conception leads to interventions that are not only medical but also psycho-social (for example, psychotherapy, psycho-education and rehabilitation). Mental disorder, for its part, is defined as "clinically significant conditions characterized by alterations in thinking, mood (emotions) or behavior associated with personal distress and/or impaired functioning" (WHO, 2001, p. 21). Mental disorder is generally classified as "common or moderate" or "severe." Generally, common mental disorders are viewed as the main focus of primary mental healthcare (Bower & Gilbody, 2005).

The major common mental disorders are mood disorders and anxiety disorders. One of the most widespread mood disorders is major depression. Alcohol use is also quite common. According to the Canadian Community Health Survey (CCHS), the incidence of major depression for a given year is 4.5%, and for mood disorders as a whole 4.9% (Statistics Canada, 2002). International surveys suggest, however, that the incidence of mood disorders, for a given year, is estimated at 9.5% in the United States (Kessler et al., 2005), 8.5% in France, 6.9% in Netherlands, and only 3.6% in Germany, for instance (Demyttenaere et al., 2004). According to the CCHS, the incidence of anxiety disorders in a given year was 1.6% for panic disorders, 0.7% for agoraphobia, and 3.0% for social anxiety disorders, and 4.7% as a whole (Statistics Canada, 2002). International surveys suggest that the overall incidence of anxiety disorders is 18.1% yearly in the United States (Kessler et al., 2005), 12% in France, 8.8% in Netherlands, and 6.2% in Germany (Demyttenaere et al, 2004). In the Epidemiological Catchment Area Study (Regier et al., 1990), the lifetime incidence for alcohol and drug abuse in the population was evaluated at 17%. The CCHS reported that an estimated 4.6 to 1.9% of the Quebec population experience mild to serious alcohol consumption problems yearly (Statistics Canada, 2002).

The most prevalent serious mental disorders are schizophrenia, bipolar disorder, and delirious disorder. Patients with serious mental disorder usually differ substantially from patients with common mental disorder. Serious mental disorder patients (2 to 3% of the population) are generally unemployed and need considerable help in many biopsychosocial domains on a long-term basis (Nelson, 2006). Patients with common mental disorders are generally employed (or on sick leave when ill); their problems are often less disabling though they may be recurrent, relapse or become chronic. In a systematic needs-assessment literature review (Joska & Flisher, 2005), patients with mental disorder are reported to experience between 3.3 and 8.6 needs, depending on their mental disorder profile; patients with less severe diagnostics usually have fewer needs than patients with mild or moderate mental disorder. Psychotic symptoms, company, daytime activities and psychological distress are usually the domains with the highest incidence of needs (Hansson et al., 2001). Unmet needs are more predominant in needs domains related to interpersonal relations like company, intimate relationships, and sexual expression (Middelboe et al., 2001).

The incidence of mental disorder is higher among adults (aged 18 to 64). However, the first manifestations of mental disorder often occur in adolescence and early adulthood. According to the Canadian Community Health Survey (CCHS), 47.9% of adults from 45 to 64 years, and 34.1% of seniors have indicated that their mental disorder appeared before the age of 25 (Government of Canada, 2006). On average, common mental disorder is more widespread among women than men. Depression and anxiety in particular are more prevalent among women. However, addictions and antisocial personality disorders are more common among men. Serious mental disorders, like schizophrenia, are as frequent in men as in women, but men usually develop this mental disorder earlier than women

(Mueser & McGurk, 2004). Moreover, a significant proportion of the population is affected by more than one mental disorder (particularly concurrent anxiety and depressive disorders). In a study by Kessler and colleagues (2005), out of an overall incidence of 26.2% for mental disorder in a given year, 14.4% of the sample had a single mental disorder, 5.8% had two types of mental disorder, and 6.0% had at least three types of mental disorder. The recurring nature of mental disorder makes managing these problems more complex. Lloyd and colleagues (1996) followed a cohort of patients with mental disorder treated in general practice: they noted that after 11 years 54% still had specific problems and 37% had had other episodes of illnesses likely associated with chronic mental disorder. It has also been reported that more than 75% of patients with depression relapse or experience recurrence (Howell et al. 2008); this finding substantiates the relevance of close monitoring and long-term approaches to care.

The magnitude of co-morbid conditions associated with mental disorders (more frequent with increasing age) is very high. The combination of concurrent problems can result in a more negative prognosis and make it less likely that a person will stick to a particular medical regimen. For example, according to the Canadian Community Health Survey (CCHS), 66% of Canadians suffering from depression in the past 12 months also present at least one chronic condition (Schmitz et al., 2007). The most common physical concurrent problems related with mental disorder are cardiovascular, gastrointestinal, and lung diseases, diabetes, and neurological disorders (for example, Parkinson's disease or epilepsy) (Jones et al., 2004). Concurrent substance abuse problems were also found in about 15 to 50% of individuals with serious mental disorder, especially bipolar disorder (Skinner et al., 2004). Nearly 60% of homeless individuals (Weinreb et al., 2005) and from 15 to 35% of individuals with intellectual disabilities may also suffer from mental disorder (*Ministère de la Santé et des Services sociaux du Québec*, 2006). In addition, suicide is from 10 to 20% more prevalent in individuals who have schizophrenia or who have had depression or an anxiety disorder (Statistics Canada, 2002).

It is worth noting that the incidence of mental disorder may vary significantly from one study to another, depending on the country where the survey was conducted, types of mental disorder included in the survey (for instance, most serious disorders and personality disorders are not included), measurement instruments employed (survey, database or administrative records), and types of population studied (general population or clinical sample). DSM-IV and ICD-10 are the most widely used diagnostic systems. As regards anxiety disorders, Kessler and colleagues (2010, p. 31) have suggested that "the current DSM and ICD definitions might substantially under-estimate the proportion of the population with a clinically-significant anxiety condition." Finally, although diagnosis is an important factor for service planning, a more comprehensive view of individuals is necessary to establish appropriate service offerings (for example, social support, socioeconomic profile, and history of illness).

3.2 Determinants of service utilization of patient with mental disorders

In general, mental health service utilization is most closely associated with needs-related factors, such as having the following diagnoses: schizophrenia (Leaf et al., 1985); major depression (Leaf et al., 1985); anxiety disorders (Leaf et al., 1985); antisocial behavior (Leaf et al., 1985); and maternal history of mental disorder (Mojtabai et al., 2002). Previous studies have reported that severe mental disorder cases were associated with more intensive service utilization than mildly severe or moderate cases (Tempier et al., 2009; Wang et al., 2007).

Number of diagnoses or needs and concurrent disorders are positively associated with higher service utilization. Individuals with concurrent mental disorder and substance abuse usually reported the highest utilization rates, and the least favorable self-perception/assessment of good health (Rush et al., 20010). Substance abuse alone is related to very low service utilization (Tempier et al., 2009). Attitudes and beliefs regarding mental disorder and treatment also play a role in service utilization. High rates of health service use have been found among individuals who consider their mental health to be poor (Leaf et al., 1985). Generally, the more serious the mental disorder diagnosis and its symptoms are and the greater the number of serious needs and co-morbid health conditions, the greater is the use of services and the poorer the prognosis.

Socio-demographic factors are also closely related to service utilization. Age, gender, marital status, education, country of birth, and race/ethnicity are important determinants of service utilization among individuals with mental disorder. Several studies have found that younger (18 to 24) and older (65 and up) individuals are less likely to use services than participants aged 25 to 64 (Wang et al., 2005a; Kessler et al., 2001). Females are the most frequent users of health services, principally of general practitioners; men are more likely to seek specialized services (Vasiliadis et al., 2007; Carr et al., 2003; Narrow et al., 2000). Generally, studies have found that persons who were previously or currently married used services more often than bachelors (Vasiliadis et al., 2007; Wang et al., 2005b; Bebbington et al., 2000; Parslow & Jorm, 2000). Individuals with more education (Vasiliadis et al., 2007; Leaf et al., 1985) also use health services significantly more often than less well-educated persons, despite the higher incidence of mental disorder among the latter (Olfson et al., 2002). Individuals with more elevated socio-economic status tend to use specialized services more assiduously, particularly psychiatric and psychological care, even among individuals with comparable insurance coverage (Wang et al., 2000; Hendryx & Ahern, 2001; Alegria et al., 2000). With regard to country of birth, race, and ethnicity, studies found that Caucasians are more likely to use health services than Blacks or immigrants (Vasiliadis et al., 2007; Hatzenbuehler et al., 2008; Keyes et al., 2008).

Professional and social support (including family and friends) also plays a role (Lemming & Calsyn, 2004; Bonin et al., 2007). Social support can be positively or negatively associated with service utilization for mental healthcare reasons (Carr et al., 2003; Pescosolido et al., 1998; Albert et al., 1998). Some social networks help individuals to recognize their problems and seek aid from health providers; other networks tend not to encourage members to seek help, thereby constituting a barrier to accessibility (Howard et al., 1996). Perceived barriers to accessibility to care are negatively associated with service utilization (Leaf et al., 1985). Access to a regular source of medical care (or continuity of care) is positively associated with service utilization (Leaf et al., 1985). Compared to users of primary care only, individuals who sought both primary and specialized care for a mental disorder presented more mental disorders and lower quality of life. Individuals using only specialized healthcare received significantly less social support than persons using primary care exclusively and lived in neighborhoods with a high proportion of rental housing (Fleury et al., 2011). Generally, a positive response to pharmacotherapy, compliance with drug treatment, low number of acute-care hospitalizations, and satisfactory outpatient services play a central role in the patient recovery process (Casper & Donaldson, 1990; Breier et al., 1991; Korkeila et al., 1998). Lastly, failure to seek treatment or abandoning treatment is often explained by the belief that a mental health disorder will resolve on its own and by the fear of being stigmatized (Fournier et al., 2007). Denial of illness is also very frequent among heavy users of mental healthcare services, which impedes their recovery (Kent et al., 1995; Kent & Yellowlees, 1995).

3.3 Mental health primary care reforms and best practices

In Canada (including Quebec), as in other industrialized countries, major reforms are underway to reinforce primary care and collaboration among providers. Led by the Government of Canada with the *Health Transition Funds*, major grants were distributed between 2000 and 2006 to support primary healthcare transformation at the provincial level (Bergman, 2007) as health and social services are a provincial jurisdiction in Canada. In 1997, the College of Family Physicians of Canada and the Canadian Psychiatric Association produced a joint position paper on shared mental healthcare in Canada (Kates et al., 1997). These initiatives encouraged reform within the primary mental healthcare system. In Canada, as in other countries such as the United Kingdom and Australia, strengthening primary mental healthcare and integration between providers are key issues (Bosco, 2005).

Mental primary healthcare reforms are designed to improve access, continuity and quality of care, and the management of mental disorder. Reforms target general practitioners' modes of practice and payment. General practitioners are increasingly encouraged to work in group practice and multidisciplinary settings. In Canada, 60% of general practitioners work in private physician-run clinics, and a minority (8.3%) in public governance models such as community care centers (College of Family Physicians of Canada, 2004); 23% work in solo practice, 51% in group practices, and 24% in multidisciplinary team practices (College of Family Physicians of Canada, 2008). In 2007, about 39% of Canadians 18 and over said they had access to an interdisciplinary team of primary care providers (Khan et al., 2008). A large number of general practitioners in Canada and the U.S. are deserting primary care; in addition, recruitment in family medicine school is more difficult than in other countries. About 40% of general practitioners work partly in hospitals, and the same proportion in walk-in clinics (College of Family Physicians of Canada, 2004). In Quebec, this situation has produced a considerable impact. Close to 25% of the population in the province lack a family physician; accordingly, patient volume at walk-in clinics is high. One study (Haggerty et al., 2004) estimated that walk-in clinics were a regular source of care for 60% of patients in some regions of Quebec. However, there is worldwide upswing in the number of general practitioners working in group and multidisciplinary settings or public governance models (McAvoy & Coster, 2005; Bourgueil et al., 2007).

In current primary care reforms, patient rostering is also promoted. Financial incentives are geared toward patient rostering, but also toward targeted disease detection rates and patient outcomes (as in the United Kingdom) or the management of patient with complex or severe illnesses who are rostered (as in Quebec and Ontario). In opposition to fees for services, other payment structures such as salary, hourly fees or mixed compensation modes are also actively encouraged, especially for the management of complex or chronic care patients (the United Kingdom, Spain, and Italy have developed these models). In Canada (similarly to the United States, France and Germany), general practitioners are paid mainly through fees for services (about 73%), but also partly through salary in community care centers or an hourly fee in hospitals. Over the years, in Canada the number of general practitioners working outside fees for services has increased; this also seems to be a trend at the international level (Simonet, 2009).

Well-designed reform of primary mental healthcare embraces the full continuum of care, focusing on comprehensive patient needs and better integration between providers. Access to increasingly systematic and proactive psychosocial follow-up services, psychotherapy (especially cognitive behavioral therapy), and patient self-management are central developments within current reforms. Incentives promoting implementation of best practices and innovations are also in place. Specifically, in order to help general practitioners manage patients with mental disorder more effectively, efforts are being made to develop approaches, instruments or guidelines, and collaborative care models with demonstrated efficacy. Models of optimally effective mental healthcare encompass a broad range of management and clinical tools, including: stepped care, shared care, case management, patient self-management, psychometric diagnostic tools for increasing screening, clinical protocols or evidence-based treatment guidelines, continuous education, and computerized management systems (Craven & Bland, 2006). They are part of coherent integrated organizational models such as the chronic care model, integrated service networks or patient-centered medical home approaches. These care models acknowledge the considerable interdependence among providers. Optimally effective integrated care models are also supported by major government mental healthcare policy initiatives (Smith, 2009).

Overall, compared with services as usual, coherent and integrated care models encompassing multimodal strategies have demonstrated better clinical outcomes, more efficient use of resources, and enhanced patient experience of seeking and receiving care, especially in the case of patients with chronic or complex problems such as major depression (Kates et al., 2011; Katon et al., 2007; Williams et al., 2007; Smith 2009). The availability of evidence varies according to the models or strategies studied (for example, shared care, clinical protocols) and types of clientele (severe depression being the illness mainly studied in primary mental healthcare). Generally, the quantity and quality of evidence is limited in most models and strategies. It is unclear which patient profiles as targeted by reform would lead to the best income; therefore, more research is required (Walters et al., 2008). In addition, even if major progress has been realized in the past decade, most of the models or multimodal strategies cited above are in the early stage of implementation, as is the case in Canada and Quebec (Kates et al., 2011; Pawlenko, 2005). According to Walters and colleagues (2008), the challenge ahead is to define which component of complex multimodal interventions are important and for which patient profiles and determine how well they can be incorporated into different primary care integrated models.

Integrated care models or multimodal strategies are not incompatible with one another and can easily be combined. They illustrate approaches and strategies designed to: (1) improve general practitioners' ability to manage mental disorder, including patient self-management support; (2) reinforce support and coordination between general practitioners and specialized care professionals; (3) extend biopsychosocial services through greater collaboration with psychosocial teams and more services supplied in the community (on an outpatient basis); (4) transfer patients to specialized care during crisis periods with subsequent follow-up by a general practitioner and other psychosocial practitioners in the community as needed; or (5) organize overall care network more efficiently for improved healthcare provision, efficiency, and outcomes.

One of the best-known models, extensively studied and increasingly implemented for several illnesses (for example, hypertension, congestive heart failure, diabetes, and depression) is the chronic care model (Wagner et al., 2001). With its focus on improving general practitioners' clinical practice and team collaboration, the chronic care model also encompasses holistic care. It revolves around: (1) organization of services and delivery; (2)

patient self-management support; (3) clinical decision support; (4) clinical information systems development; (5) use of community resources; and (6) community-inclusive healthcare organization (Bodenheimer et al., 2002). Contrary to the chronic care model, integrated service networks (also known as organized delivery systems, integrated delivery systems, and disease management) focuses on the organization of the full network of care spectrum for patients needs, including coordination of the functional or administrative, clinical and medical components of the care process (Fleury, 2006). Integrated service networks are defined as a set of autonomous organizations that distribute a continuum of coordinated services to a defined population (Shortell et al., 1994). These organizations are held financially and clinically accountable for achieving efficient results and improving the health and well-being of the population they serve. Integrated service networks are based on an acknowledgment of considerable interdependence among players and organizations, usually developed in local settings (for the purposes of feasibility). As for the patient-centered medical home approach, it is designed to provide comprehensive primary care services for patients. It was first applied to children with special healthcare needs, but has since been extended to adults as well. It focuses on the general practitioner-patient relationship (including, when appropriate, the patient's family), patient rostering, continuity, and access to care (Cruickshank, 2010). This approach emphasizes the right of patients to be managed by a general practitioner who acts as a coordinator of a multidisciplinary team of healthcare professionals (a challenge in settings where there is a shortage of general practitioners). Leading physician groups in the United States and Canada have endorsed this model as a means of improving primary healthcare (College of Family Physicians of Canada, 2009). Compared with integrated service networks (which focus on the macro level) and the chronic care model (meso level), the patient-centered medical home approach targets the micro level of care.

Stepped care implies a progression from light to intensive treatment or to low-cost community-based treatment before high-cost institutional or specialized services according to patient need profiles (Seekles et al., 2009). The selection of treatment steps depends on patient profiles (for example, the severity of patients' illness, their socio-demographic characteristics, and social support). Stepped care simplifies the patients' care pathways, promotes their active engagement toward recovery and prevention of relapse, and uses limited resources to the greatest effect for a population-wide level of care. Treatments are monitored systematically; if they do not lead to adequate results, stepping-up is recommended. Stepped care is particularly relevant for minor disorders, without adverse consequences, and when a set of treatment alternatives coexist. In such cases, it initially relies on less expensive interventions such as self-help approaches, bibliotherapy, computerized treatments, including lifestyle changes, problem-solving, psycho-education, and motivational interviewing. When combined with previous interventions, minimal telephone follow-up for assistance in attainment of or adherence to medication is usually perceived to be more effective. If needed (as ulterior steps), brief individual or group therapy may be required, usually based on cognitive behavioral therapy (Walters et al., 2008) or more extensive and specialized care. For instance, the best-practice treatment recommendation for depression in use at the National Institute for Health and Clinical Excellence (NICE, United Kingdom) includes five treatment steps (Tylee, 2006). In Step 1, patients with mild depression are fully managed by general practitioners (early detection is also greatly encouraged). In Step 5, patients with severe depression presenting risk of dangerousness or suicide are managed by a specialized psychiatric care team.

Shared care involves coordination among general practitioners, psychiatrists, mental healthcare resources, and the voluntary sector (for example, food bank, self-support groups). In its early implementation stage, it focused primarily on general practitioners and psychiatrist collaborations. Now, it has been extended to psychosocial mental healthcare professionals (including the voluntary sector) and is referred to increasingly as "collaborative care" (Kisely & Campbell, 2007; Kates et al., 2011). Several taxonomies of shared-care models coexist. The most commonly cited are the shifted outpatient, community consultation-liaison, and attachment models (Craven & Bland, 2006). The shifted outpatient scheme, which has been broadly implemented, involves general practitioners remaining in their practices and referring patients to psychiatric teams in outpatient clinics. The two other models have been less extensively deployed. In community consultation-liaison, psychiatric consultations are provided to general practitioners to help them manage difficult patients or advise them on best practices. The attachment scheme is built on the previous model and involves part-time psychiatrists and psychosocial mental health professionals assigned to general practitioners' clinics. In Bower and Gilbody (2005), another interesting model of "quality improvement in primary care mental health" is presented with two components related to shared care: consultation-liaison and collaborative care. The former includes strategies designed to improve general practitioners' training in mental healthcare and referral to specialized care when needed (minority of cases); here, training is provided by mental healthcare specialists. The latter is built on the previous component and features the addition of case managers who liaise with general practitioners and mental healthcare specialists. Overall, the different models of shared care developed to date vary with regard to the intensity of assistance provided to general practitioners by psychiatrists and other psychosocial mental healthcare professionals. Best models depend on the context (for example, practice settings, network organization of care) and patient profiles. Shared-care component models can include the following: (1) informal care support for general practitioners by psychiatrists; (2) "specialized mental health general practitioners" – i.e., general practitioners are both trained in physical medicine and psychiatry; (3) formal and more rapid referral process and efficient telephone support from psychiatrists; and (4) onsite mental healthcare specialists into the general practitioners' surgeries, which imply general practitioners' consultations with mental healthcare specialists (psychiatrists or other psychosocial professionals such as case managers), patients' consultations with psychiatrists or both general practitioners and psychiatrists, and linking patients with case managers, including follow-up with a general practitioner (Morden et al., 2009).

As the mental healthcare literature reveals, a key feature of shared-care models is the increasingly important role played by case managers, a source of systematic and proactive psychosocial follow-up, which involves screening, patient psycho-education, subsequent treatment (including drug adherence), and patient self-management techniques. Assigning case managers to patients with mental disorder has been advocated as a means of reducing hospital admissions, promoting community-based care, and enhancing patient quality of life (Fitzpatrick et al., 2004). According to Fleury and colleagues (2010b), the presence of a case manager was the most significant variable associated with the use of primary care services by individuals with serious mental disorder (mainly schizophrenia). Case managers (offering personalized follow-up arrangements) are increasingly called on to play a major role in connecting patients with services in appropriate and cost-effective ways to fulfill patient needs at, increasingly, the offices of general practitioners.

Another development in current mental healthcare reforms is the reinforcement of access to psychotherapy as an alternative to drug treatment or a form of complementary care designed to meet the comprehensive needs of patients. Some patients have strong resistance to psychopharmacological treatment (for example, fear for stigmatization, side effects or dependency), particularly when drugs are taken for a long period (Howell et al., 2008). The use of psychotherapy compared to medication is also found to be more effective in the long term; however, the latter results in more rapid patient recovery (Howell et al., 2008). When compared to practices in several developed countries such as Australia, the United Kingdom, the Netherlands, and other nations in Europe (Hakkaart-van Roijen et al., 2006), non-pharmacological treatment in primary care Canada for common mental disorder is more limited (Myrrh & Payne, 2006). In 2001, approximately 80% of consultations with psychologists were within the private system, with a proportion of costs covered by private insurance or out-of pocket spending (Moulding et al., 2009). In Quebec, however, psychosocial services have been considerably reinforced in community care centers for the management of common mental disorder. The reform launched in 2005 was designed to develop a mental healthcare team of 20 full-time psychosocial professionals along with two general practitioners assigned to each team for a total population of 80,000 adult patients. Over the past decade, major initiatives have been undertaken in Australia (*Outcomes in Mental Health Care Program*, 2001; *Better Access*, 2006, as cited in Howell et al., 2008) and the United Kingdom (*Improving Access for Psychological Therapies* program, 2007, as cited in Clark et al., 2009) to provide people who suffer from mental disorder with more streamlined access to psychotherapy as an alternative or complement to pharmacological treatment. In the United Kingdom, close to 10,000 new therapists have been assigned to operate the mental healthcare system, under the close supervision of psychologists and psychiatrists (Mykletun et al., 2010). As part of these initiatives, improving mental healthcare training (for general practitioners and psychosocial professionals especially in the area of cognitive behavioral therapy) and collaboration between practitioners were key reform features. Recent studies show that enhanced access to psychosocial care in the treatment of mental disorder and closer cooperation among general practitioners and psychologists resulted in improved patient care, positive patient outcomes, and greater satisfaction among general practitioners, without increasing healthcare costs (Clark et al., 2009; Layard et al., 2007; Chomienne et al., 2010).

In all aforementioned models or strategies of current primary mental healthcare reform, patient self-management is a key orientation. It is a core component of the chronic-care model, the patient-centered medical home approach, stepped care, and psychosocial intervention. In the Canadian province of British Columbia, for example, 700 general practitioners were recently trained to apply this approach in their practice (Bilsker, 2010). Patient self-management includes self-help materials, bibliotherapy, and interactive web programs based on psychological treatment. It aims to provide information on diseases and treatment options, but also on practices designed to foster lifestyle changes, effective problem-solving, and improvement-oriented motivational behavior. It enhances participation in care process and patient empowerment. Increasingly, research underscores the importance of patient choice and engagement in improving treatment outcomes (Kisely & Campbell, 2007). Patient self-management is also perceived to be cost-effective; it can be easily implemented at a population-wide level, targeting mild and early cases of mental disorder. It is proving increasingly effective; however, more research is needed. It can be promoted as a first step in the care of patients with mild mental disorder or encouraged as a treatment strategy in a comprehensive care package for more complex cases.

At last, other strategies worth mentioning for reforming the primary mental healthcare system are evidence-based treatment guidelines or screening tools, continuous education, and computerized management systems. Since the 1990s, there has been an increase in the number of clinical guidelines. While many efforts have been made to standardize and promote best clinical practices, studies generally reveal the difficulty of implementing them in actual practice settings, the low rates of treatment adherence, and the slight (if any) improvement in patient outcomes produced by both guidelines and screening tools (Collins et al, 2006; Walters et al., 2008; Seekles et al., 2009). Inadequate implementation is partly explained by the fact that such intervention does not always closely correspond to the problems faced by general practitioners (van Rijswijk et al., 2009). Walter and colleagues (2008) have suggested reserving screening tools to high-risk groups (for example, patients with chronic physical illness, unemployed or experiencing bereavement). Since the production of guidelines has resulted in a great of duplication of efforts, a new trend has developed, namely, to adapt gold standard quality tools (such as the ones designed by the National Institute for Health and Clinical Excellence (NICE) in the United Kingdom) to the local context to organize services (Fervers et al., 2006). Research also reveals that continuous education or training does not always lead to outstanding results; in fact, training is often reported as being ineffective (Mykletun et al., 2010). In their review of training practices, Bower and Gilbody (2005, p. 841) reported the following paradox: "Training that is feasible within current educational structures (such as guidelines and short training courses) is not effective, whereas more intensive training is effective but may not be feasible." Cross-training is an example of effective learning. It involves the presence of various professionals working in the same field (for example, mental healthcare) in a local territory. It consists as a leaning strategy which integrates a set of interrelated techniques (for example, clarification, observation, and personal rotation) patterning to a specific topic, enabling the emergence of inter-positional knowledge of partners and community of practice (Perreault et al., 2009). Overall, clinical standardized screening or guidelines and training are effective when used as part of a comprehensive care package and management program that is continually updated.

Computerized management systems, especially electronic medical records, are also central to healthcare system reform, but have been found to be effective only if they include a broad range of features and are integrated within a coherent knowledge-management structure. Features may include: access to test results; drugs registration; patient history and clinical profile; and formal referral procedure. List of patients may also be produced for more effective management (for example, by illness, prescribed medication, specific risk profiles), for preventive measure or screening, or for follow-up or subsequent treatment. Guidelines designed to foster knowledge transfer or support clinical decision-making may also be integrated (Dorr et al., 2007; *Commissaire à la Santé et au Bien-être*, 2010). Computerized management systems have been reported to improve access to test results, referrals, and claims processing; improve staff time-management leading to greater productivity; reduce the number of return visits to emergency rooms; decrease the incidence of misdirected referrals and, consequently, the number of follow-up visits with specialists (Fontaine et al., 2010). In comparison to countries such as the United Kingdom, New Zealand, and Australia, the implementation of such electronic systems in Canada and the United Stated has been very slow. In both countries, about 20% of physicians have reported using such electronic systems (comprising only some of the features mentioned above) (*Commissaire à la Santé et au Bien-être*, 2010; Fontaine et al., 2010). Few patients are also able to communicate by e-mail directly with their general practitioners (The Commonwealth Fund, 2008 as cited in *Commissaire à la Santé et au Bien-être*, 2009). There are numerous challenges associated with the deployment of electronic systems, which account for the lagging development, including (to mention only few hindering factors): their complexity combined with a quickly evolving environment in which knowledge is constantly being produced; the fact that the healthcare system is segmented; substantial funding requests and changes to practices; and the potential of disclosing personal and confidential information unwittingly. Finally, while the challenge of implementing electronic medical records is significant, all the strategies and models described above do not stand alone, they must be integrated in a coherent primary care package and organized service structure, which are undergoing sweeping changes in hopes of improving both systems and patient outcomes (Upshur & Weinreb, 2008).

4. Results of the two research projects on Quebec general practitioners

4.1 Socio-demographic profile of general practitioners participating in the two studies
Of the 1,415 targeted general practitioners, 353 were excluded since they had retired or moved to another area or could not be reached either by phone or e-mail. Subsequently, 37 questionnaires were excluded as they were not duly completed. The final sample comprised 398 subjects for a response rate of 41%. The sample was compared to non-responding general practitioners for gender distribution, which yielded a non-significant result ($\chi 2=3.44$; df=1; P=0.0637). Comparisons were also made between the study sample and Quebec's general practitioner population as a whole, regarding gender, age, clinical practice settings, territory of practice, income level from fees for services, and volume of patients with mental disorder. No significant difference was found in any of these comparisons. When data were available, comparisons were made between the general practitioner population in Quebec and Canada. Significant differences were found between the study sample (n=398) and Canadian general practitioners only regarding gender (51.3% female in the sample vs 36.7% for Canadian general practitioners; Chi-square: 3.98; P value: 0.046) and income from fees for services (65% vs 51%, Chi-square: 4.02; P value: 0.045) (Pong, 2005; College of Family Physicians of Canada, 2007). In addition, the two samples, namely, 398 general practitioners in the initial study (quantitative investigation) and 60 general practitioners in the subsequent study (qualitative investigation), were compared for key parameters: age, sex, and fee-for-service income. No significant differences were found. However, the sample that included 60 general practitioners earned a great deal less income from service fees than Quebec's general practitioner population as a whole.

4.2 General practitioner management of patients with mental disorders (clinical and collaborative practices)
According to the Quebec public register for all general practitioner medical acts (known as the RAMQ database), 15% of the Quebec population aged over 18 consulted a general practitioner for a mental disorder. The survey of 398 general practitioners (20% of Quebec's general practitioner population) also revealed the high incidence of mental disorder-related consultations in general practitioners' surgeries. About one quarter of all medical visits were associated with mental healthcare – either reported as a medical act or diagnosis in both the RAMQ database and the survey. Most visits related to a mental disorder were associated specifically with depression or anxiety. Individuals with mental disorder were found to consult general practitioners twice as often (12 visits annually) as individuals without

mental disorder (6 visits annually). In the survey, the continuity of care provided by general practitioners was investigated (number of visits per year to a "family physician" for treatment of a mental disorder). Common mental disorder cases were seen on average nine times per year, and serious mental disorder six times.

General practitioners generally used their clinical intuition, experience, and the DSM-IV to detect and diagnose mental disorder. Standardized scales or questionnaires were used infrequently (reserved essentially for specific or complex cases). Occasionally, these instruments were used to persuade patients who did not recognize their disorder and shepherd them into the care process. Few general practitioners considered using these tools to monitor mental healthcare outcomes. Almost all general practitioners reported managing patients with common mental disorder on a continual basis and felt confident in adequately treating these cases. The situation was reversed for serious mental disorder; very few general practitioners mentioned treating them on a regular basis; generally, they did not felt confident enough to take them on. In general, basic treatment for mental disorder offered by general practitioners was medication and support therapy – very few used best-practice treatment guidelines. General practitioners who managed more patients with serious disorders shared the following profile: they had more training in mental health; they had practiced in psychiatric settings; they were practicing in community care centers (where multidisciplinary teams were available onsite, and general practitioners were paid on a salary basis); they practiced more in rural and semi-urban territories (where psychiatrists were less numerous). General practitioners also estimated that they managed, on a regular basis, 71% of the patients with common mental disorder who consulted them, as compared with 34% of individuals with serious mental disorder.

General practitioners were also found to practice mostly in solo (on an individual basis little collaboration from other medical or psychosocial professionals). They reported that they benefitted from few formal collaboration practices (for example, shared care) in the management of patients with mental disorder. Moreover, they believed the quality of the mental healthcare system to be quite poor; consequently, they supported reforms designed to enhance primary integrated care. Referral was the strategy they used most often in response to the diverse needs of patients with mental disorder. In their estimation, general practitioners referred 17% of their patients with common mental disorder to mental healthcare resources (including 31% of patients to psychologists in private practice; 20% to psychosocial professionals in community care centers; 13% to psychiatrists). They also referred 71% of patients with serious mental disorder (mainly to psychiatric facilities and emergency rooms). More than 50% of the general practitioners also reported that they had no contact (face-to-face or telephone interaction) with any one of the following mental healthcare resources: psychiatrists, community care centers, psychologists in private practice, the voluntary sector, or detox centers.

4.3 Enabling and hindering factors in the management of patients with mental disorder

Enabling factors in general practitioners' management of patients with mental disorder were as follows: (1) considerable interest in the management of mental disorder; (2) personal skills such as listening and empathy; (3) working in an interdisciplinary practice setting, especially community care centers (where general practitioners also are paid by salary or hourly fee); (4) high volume of patients with mental disorder with no complex or recursive profiles (allowing physicians to consolidate knowledge); (5) training in the treatment of mental disorder (academic settings and continuing education); (6) limited access to psychiatric care (which compels general practitioners to manage patients with mental disorder); and (7) patient rostering (encouraging continuity of care by general practitioners). Interprofessional collaboration with general practitioners was strengthened when: (1) general practitioners worked mainly in community care centers; (2) they had practiced or were currently practicing in psychiatric care facilities; (3) they have developed strong informal networks (that is, personal relationships with mental healthcare resources), thereby bypassing long waiting time and gaining prompt access to the formal mental healthcare network; (4) they were practicing in healthcare networks where shared care (or collaborative care) was developed, including evaluation liaison modules (the latter is a referral process to specialized mental disorder services that general practitioners can use, usually deployed through university-affiliated psychiatric facilities in Quebec).

Several hindering factors associated with general practitioners' management of mental disorder were found: (1) significant lack of mental healthcare resources in the Quebec healthcare system; (2) long waiting time for access to mental healthcare, especially psychiatric care (60 days' wait on average in Quebec) and psychotherapy at community care centers (where it is free of charge, covered by the public healthcare system); (3) insufficient knowledge of waiting time for access to services, which impedes care management; (4) limited psychotherapy sessions (either in community care centers (public system) or in the private system through insurance coverage); (5) great difficulty communicating with mental healthcare resources; (6) low availability of general practitioners given the shortage of family physicians in Quebec as healthcare demand increases; (7) inappropriate remuneration or incentives offered to general practitioners for the management of mental disorder (especially troublesome in this regard are fees for services, which fail to compensate for longer and frequent patient visits and also fail to take into account the importance of collaboration with mental healthcare resources which are not remunerated); (8) bureaucracy and inefficiency of referral and collaboration procedures; (9) instability of healthcare resources, especially the high turnover of professionals as Quebec undergoes healthcare reforms; (10) training that does not favor interprofessional collaboration; and (11) complexity of patient profiles and management of mental disorder (for example, the need to treat concomitant illnesses along with mental disorder; general practitioners' emotional involvement or investment in the care of patients with mental disorder; frequency of follow-ups with insurance companies when patients take sick leave). Even though psychiatric access has been facilitated in some Quebec healthcare networks, general practitioners still deplore the absence of: stepped care when patients need it; continuous support from psychiatrists, especially when recommendations provided by psychiatrists to general practitioners do not lead to expected results or when patients' health does not warrant their transfer back to their general practitioner; psychiatric care in the evening and on weekends; and access to psychiatrists for semi-urgent cases (urgent cases were rapidly seen at emergency rooms).

4.4 General practitioner strategies and recommendations to improve the management of mental disorders

To bypass the negative impacts of mental disorder management on their practice, general practitioners have suggested the following strategies: optimizing their informal collaborative networks; plan longer and more numerous consultations ("one problem per consultation solution"), particularly at the beginning and the end of the day; reserve time slots for potential patient crises (or emergency situations), walk-in clinics being ideal for these situations; and provide self-referral to other, more appropriate practice settings for the treatment of mental disorder (as a result, general practitioners would see patients in varied settings, including community care centers, in accordance with the current trend of general practitioners working in several settings). Effective incentives for the management of mental disorder and maintenance of collaboration were also highlighted as desirable developments. General practitioners were all in favor of increasing access to psychiatrists and psychotherapy. The latter, especially cognitive behavioral therapists, associated with medication, stood out as a best-practice option in the management of common mental disorder. More intensive contact between general practitioners and psychosocial professionals, especially psychologists, was promoted in the form of brief reports or telephone follow-ups designed to clarify treatment objectives, propose approaches, and forecast the length of therapy. Shared care led by psychiatrists was also identified as a key strategy to strengthen the treatment of more complex cases of common mental disorder (for example, when medication or treatment does not work, recurrent cases, and crisis situations) or serious mental disorder. One monthly visit to the general practitioner and weekly telephone support from psychiatrists when needed were recommended. Training sessions every three months, involving case studies with various mental healthcare professionals (for example, psychologists and social workers), under the leadership of psychiatrists in local service networks was also highly recommended, as these were considered to foster knowledge on mental disorder and favor networking or the creation and maintenance of a community of practice among professionals.

General practitioners have also recommended the integration of nurses with sufficient experience in the treatment of mental disorder into their work settings. Nurses' role would be to prioritize patients to be seen, collect relevant information on patient profiles (for example, social support, life habits, medical record), offer psycho-education services (involving links with the family when appropriate), strengthen drug adherence, and provide case management for more complex mental disorder cases. Collaboration with social workers (rather than nurses) was preferred for the treatment of patients with serious mental disorder given these patients' need for rehabilitation and life-skill learning. According to general practitioners, the voluntary sector and detox centers should be further integrated into the primary care system; accordingly, mental healthcare teams in community care centers would coordinate patient care with these partners. The inclusion of diverse mental healthcare professionals in general practitioner settings was recommended as an initial reform in family medicine groups and network clinics, where rostering of patients exists and nurses are already on the payroll. The integration of mental healthcare professionals in general practitioner offices was perceived as a key issue for improving the management of mental disorder. This strategy would enhance the efficiency of the mental healthcare system, screening of patients, and prevention of mental disorder. It would lead to more appropriate responses to patient needs on an ongoing basis, thereby reducing hospitalization and emergency-room visits and favoring patient recovery. Finally, the integration of mental healthcare professionals was seen to be an appropriate solution to relieve the pressure on general practitioners with respect to patient follow-up and help to attenuate the shortage of family physicians (calling on mental healthcare professionals for cases of mental disorder would free up general practitioners and allow them to see an increasing number of new patients).

5. Discussion

As mentioned above, general practitioners are consulted more frequently for mental disorder problems than other healthcare professionals (Heymans, 2005: Walters et al., 2008). According to the Canadian Community Health Survey (CCHS, Statistics Canada, 2002; Lesage et al., 2006), 5% of the Quebec population aged over 18 consulted a general practitioner for a mental disorder problem (which is almost the same percentage in the United States; Vasiliadis et al., 2007). In the Quebec public register (RAMQ database), we found that figure to 15%. The gap between the population survey (5%) and the database (15%) may be explained by an underestimation in the population survey of the number of patient visits to general practitioners for mental disorder problems and the high volume of patient visits to general practitioners for concurrent physical problems or conditions (for example, chronic problems or substance abuse) as reflected in the database. In addition, the figure of 15% includes mental disorder diagnoses and clinical acts; the latter showing an upward trend in recent years. This trend is interesting and parallels the increase in drug prescriptions in the recent years. There has been an upsurge in prescriptions in Quebec even in cases where there was no specific diagnosis of mental disorder (*Conseil du médicament*, 2011). In the United States, the annual incidence of antidepressant treatment increased from 2.2% in 1990-1992 to 10.1% in 2001-2003 (Mojtabai, 2008); in New Zealand, from 7.4% in 2004-2005 to 9.4% in 2006-2007 (Exeter et al., 2009); in Italy, from 5.1% in 2003 to 6.0% in 2004 (Trifiro et al., 2007); and in Quebec, from 8.1% in 1999 to 14.9% in 2009 (*Conseil du médicament*, 2011). Generally, it should be noted that there is no gold standard in the measurement of mental healthcare service use (surveys, database or administrative records are all used to gauge service utilization). Individuals with a mental illness may systematically under-or over-report their service use (Rhodes & Fung, 2004); therefore, comparing results from different tools or strategies is of interest and value.

There are mixed findings with regard to general practitioners' preparation and confidence in taking on patients with common mental disorder (Bathgate et al., 2001; Krupinski & Tiller, 2001). Similarly to our research, recent studies (Rockman et al., 2004; Wright et al., 2005; see also Fleury et al., 2009) show that general practitioners are comfortable treating most cases of common mental disorder, but experience difficulty treating personality disorders, eating disorders, substance-abuse disorders, and young patient with mental disorder. For substance abuse co-morbidity and some cases of refractory and recursive common mental disorder, general practitioners also expressed a need for psychiatric expertise for evaluation and diagnosis, medication follow-up, and specialized intervention: generally, these are the three reasons that are reported in the literature for referral to psychiatric services (Rockman et al., 2004). Some studies have cast doubt on the ability of general practitioners to diagnose and treat more complex forms of mental disorder, particularly major depression with suicidal tendency, schizophrenia, and bipolar disorder (Wright et al., 2005). In our research, few general practitioners managed patients with serious mental disorder on a consistent basis. A parallel random cohort study of 140 patients with serious mental disorder released from hospital 12 months before the survey and living in five of Quebec's administrative health regions (Fleury et al., 2010b) showed that 93% of patients were followed by a psychiatrist, 84% by a case manager, and only 50% by a general practitioner. There are many reasons explaining why only a minority of general practitioners manage patients with severe mental disorder. Such patients are deemed to be more difficult to treat and require more care, time, and frequent visits (Balanchandra et al., 2005; Kisely et al., 2006). Often, they have concurrent diagnoses (for example, substance abuse) and interrelated physical or social problems (Iacovides et al., 2008; Jones et al., 2008). General practitioners either consider these disorders too specialized for routine primary care, deeming their skills and experience inadequate for effective diagnosis and treatment, or they position themselves as complementary to specialized care, treating what are essentially physical problems (Lester et al., 2005; Lockhart, 2006). None of these findings suggest that general practitioners should be removed from the treatment equation for these patients. Patients with serious mental disorder are in great need of adequate physical care and mental health follow-up as they face higher risks of interrelated morbidity. Moreover, as psychiatric teams are generally located in urban settings, general practitioners are often the sole available source of care. This is the case in Quebec where almost half of the psychiatrists practice in the Montreal metropolitan area, and where in more remote regions, specialized care is scarce (Lafleur, 2003). Best practices for serious mental disorder management usually include more comprehensive care packages delivered by multidisciplinary teams on a longitudinal basis (Slade et al., 2005; Lester et al., 2005) . As a result, the care pathway for patients with serious mental disorders involves greater collaborative care (especially links between primary and specialized care), since it entails more frequent referrals.

However, general practitioners working in Quebec community care centers (paid by salary) perceived themselves as able to treat patients with more complex mental disorder. Previous studies (Geneau et al., 2007, 2008) have highlighted the key role played by community care centers (or multidisciplinary settings) in the treatment of complex cases involving both physical and mental illness, which are generally associated with dimmer prognoses. Family medicine groups and network clinics, promoting physician group practice and involving nurses, can also play a key role in the treatment of more complex mental healthcare cases. However, our study, similarly to others (*Ministère de la Santé et des services sociaux du Québec*, 2009a; 2009b), did not find evidence of this. Nurses with training in the treatment of mental disorder should be recruited, and targeted outcomes in mental health should be introduced.

Our findings show that general practitioners refer patients with mental disorder according to diagnosis, that is, common mental disorder or severe mental disorder, the former being less frequently referred. In fact, most patients with common mental disorder are treated by general practitioners, without significant referral to other mental healthcare providers. In the international literature (Valenstein et al., 1999; Younes et al., 2005; Grembowski et al., 2002), referral rates between general practitioners and mental healthcare resources range from 4 and 23% of patients with mental disorder. More considerable variations are reported for contacts, with 9 to 65% of general practitioners estimated to have some contact with mental healthcare providers (Craven & Bland, 2006). Compared to contact (for example, shared-care initiatives, face-to-face or telephone follow-up), referral is difficult to interpret when gauging the effectiveness of clinical practice since it does not provide information regarding failures to refer and does not distinguish between useful and unnecessary referral. Patients may be harmed if referral occurs too late, and delays may make major treatment necessary in later stages. A large number of referrals also may be interpreted as patient transfers (Coulter, 1998). In the referral process, concurrent treatment may be parallel rather than collaborative. Patients may fail to follow through with referral, without their general practitioners' knowledge (Valenstein et al., 1999). In the Canadian Community Health Survey for instance, close to 50% of the population who saw a general practitioner for mental a disorder also concurrently used the services of another healthcare professional

(Lesage et al., 2006) – this proportion is much higher than the figures reported by general practitioners (even if the number of patient from referral and contact are included). In a study conducted in a Montreal catchment area where 2,443 individuals were surveyed, 406 (17%) experienced at least one mental disorder episode in the 12 months before their participation in the study. Among this subset, 212 (52%) reported at least one episode of healthcare service use. Most participants consulted general practitioners (63%), psychiatrists (58%) and psychologists (32%), and 20% consulted with at least four types of professionals (Fleury et al., in revision). In light of general practitioners' reports with respect to patient referral, these two studies raise serious questions regarding general practitioners' knowledge of the "parallel care" their patients seek.

For Rothman and Wagner (2003), non-physicians play a significant role in most successful treatments of chronic illness. Our research found that general practitioners mainly referred patients with common mental disorder to psychologists in private practice, followed by psychosocial resources in community care centers, and, finally, psychiatrists. The major role played by psychologists (or other well-trained psychosocial professionals) in treating patients with common mental disorder has been abundantly reported (Parslow & Jorm, 2000; Grenier et al., 2008). General practitioners in our research recommended joint psychotherapy and medication for most of their patients with mental disorder, suggesting that they recognized the limited effectiveness of a pharmacology-only approach. Some patients also prefer psychotherapy instead of medication (van Rijswijk et al., 2009). Moreover, as already said, compliance to medication being generally poor in those patients (*Conseil du Médicament*, 2011; Seekles et al., 2009), there is a great need to reinforce psycho-educational or patient-centered approaches. Psychiatrists, also viewed as key partners, were essential to the management of more difficult cases of mental disorder and knowledge transfer. Similarly to other studies (van Rijswijk et al., 2009), general practitioners recommended a key role for nurses, but with some reservation. The serious shortage of nurses in the Quebec healthcare system (as in several other countries, WHO, 2006) would undoubtedly hamper efforts to foster their participation in mental healthcare. Contrary to other Canadian provinces and some other countries, mental healthcare nursing is not a recognized specialty in Quebec (Canadian Institute for Health Information, 2008, 2010). Moreover, the number of hours dedicated to mental healthcare training in nursing school is low (and has steadily been decreasing in recent years) (*Ordre des infirmières et infirmiers du Québec*, 2009). As a result, nurses in the province may not always be appropriately equipped to play an extensive role in primary mental healthcare.

In our research, as in the literature, different factors were found that may account for general practitioners' decision to treat patients with mental disorder: (1) environment (international trends, mental healthcare policies); (2) macro-organizational features and reforms (collaborative care, access to resources); (3) practice settings (remuneration by salary, internal professional collaboration, volume of patients with mental disorder); (4) general practitioners' individual characteristics (training and background in mental healthcare, informal networks, interests and confidence in treating mental disorder); and (5) patient management profiles (attitudes, illness severity, prognoses).

In efforts to improve primary care in Quebec, particularly regarding mental disorder, the following initiatives have been deployed: family medicine groups; network clinics; and shared care, including the consolidation of mental health psychosocial teams and introduction of single access points in community care centers within each local network. Single access points serve as a standardized and coordinated referral procedure to psychosocial services (patient self-referral or general practitioner referral) in all local networks, at community care centers (where psychosocial services are covered by the public system) or to psychiatric services in hospital settings, when patients require specialized care. Our results showed that the Quebec reform has not yet significantly improved the mental healthcare system, as quality of care was regarded to be quite poor and care collaboration as being severely underdeveloped. This state of affairs is due in part to the modest progress made in implementing current reforms (for example, very little development of shared care, understaffed psychosocial teams at community care centers, and inadequate operation of single access points). Findings of poor mental healthcare quality unfortunately are not specific to Quebec; numerous studies (Pawlenko, 2005; Nolan & Badger, 2002) have found similar results in other countries; however, recent efforts in some countries, for example, the United Kingdom and Australia to bring about improvements in this regard have been noted (Hickie & Groom, 2002; Lester et al., 2004). Repeated mention of insufficient collaboration among providers, particularly psychiatrists and general practitioners, can be found in the literature (Bambling et al, 2007; Cunningham, 2009). Upshur and Weinreb (2008) have indicated that partial implementation of shared-care initiatives does not usually produce substantive outcomes. Key elements for development of effective shared care, as per the literature (Kringos et al., 2010; Upshur & Weinreb, 2008), include: the development of electronic medical records; physician leadership; incentives for inter-professional collaboration and management of complex patient profiles; team vision; recognition of diversified expertise requirements; absence of hierarchical structures among professionals; adequate space and locations; effective management and clinical skills; strong commitment to innovation and patient empowerment; and established clinical relationships. To improve the quality of mental healthcare services, other recurring issues to pay attention to are: long waiting times for psychiatric care or psychotherapy at no charge; limited primary-care team practice; general practitioners' limited training or experience with effective team practice (Rothman & Wagner, 2003); inappropriate modes of remuneration; and lack of financial incentives for general practitioners to manage patients with mental disorder (Collins, 2006; Morden et al., 2009). General practitioners' busy schedules and the competing demands of other patients are other contributing factors (Starfield, 1998; Craven & Bland, 2006). The historical separation between psychiatry and primary care (Crews et al., 1998) may also explain general practitioners' reluctance to take on patients with mental disorder, especially among those who may consider hospital psychiatric teams to be more appropriate. In addition, the length of visits, essentially designed for general practitioners to prescribe medication and provide quick support therapy, was found to be too brief to permit optimal management of mental disorder. Consequently, in the light of the foregoing, implementing strategies to enhance general practitioners' management of mental disorder represents a considerable challenge.

6. Conclusion

On the whole, our research studies found that general practitioners welcomed opportunities to manage patients with common mental disorder; however, they also faced a number of obstacles, including: healthcare system fragmentation; lack of communication, resources, and clinical tools; the prevalence of solo practice; and unsuitable modes of payment. In Quebec, as in most other jurisdictions, reforms are under way, but best practices such as patient self-management, stepped-care therapy, and shared care are as yet underdeveloped.

General practitioners worked mainly in solo practice and relied on their clinical intuition with little clinical or collaborative support. Psychosocial resources, such as cognitive behavioral therapy, are not sufficiently widespread, which too often compelled general practitioners to turn to pharmacological solutions as the only affordable option for patients. In light of current reforms and best-practice recommendations, our research advocates, as a stepped-care approach to system change, increased access to psychologists and psychiatrists as in other countries (for example, the United Kingdom and Australia) in efforts to implement further biopsychosocial modes of treatment and strengthen collaborative care. Development of a network of general practitioners in multidisciplinary settings with more specialized knowledge of mental disorder would prove beneficial in the treatment of more complex cases. Specialized resources for the treatment of substance abuse (given the incidence of concomitant disorders) and greater participation by the voluntary sector also represent desirable developments. In addition, rostering of patients and salary-based or hourly-fee compensation should be promoted. Continuing education and case discussion in local networks with psychiatrists and multidisciplinary resources are also recommended as they favor skill and network development, respectively. Government policy, implementation incentives, and support mechanisms must drive reforms, enabling general practitioners to play a significant role in the management of mental disorders and bolstering integrated biopsychosocial approaches. Finally, a culture of collaboration has to be encouraged as comprehensive services and continuity of care are key recovery factors of patients with mental disorder. Collaborative care, an extended role for psychosocial resources, and more efficient mental primary care organization should lead to expanded caseloads for general practitioners and better access to services for patients with mental disorder.

7. Acknowledgment

The research was funded by the Canadian Institute of Health Research (CIHR), *Fonds de la recherche en santé du Québec* (FRSQ) and other decision-making partners. We would like to thank all the grant agencies, partners, and general practitioners who took part in the research project. In addition, we would like to underscore the contribution of our project co-researchers: Drs Jacques Tremblay, Jean-Marie Bamvita, Lambert Farand, Denise Aubé, Alain Lesage, and Armelle Imboua.

8. References

Albert, M., Becker, T., McCrone P. & Thornicroft, G. (1998). Social networks and mental health service utilisation. A literature review. *International Journal of Social Psychiatry*, Vol. 44, No. 4, (Winter 1998), pp. 248-266, ISSN 0020-7640

Alegria, M., Bijl, R.V., Lin, E., Walters, E.E. & Kessler, R.C. (2000). Income differences in persons seeking outpatient treatment for mental disorders: a comparison of the United States with Ontario and the Netherlands. *Archives of General Psychiatry*, Vol. 57, No. 4, (April 2000), pp. 383-391, ISSN 0003-990X

Bachrach, L.L. (1996). Psychosocial rehabilitation and psychiatry: what are the boundaries? *Canadian Journal of Psychiatry*, Vol. 41, No. 1, (February 1996), pp. 28-35, ISSN 0706-7437

Balanchandra, K., Sharma, V., Dozois, D. & Bhayana, B. (2005). How bipolar disorders are managed in family practice: self-assessment survey. *Canadian Family Physician*, Vol. 51, No. 4, (April 2005), pp. 534-535, ISSN 0008-350X

Bambling, M., Kavanagh D., Lewis G., King, R., King, D., Shurk, H., Turpin, M., Gallois, C. & Bartlett, H. (2007). Challenges faced by general practitioners and allied mental health services in providing mental health services in rural Queensland. *Australian Journal of Rural Health*, Vol. 15, No. 2, (April 2007), pp. 126-130, ISSN 1038-5282

Bathgate, D., Bermingham, B., Curtis, D. & Romans, S. (2001). The view of Otago urban and rural General Practitioners on mental health services. *New Zealand Medical Journal*, No. 114, No. 1134, (June 2001), pp. 289-291, ISSN 0028-8446

Bebbington, P., Meltzer, H., Brugha, T.S., Farrell, M., Jenkins, R., Ceresa, C. & Lewis, G. (2000). Unequal access and unmet need: neurotic disorders and the use of primary care services. *Psychological Medicine*, Vol. 30, No. 1-2, (February-May 2000), pp. 1359-1367, ISSN 0033-2917

Bergman, J.S. (2007). *Primary Health Care Transition Fund. Evaluation and evidence.* Health Canada, Ottawa, Canada

Bilsker, D. (2010). Supported self-management: Maximizing the impact of primary mental heath care. *Quintessence*, Vol. 2, No. 1 (January 2010). Available from: www.qualaxia.org/mental-health-information/quintessence.php?lg=en

Bodenheimer, T., Wagner, E.H. & Grumbach, K. (2002). Improving primary care for patients with chronic illness. *Journal of American Medical Association*, Vol. 288, No. 14, (October 2002), pp. 1775-1779, ISSN 0098-7484

Bonin, J.P., Fournier, L. & Blais, R. (2007). Predictors of mental health service utilization by people using resources for homeless people in Canada. *Psychiatric Services*, Vol. 58, No. 7, (July 2007), pp. 936-941, ISSN 1075-2730

Bosco, C. (2005). *Health human resources in collaborative mental health care. A discussion on overcoming the human resource barriers to implementing collaborative mental health care in Canada.* Canadian Collaborative Mental Health Initiative, ISBN 1-896014-82-8, Mississauga, Ontario.

Bourgueil, Y., Marek, A. & Mousquès, J. (2007). Médecine de groupe en soins primaires dans six pays européens, en Ontario et au Québec : quels enseignements pour la France? *Questions d'économie de la santé*, No. 127, (November 2007), pp. 1-8, ISSN 1238-4769

Bower, P. & Gilbody, S. (2005). Stepped care in psychological therapies: access, effectiveness and efficiency. Narrative literature review. *British Journal of Psychiatry*, No. 186, (January 2005), pp. 11-17, ISSN 0007-1250

Bower, P. (2002). Primary care mental health workers: models of working and evidence of effectiveness. *British Journal of General Practice*, Vol. 52, No. 484, (November 2002), pp. 926-933, ISSN 0960-1643

Breier, A., Schreiber, J.L., Dyer, J. & Pickar, D. (1991). National Institute of Mental Health longitudinal study of chronic schizophrenia. Prognosis and predictors of outcome. *Archives of General Psychiatry*, Vol. 48, No. 3, (March 1991), pp. 239-248, ISSN 0003-990X

Canadian Institute for Health Information. (2010). *Infirmières réglementées: tendance canadienne, de 2005 à 2009.* Canadian Institute for Health Information, ISBN 978-1-55465-828-2, Ottawa, Canada

Canadian Institute for Health Information (2008). *Les dispensateurs de soins de santé au Canada, de 1997 à 2006 - Guide de référence*. Canadian Institute for Health Information, ISBN 978-1-55465-318-8, Ottawa, Canada

Carr, V.J., Johnston, P.J., Lewin, T.J., Rajkumar, S., Carter, G.L. & Issakidis, C. (2003). Patterns of service use among persons with schizophrenia and other psychotic disorders. *Psychiatric Services*, Vol. 54, No. 2, (February 2003), pp. 226-235, ISSN 1075-2730

Casper, E.S. & Donaldson, B. (1990). Subgroups in the population of frequent users of inpatient services. *Hospital & Community Psychiatry*, Vol. 41, No. 2, (February 1990), pp. 189-191, ISSN 0022-1597

Chomienne, M.H., Grenier, J., Gaboury, I., Hogg, W., Ritchie, P. & Farmova-Haynes, E. (2010). Family doctors and psychologists working together : doctor's and patients' perspectives. *Journal of Evaluation in Clinical Practice*, Vol. 17, No. 2, (April 2010), pp. 282-287, ISSN 1356-1294

Clark, D.M., Layard, R., Smithies, R., Richards, D.A., Suckling, R. & Wright, B. (2009). Improving access to psychological therapy: Initial evaluation of two UK demonstrations sites. *Behaviour and Research Therapy*, Vol. 43, No. 3, (November 2009), pp. 910-920, ISSN 0005-7967

College of Family Physicians of Canada (2009). *Patient-centred primary care in Canada: Bring it on home*. College of Family Physician of Canada, Mississauga, Ontario

College of Family Physicians of Canada (2008). *Soutenir les effectifs futurs en médecine familiale au Canada. En fait-on assez aujourd'hui pour se préparer pour demain?* College of Family Physician of Canada, Mississauga, Ontario

College of Family Physicians of Canada (2007). *National Physician Survey*. Available from: www.nationalphysiciansurvey.ca/nps/2007_Survey/2007nps-e.asp

College of Family Physicians of Canada (2004). *National Physician Survey*. Available from: www.nationalphysiciansurvey.ca/nps/2004_Survey/2004results-e.asp

Collins, K. A., Wolfe, V.V., Fisman, S., DePace, J. & Steele, M. (2006). Managing depression in primary care: community survey. *Canadian Family Physican*, Vol. 52, No. 7, (July 2006), pp. 878-879, ISSN 0008-350X

Commissaire à la Santé et au Bien-être (2010). *Rapport d'appréciation de la performance du système de santé et de services sociaux 2010 : Adopter une approche intégrée de prévention et de gestion des maladies chroniques : recommandations, enjeux et implication*. Gouvernement du Québec, ISBN 978-2-550-58277-4, Québec, Québec

Commissaire à la Santé et au Bien-être (2009). *L'expérience de soins des personnes présentant les plus grands besoins de santé : le Québec comparé. Résultats de l'enquête internationale sur les politiques de santé du Commonwealth Fund de 2008*. Gouvernement du Québec, ISBN 978-2-550-57271-8, Québec, Québec

Conseil du Médicament. (2011). *Portrait de l'usage des antidépresseurs chez les adultes assurés par le régime d'assurance médicaments du Québec*. Gouvernement du Québec, ISBN 978-2-550-60457-0, Québec, Québec

Coulter, A. (1998). Managing demand at the interface between primary and secondary care. *British Medical Journal*, Vol. 316, No. 7149, (June 1998), pp. 1974-1976, ISSN 0959-8138

Craven, M. & Bland R. (2006). Better practices in collaborative mental health care: an analysis of the evidence base. *Canadian Journal of Psychiatry*, Vol 51, No. 6, (May 2006) pp. 7s-72s, ISSN 0706-7437

Crews, C., Batal, H., Elasy, T., Casper, E. & Mehler, P.S. (1998). Primary care for those with severe and persistent mental illness. *Western Journal of Medicine*, Vol. 169, No. 4, (October 1998), pp. 245-250, ISSN 0093-0415

Cruickshank, J. (2010). The patient-centered medical home approach to improve dyslipidemia outcomes. *Journal of the American Osteopathic Association*, Vol. 110, No. 4, Suppl 5, (April 2010), eS3-5, ISSN 0098-6151

Cunningham, P.J. (2009). Beyond parity: primary care physicians' perspectives on access to mental health care. *Health Affairs*, Vol. 28, No. 3, (May-June 2009), pp. w490-501, ISSN 1544-5208

Demyttenaere, K., Bruffaerts, R., Posada-Villa, J., Gasquet, I., Kovess, V., Lepine, J.P., Angermeyer, M.C., Bernet, S., de Girolamo, G., Morosini, P., Polidori, G., Kikkawa, T., Kawakami, N., Ono, Y., Takeshima, T., Uda, H., Karam, E.G, Fayyad, J.A., Karam, A.N., Mneimneh, Z.N., Medina-Mora, M.E., Borges, G., Lara, C., de Graaf, R., Omel, J., Gureje, O., Shen, Y., Huang, Y., Zhang, M., Alonso, J., Haro, J.M., Vilagut, G., Bromet, E.J., Gluzman, S., Webb, C., Kessler, R.C., Merikangas, K.R., Anthony, J.C., Von Korff, M.R., Wang, P.S., Brugha, T.S., Aguilar-Gaxiola, S., Lee, S., Heeringa, S., Pennell, B.E., Zalavsky, A.M., Ustun, T.B., Chatterji, S. & WHO World Mental Heath Survey Consortium (2004). Prevalence, severity, and unmet need for treatment of mental disorders in the World Health Organization World Mental Health Surveys, *Journal of the American Medical Association*, Vol. 291, No. 21, (June 2004), pp. 2581-2590, ISSN 0098-7484

Desjardins, Y. (2011). Strengthening primary care: A priority. *Qmentum Quarterly: Quality in Health Care*, Vol. 3, No. 1, (May 2011), pp. 10-12, 1918-039X

Dorr, D., Bonner, L.M., Cohen, A.N., Shoai, R.S., Perrin, R., Chaney, E. & Young, A.S. (2007). Informatics systems to promote improved care for chronic illness: A literature review. *Journal of the American Medical Informatics Association*, Vol. 14, No. 2, (March-April 2007), pp. 156-163, ISSN 1067-5027

Exeter, D., Robinson, E. & Wheeler, A. (2009). Antidepressant dispensing trends in New Zealand between 2004 and 2007. *Australian and New Zealand Journal of Psychiatry*, Vol. 43, No. 12, (December 2009), pp. 1131-1140, ISSN 0004-8674

Fervers, B., Burgers, J., Haugh, M.C., Latreille, J., Mlika-Cabanne, N., Paquet, L., Coulombe, M., Poirier, M. & Burnand, B. (2006). Adaptation of clinical guidelines: literature review and proposition for a framework and procedure. *International Journal for Quality in Health Care*, Vol. 18, No. 3, (June 2006), pp. 167-1776, ISSN 1353-4505

Fitzpatrick, N.K., Shah, S., Walker, N., Nourmand, S., Tyrer, P.J., Barnes, T.R., Higgitt, A. & Hemingway, H. (2004). The determinants and effect of shared care on patient outcomes and psychiatric admissions – an inner city primary care cohort study. *Social Psychiatry and Psychiatric Epidemiology*, Vol. 39, No. 2, (February 2004), pp. 154-163, ISSN 0933-7954

Fleury, M.-J., Grenier, G., Bamvita, J.M., Perreault, M. & Caron, J. (Revision). Determinants of the utilization of diversified types of professionals for mental health reasons in a Montreal catchment area. *Community Mental Health Journal*, ISSN 1573-2789

Fleury, M.-J., Grenier, G., Bamvita, J.M., Perreault, M. & Caron, J. (2011). Determinants associated with the utilization of primary and specialized mental health services. *Psychiatric Quarterly*. (May 2011), [Epub ahead of print], ISSN 1573-6709

Fleury, M.-J., Bamvita, J. M., Farand, L., Aubé, D., Fournier, L. & Lesage, A. (2010a). GP group profiles and involvement in mental health care. *Journal of Evaluation in Clinical Practice*. (November 2010), [Epub ahead of print], ISSN 1365-2753

Fleury, M.-J., Grenier, G., Bamvita, J.-M. & Caron, J. (2010b). Professional service utilization among patients with severe mental disorders. *BMC Health Services Research*, Vol. 10, (May 2010), p. 141, ISSN 1472-6963

Fleury M.-J., Bamvita, J.M. & Tremblay J. (2009). Variables associated with general practitioners taking on serious mental disorder patients. *BMC Family Practice*, Vol. 10, No. 1, (June 2009), pp. 41, ISSN 1471-2296

Fleury, M.-J., Bamvita, J.M., Farand, L. & Tremblay, J. (2008). Variables associated with general practitioners taking on patients with common mental disorders. *Mental Health in Family Medicine*, Vol. 5, No. 3, (September 2008), pp. 149-160, ISSN 1756-834X

Fleury, M.-J. (2006). Integrated Service Networks: The Quebec Case. *Health Services Management Research*, Vol. 19, No. 3, (August 2006), pp. 153-165, ISSN 0951-4848

Fontaine, P., Ross, S.E., Zink, T. & Schilling, L.M. (2010). Systematic review of health information exchange in primary care practices. *Journal of the American Board of Family Medicine*, Vol. 23, No. 5, (September-October 2010), pp. 665-670, ISSN 1557-2625

Fournier, L., Aubé, D., Roberge, P., Lessard, L., Duhoux, A., Caulet, M. & Poirier, L.R. (2007). *Vers une première ligne forte en santé mentale : Messages clés de la littérature scientifique*, Institut national de santé publique du Québec, Québec, Canada

Gask, L., Rogers, A., Campbell, S. & Sheaff, R. (2008). Beyond the Limits of Clinical Governance? The Case of Mental Health in English Primary Care. *BMC Health Services Research*, Vol. 8, No. 63, (March 2008), pp. 1-10, ISSN 1472-6963

Geneau, R., Lehoux, P., Pineault, R. & Lamarche, P. (2008). Understanding the work of general practitioners: a social science perspective on the context of medical decision making in primary care. *BMC Family Practice*, Vol. 9, (February), p. 12, ISSN 1471-2296

Geneau, R., Lehoux, P., Pineault, R. & Lamarche, P.A. (2007). Primary care practice a la carte among GPs: using organizational diversity to increase job satisfaction. *Family Practice*, Vol. 24, No. 2, (April 2007), pp. 138-144, ISSN 0263-2136

Government of Canada (2006). *The Human Face of Mental Health and Mental Illness in Canada*. Public Works and Government Services, Ottawa, Canada, ISBN 0-662-72356-2

Grembowski, D., Martin, D. & Patrick, D.L., Diehr, P. Katon, W., Williams, B., Engelberg, R., Novak, L., Dickstein, D., Devo, R. & Goldberg, H.I. Managed Care, Access to mental health specialists, and outcomes among primary care patients with depressive symptoms. *Journal of General Internal Medicine Subscribers*, Vol. 17, No. 4, (April 2002), pp. 258-269, ISSN 1535-1497

Grenier, J., Chomienne, M.H., Gaboury, I., Ritchie, P. & Hogg, W. (2008). Collaboration between family physicians and psychologists: what do family physicians know about psychologists' work? *Canadian Family Physician*, Vol. 54, No. 2, (February 2008), pp. 232-233, ISSN 0008-350X

Hakkaart-van Roijen, L., van Straten, A., Maiwenn, A. Rutten, F. & Donker, M. (2006). Cost-utility of brief psychological treatment for depression and anxiety. *British Journal of Psychiatry*, Vol. 188, No. 4, (April 2006), pp. 323-329, ISSN 0007-1250

Haggerty, J., Pineault, R., Beaulieu, M.D., Brunelle, Y., Goulet, F., Rodrigue, J. & Gauthier, J. (2004). *Continuité et accessibilité des soins de première ligne au Québec: barrières et facteurs facilitants*. Fondation canadienne de la recherche sur les services de santé (FCRSS), ISBN 2-9807566-6-0, Ottawa, Canada

Hansson, L., Vinding, H.R., Mackeprang, T., Sourander, A., Werderlin, G., Bengtsson-Tops, A., Bjarnason, O., Dybbro, J., Nilsson, L., Sandlund, M., Sorgaard, K. & Middelboe, T. (2001). Comparison of key worker and patient assessment of needs in schizophrenic patients living in the community: a Nordic multicentre study. *Acta Psychiatrica Scandinavica*, Vol. 103, No. 1, (January 2001), pp. 45-51, ISSN 0001-690X

Hatzenbuehler, M.L., Keyes, K.M., Narrow, W.E., Grant, B.F. & Hasin, D.S. (2008). Racial/ethnic disparities in service utilization for individuals with co-occurring mental health and substance use disorders in the general population: results from the epidemiological survey on alcohol and related conditions. *Journal of Clinical Psychiatry*, Vol. 69, No. 7, (July 2008), pp. 1112-1121, ISSN 0160-6689

Hendryx, M.S. & Ahern, M.M. (2001). Access to mental health services and health sector social capital. *Administration and Policy in Mental Health*, Vol. 28, No. 3, (January 2001), pp. 205-217, ISSN 0894-587X

Heymans, I. (2005). *Argumentaire pour un système de santé fondé sur les soins de santé primaires et pour le soutien au développement de centres de santé intégrés*. Fédération des maisons médicales et des collectifs de santé francophones, Vereniging van Wijkgezondheidscentra.

Hickie, I. & Groom, G. (2002). Primary care-led mental health service refom: an outline of the better outcomes in mental health care initiatives. *Australasian Psychiatry*, Vol. 10, No. 4. (December 2002), pp. 376-382, ISSN 1440-1665

Howard, K.I., Cornille, T.A., Lyons, J.S., Vessey, J.T., Lueger, R.J. & Saunders, S.M. (1996). Patterns of Mental Health Service Utilization. *Archives of General Psychiatry*, Vol. 53, No. 8, (August 1996), pp. 696-703, ISSN 0003-990X

Howell, C., Marshall, C., Opolski, M. & Newbury, W. (2008). Management of recurrent depression. *Australian Family Physician*, Vol. 37, No. 9, (September 2008), pp. 704-708, ISSN 0300-8495

Iacovides, A. & Siamouli, M. (2008). Comorbid mental and somatic disorders: an epidemiological perspective. *Current Opinion in Psychiatry*, Vol. 21, No. 4, (July 2008), pp. 417-421, ISSN 0951-7367

Jones, B.J., Gallagher, B.J. 3rd, Pisa, A.M. & McFalls, J.A. jr (2008). Social class, family history and type of schizophrenia. *Psychiatry Research*, Vol. 159, No. 1-2, (May 2008), pp. 127-132, ISSN 0165-1781

Jones, D.R., Macias, C., Barreira, P.J., Fisher, W.H., Hargreaves, W.A. & Harding, C.M. (2004). Prevalence, severity, and co-occurence of chronic physical health problems of persons with serious mental illness. *Psychiatric Services*, Vol. 55, No. 11, (November 2004), pp. 1250-1257, ISSN 1075-2730

Joska, J. & Flisher, A.J. (2005). The assessment of need for mental health services. *Social Psychiatry and Psychiatric Epidemiology*, Vol. 40, No. 7, (July 2005), pp. 529-539, ISSN 0933-7954

Kates, N., Mazowita, G., Lemire, F., Jayabarathan, A., Bland, R., Selby, P., Isomura, T., Craven, M. Gervais, M. & Audet, D. (2011). The evolution of collaborative mental health care in Canada: A shared vision for the future. *Canadian Journal of Psychiatry*, Vol. 56, No. 5, Suppl. 10, (May 2011), pp. 1-10, ISSN 0706-7437

Kates, N., Craven, M., Bishop, J., Clinton, T., Kraftcheck, D., Leclair, K., Leverette, J., Nash, L. & Turner, T. (1997). Shared mental health care in Canada. *Canadian Journal of Psychiatry*, Vol. 42, No 38, Suppl. 12 (November), pp. 877-888, ISSN 0706-7437

Katon, W., Lin, E.H. & Kroenke, K. (2007). The association of depression and anxiety with medical symptom burden in patients with chronic medical illness. *General Hospital Psychiatry*, Vol. 29, No. 2, (March-April 2007), pp. 147-155, ISSN 0163-8343

Katz, A., Glazier, R.H. & Vijayaraghavan, J. (2009). *The health and economic consequences of achieving a high-quality primary healthcare system in Canada. Applying what works in Canada closing the Gap.* June 26 2011, Available from: www.chsrf.ca/Libraries/Primary_Healthcare/11498_PHC_Katz_ENG_FINAL.sflb.ashx

Kent, S., Fogarty M. & Yellowlees, P. (1995) A review of studies of heavy users of psychiatric services. *Psychiatric Services*, Vol. 46, No. 12, (December 1995), pp. 1247-1253, ISSN 1075-2730

Kent, S. & Yellowlees, P. (1995). The relationship between social factors and frequent use of psychiatric services. *Australian and New Zealand Journal of Psychiatry*, Vol. 29, No. 3, (September 1995), pp. 403-408, ISSN 0004-8674

Kessler, R.C., Ruscio, A.M., Shear, K. & Wittchen, H.U. (2010). Epidemiology of anxiety disorders. *Current Topics in Behavioral Neurosciences*, Vol. 2 (2010), pp. 21-35, ISSN 1866-3370

Kessler, R.C., Chiu, W.T., Demler, O. & Walters, E.E. (2005). Prevalence, severity and comorbidity of 12-Month disorders in the National Comorbidity Survey Replication. *Archives of General Psychiatry*, Vol. 62, No. 6, (June 2005), pp. 617-627, ISSN 0003-990X

Kessler, R.C., Berglund, P.A., Bruce, M.L., Koch, J.R., Laska, E.M., Leaf, P.J., Mandersheid, R.W., Rosenheck, R.A., Walters, E.E. & Wang, P.S. (2001). The prevalence and correlates of untreated serious mental illness. *Health Services Research*, Vol. 36, No. 6 Pt. 1, (December 2001), pp. 987-1007, ISSN 0017-9124

Keyes, K.M., Hatzenbuehler, M.L., Alberti, P., Narrow, W.E., Grant, B.F. & Hasin, D.S. (2008). Service utilization differences for Axis I psychiatric and substance use disorders between white and black adults. *Psychiatric Services*, Vol. 59, No. 8 (August 2008), pp. 893-901, ISSN 1075-2730

Khan, S. C., McIntosh, C., Sanmartin, C., Watson, D., & Leeb, K. (2008). *Primary Health Care Teams and their impact on processes and outcomes of care.* Statistics Canada. Health Research Working Paper Series. Available from: www.statcan.gc.ca/pub/82-622x/82-622-x2008002-eng.htm

Kirby, M. J. L. (2006). *Out of the Shadows at Last* (Report). The Senate of Canada, Ottawa, Canada, June 27 2011. Available from: www.parl.gc.ca/Content/SEN/Committee/391/soci/rep/pdf/rep02may06part1-e.pdf

Kisely, S. & Campbell, L.A. (2007). Taking consultation-liaison psychiatry into primary care. *International Journal of Psychiatry in Medicine*, Vol. 37, No. 4, pp. 383-391, ISSN 0091-2174

Kisely, S., Duerden, D., Shaddick, S. & Jayabarathan, A. (2006). Collaboration between primary care and psychiatric services: does it help family physicians? *Canadian Family Physician*, Vol. 52, (July 2006), pp. 876-877, ISSN 0008-350X

Korkeila, J.A., Lehtinen, V., Tuori, T. & Helenius, H. (1998). Frequently hospitalised psychiatric patients: a study of predictive factors. *Social Psychiatric and Psychiatric Epidemiology*, Vol. 33, No. 11, (November 1998), pp. 528-534, ISSN 0933-7954

Kringos, D.S., Boerma, W.G., Hutchinson, A., van der Zee, J. & Groenewegen, P.P. (2010). The breadth of primary care: a systematic literature review of its core dimensions. *BMC Health Services Research*, Vol. 10, (March 2010), pp. 65, ISSN 1472-6963

Krupinski, J. & Tiller, J.W. (2001). The identification and treatment of depression by general practitioners. *Australian and New Zealand Journal of Psychiatry*, Vol. 35, No. 6, (December 2001), pp. 827-832, ISSN 0004-8674

Lafleur, P-A. (2003). Le métier de psychiatre au Québec. *L'information psychiatrique*. Vol. 79, No. 6, (June 2003), pp. 503-510, ISSN 0020-0204

Layard, R., Clark, D., Knapp, M. & Mayraz (2007). Cost-benefit analysis of psychological therapy. *National Institute Economic Review*, No. 2002, (October 2007), pp. 90-98, ISSN 0027-9501

Leaf, P.J., Livingston, M.M., Tischler, G.L., Weissman, M.M., Holzer, C.E. 3rd & Myers, J.K. (1985). Contact with health professionals for the treatment of psychiatric and emotional problems. *Medical Care*, Vol. 23, No. 12, (December 1985), pp. 1322-1337, ISSN 0025-7079

Lemming, M.R. & Calsyn, R.J. (2004). Utility of the behavioral model in predicting service utilization by individuals suffering from severe mental illness and homelessness. *Community Mental Health Journal*, Vol. 40, No. 4, (August 2004), pp. 347-364, ISSN 0010-3853

Lesage, A., Vasiliadis, H.-M., Gagné, M.-A., Dudgeon, S., Kasman, N. & Hay, C. (2006). *Prevalence of mental illness and related service utilization in Canada: an analysis of the Canadian Community Health Survey*. Health Canada's Primary Health Care Transition Fund, ISBN 1-869014-84-4, Mississauga: Ontario

Lester, H., Tritter, J.Q. & Sorohan, H. (2005). Patients' and health professionals' views on primary care for people with serious mental illness: focus group study. *British Medical Journal*, Vol. 330, No. 7500, (May 2005), pp. 1122-1126, ISSN 0959-8138

Lester, H., Glasby, J. & Tylee, A. (2004). Integrated primary mental health care: threat or opportunity in the new NHS? *British Journal of General Practice*, Vol. 54, No. 501, (April 2004), pp. 285-291, ISSN 0960-1643

Lloyd, K.R., Jenkins, R. & Mann, A. (1996). Long-term outcome of patients with neurotic illness in general practice. *British Medical Journal*, Vol. 313, No. 7048, (July 1996), pp. 26-28, ISSN 0959-8138

Lockhart C. (2006). Collaboration and referral practices of general practitioners and community mental health workers in rural and remote Australia. *Australian Journal of Rural Health*, Vol. 14, No. 1, (February 2006), pp. 29-32, ISSN 1038-5282

McAvoy, B.R. & Coster, G.D. (2005). General practice and the New Zealand reforms- lessons for Australia? *Australia and New Zealand Health Policy*, Vol. 2, (November 2005), pp. 26, ISSN 1743-8462

Middelboe, T., Mackeprang, T., Hansson, L., Werdelin, G., Karlsson, H., Bjarnason, O., Bengtsson-Tops, Dybbro, J., Nilsson, L.L., Sandlund, M. & Sorgaard, K.W. (2001). The Nordic study on schizophrenic patients living in the community. Subjective needs and perceived help. *European Psychiatry*, Vol. 16, No. 4, (June 2001), pp. 207-214, ISSN 0924-9338

Ministère de la Santé et des Services Sociaux du Québec (2009a). *Évaluation de l'implantation et des effets des premiers groupes de médecine de famille au Québec.* Gouvernement du Québec, ISBN 978-550-55493-4, Québec, Québec

Ministère de la Santé et des Services Sociaux du Québec (2009b). *Sondage auprès des infirmières des Groupes de médecins de famille du Québec - 2007-2008.* Gouvernement du Québec, Québec, Québec

Ministère de la Santé et des Services Sociaux du Québec (2006). *Plan d'action en santé mentale 2005-2010 - La force des liens.* Ministère de la Santé et des Services sociaux, ISBN- 13 : 978-2-550-47927-7, Québec, Québec

Mojtabai, R. (2008). Increase in antidepressant medication in the US adult population between 1990 and 2003. *Psychotherapy and Psychosomatics*, Vol. 77, No. 2 (January), pp. 83-92, ISSN 0033-3190

Mojtabai, R., Olfson, M. & Mechanic, D. (2002). Perceived need and help-seeking in adults with mood, anxiety, or substance use disorders. *Archives of General Psychiatry*, Vol. 59, No. 1, (January 2002), pp. 77-84, ISSN 0003-990X

Morden, N. E., Mistler, L.A., Weeks, W.B. & Bartels, S.J. (2009). Health care for patients with serious mental illness: family medicine's role. *Journal of the American Board of Family Medicine*, Vol. 22, No. 2, (March-April 2009), pp. 187-195, ISSN 1557-2625

Moulding, R., Grenier, J., Blashki, G., Ritchie, P., Pirkis, J. & Chomienne, M.H. (2009). Integrating psychologists into the Canadian health care system: the example of Australia. *Canadian Journal of Public Health*, Vol. 100, No. 2, (March-April 2009), pp. 145-147, ISSN 0008-4263

Mueser, K.T. & McGurk, S.R. (2004). Schizophrenia. *Lancet, Vol.* 363, No. 9426, (June 2004), pp. 2063-2072, ISSN 1745-1701

Mykletun, A., Knudsen, A.K., Tangen, T. & Overland, S. (2010). General practitioners' opinions on how to improve treatment of mental disorders in primary health care. Interviews with one hundred Norwegian general practitioners. *BMC Health Services Research*, Vol. 10, (February 2010), pp. 35, ISSN 1472-6963

Myhr, G. & Payne, K. (2006). Cost-effectiveness of cognitive-behavioural therapy for mental disorders: Implications for public health care funding policy in Canada. *Canadian Journal of Psychiatry*, Vol. 51, No. 10, (September 2006), pp. 662-670, ISSN 0706-7437

Nabalamba, A. & Millar, W.J. (2007). Going to the doctor. *Health Reports*, Vol. 18, No.1, (February 2007), pp. 23-35, ISSN 0840-6529

Narrow, W.E., Regier, D.A., Norquist, G., Rae, D.S., Kennedy, C. & Arons, B. (2000). Mental health service use by Americans with severe mental illnesses. *Social Psychiatry and Psychiatric Epidemiology*, Vol. 35, No. 4, (April 2000), pp. 147-155, ISSN 0933-7954

Nelson, G. (2006). Mental Health Policy in Canada. In *Canadian Social Policy: Issues and Perspectives* (4th ed), Westhues, A. (Ed.), pp. 245-266, Wilfrid Laurier University Press, ISBN 0889204055, Waterloo, Ontario

Nolan, P. & Badger, F. (Eds.) (2002). *Promoting collaboration in primary mental health care*, Nelson Thormes, ISBN 0-7487-5874-7, Cheltenham, United Kingdom

Olfson, M., Marcus, S.C., Druss, B. & Pincus, H.A. (2002). National trends in the use of outpatient psychotherapy. *American Journal of Psychiatry*, Vol. 159, No. 11 (November 2002), pp. 1914-1920, ISSN 0002-953X

Ordre des infirmières et infirmiers du Québec (2009). *La pratique infirmière en santé mentale. Une contribution essentielle à consolider*, Rapport du comité d'experts sur la pratique infirmière en santé mentale et en soins psychiatriques, Ordre des infirmières et infirmiers du Québec, ISBN 978-2-89229-487-3, Westmount, Québec

Ouadahi, Y., Lesage, A., Rodrigue, J. & Fleury, M.-J. (2009). Les problèmes de santé mentale sont-ils détectés par les omnipraticiens? Regard sur la perspective des omnipraticiens selon les banques de données administratives. *Santé mentale au Québec*, Vol. 34. No. 1 (Spring 2009), pp. 161-172, ISSN 0383-6320

Parslow, R.A. & Jorm, A.F. (2000). Who uses mental health services in Australia? An analysis of data from the National Survey of Mental Health and Wellbeing. *Australian and New Zealand Journal of Psychiatry*, Vol. 34, No. 6, (December 2000), pp. 997-1008, ISSN 0004-8674

Pawlenko, N. (2005). *Collaborative Mental Health Care in Primary Health Care Settings Across Canada. A Policy Review. Canadian Collaborative Mental Health Initiative*. Health Canada's Primary Health Care Transition Fund, ISBN 1-896014-78-X, Mississauga, Ontario

Perrault, M., Wiethaueper, D., Perreault, N., Bonin, J.P., Brown, T.G. & Brunaud, H. (2009). Meilleures pratiques et formation dans le contexte de continuum en santé mentale et en toxicomanie: le programme de formation croisée du sud-ouest de Montréal. *Santé mentale au Québec*, Vol. 34, No. 1, (Spring 2009), pp. 143-160, ISSN 0383-6320

Pescosolido, B.A., Gardner, C.B. & Lubell, K.M. (1998). How people get into mental health services: stories of choice, coercion and "muddling through" from "First-timers". *Social Science & Medicine*, Vol. 46, No. 2, (January 1998), pp. 275-286, ISSN 0277-9536

Provan, K.G. & Milward, B.H. (1995). Preliminary Theory of Interorganizational Network Effectiveness: A Comparative Study of Four Community Mental Health Systems. *Administrative Science Quarterly*, Vol. 40, No. 1, (March 1995), pp. 1-33, ISSN 0001-8392

Pong, R. (2005). *Répartition géographique des médecins au Canada : au-delà du nombre et du lieu*. Institut canadien d'information sur la santé, ISBN 1-55392-738-9, Ottawa, Canada

Reavley, N.J. & Jorm, A.F. (2010). The quality of mental disorder information websites: A review. *Patient Education and Counselling*, Vol. 85, No. 2, (November 2010), p.p. 216-e25, ISSN 0738-3991

Regier, D.A., Farmer, M.E., Rae, D.S., Locke, B.Z., Keith, S.J., Judd, L.L. & Goodwin, F.K. (1990). Comorbidity of mental disorders with alcohol and other drug abuse. Results from the Epidemiological Catchment Area (ECA) Study. *Journal of the American Medical Association*, Vol. 264, No. 19, (November 1990), pp. 2511-2518, ISSN 0098-7484

Rhodes, A.E. & Fung, K. (2004). Self-reported use of mental health services versus administrative records: care to recall? *International Journal of Methods in Psychiatric Research*, Vol. 13, No. 3, (August 2004), pp. 165-175, ISSN 1094-8931

Rockman, P., Salach, L., Gotlib, D., Cord, M. & Turner, T. (2004). Shared mental health care. Model for supporting and mentoring family physicians. *Canadian Family Physician*, Vol. 50, No. 3, (March 2004), pp. 397-402, ISSN 008-350X

Rothman, A.A. & Wagner E.H. (2003). Chronic Illness Management: What is the role of primary care? *Annals of Internal Medicine*, Vol. 138, No. 3, (February 2003), pp. 256-262, ISSN 0003-4819

Rush, B.R., Urbanoski, K.A., Bassani, D.G., Castel, S. & Wild, T.W. (2010). The epidemiology of co-occurring substance use and other mental disorders in Canada: Prevalence, service use and unmet needs. In *Mental disorder in Canada; an epidemiological perspective*, Cairney, J. & Streiner, D.L. (Eds.), pp. 144-169, University of Toronto Press, ISBN 978-8020-9202-1, Toronto, Buffalo, London

Savard, I. & Rodrigue, J. (2007). *Des omnipraticiens à la grandeur du Québec. Évolution des effectifs et des profils de pratique. Données de 1996-1997 à 2005-2006*. Direction de la planification et de la régionalisation – Fédération des Médecins Omnipraticiens du Québec (FMOQ), ISBN 978-550-55141-6, Québec, Canada

Schmitz, N., Wang, J., Malla, A. & Lesage, A. (2007). Joint effect of depression and chronic conditions on disability: results from a population-based study. *Psychosomatic Medicine*, Vol. 69, No. 4, (May 2007), pp. 332-338, ISSN 0333-3174

Seekles, W., van Straten, A., Beekman, A., van Marwijk, H. & Cuijpers, P. (2009). Stepped care for depression and anxiety: from primary care to specialized mental health care: a randomised controlled trial testing the effectiveness of a stepped care program among primary care patients with mood or anxiety disorders. *BMC Health Services Research*, Vol. 9, (June 2009), pp. 90, ISSN 1472-6963

Shortell, S.M., Gillies, R.R. & Anderson, D.A. (1994). The new world of managed care: creating organized delivery systems.. *Health Affairs*, Vol. 13, No. 5 (Winter 1994), pp. 46-64, ISSN 1544-5208

Simonet, D. (2009). Changes in the delivery of primary care and in private insurers' role in United Kingdom, Italy, Germany, Swittzerland and France. *Journal of Medical Marketing*, Vol. 9, No. 2, (June 2009), pp. 96-103, ISSN 1745-7904

Skinner, W., O'Grady, C., Bartha, C. & Parker, C. (2004). *Les troubles concomitants de toxicomanie et de santé mentale*, Centre de toxicomanie et de santé mentale, ISBN 0-88868-475-4, Toronto, Ontario

Slade, M., Leese, M., Cahill, S., Thornicroft, G. & Kuipers, E. (2005). Patient-rated mental health needs and quality of life improvement. *British Journal of Psychiatry*, Vol. 187, (September 2005), pp. 256-261, ISSN 0007-1250

Smith, G.C. (2009). From consultation-liaison psychiatry to integrated care for multiple and complex needs. *Australian and New Zealand Journal of Psychiatry*, Vol. 43, No. 1, (January 2009), pp. 1-12, ISSN 0004-8674

Starfield, B. (2008). The importance of Primary Health Care in Health Systems. Qatar-EMRO Primary Health Care Conference Doha, Qatar, June 27 2011. Available from: gis.emro.who.int/HealthSystemObservatory/Workshops/QatarConference/PPt%20converted%20to%20PDF/Day%202/P%20Reg%20Experiences%20and%20Innovative%20Solution/Dr%20B.%20Starfield%20-%20Importance%20of%20PC.pdf

Starfield, B., Shi, L. & Macinko, J. (2005). Contribution of primary care to health systems and health. *Milbank Quarterly*, Vol. 83, No. 3, pp. 457-502, ISSN 0887-378X

Starfield, B. (1998). Primary care visits and health policy. *Canadian Medical Association Journal*, Vol. 159, No. 7, (October 1998), pp. 795-796, ISSN 0820-3946

Statistics Canada (2002). Santé mentale et bien-être, *Enquête sur la santé dans les collectivités canadiennes de 2002 (ESCC-2002); June 27 2011. Available from*: dsp-psd.pwgsc.gc.ca/Collection/Statcan/82-617-X/82-617-XIF.html

The Commonwealth Fund (2008). *W2008 Commonwealth Fund International Health Policy Survey of Sicker adults June 29 2011,* Available from: www.commonwealthfund.org/Content/Surveys/2008/2008-Commonwealth-FundInternational-Health-Policy-Survey-of-Sicker-Adults.aspx

Tempier, R., Meadows, G.N., Vasiliadis, H.M., Mosier, K.E., Lesage, A., Stiller, A., Graham, A. & Lepnurm, M. (2009) Mental disorders and mental health care in Canada and Australia: comparative epidemiological findings. *Social Psychiatry and Psychiatric Epidemiology*, Vol. 44, No. 1, (January 2009), pp. 63-72, ISSN 0933-7954

Trifiro, G., Barbui, C., Spina, E., Moretti, S., Tari, M., Alacqua, M., Caputi, A.P., UVEC Group & Arcoraci, V. (2007). Antidepressant drugs: prevalence, incidence and indication of use in general practice of Southern Italy during the years 2003-2004. *Pharmacoepidemiology and Drug Safety*, Vol. 16, No. 5, (May 2007), pp. 552-559, ISSN 1099-1557

Tylee, A. (2006). Identifying and managing depression in primary care in the United Kingdom. *Journal of Clinical Psychiatry*, Vol. 67, Suppl. 6, (2006), pp. 41-45, ISSN 0160-6689

Tyrer, P. (2009). Are general practitioners really unable to diagnose depression? *Lancet*, Vol. 374, No. 9690, (August 2009), pp. 589-590, ISSN 0140-6736

Upshur, C. & Weinreb, L. (2008). A survey of primary care provider attitudes and behaviors regarding treatment of adult depression: what changes after a collaborative care intervention? *Primary Care Companion of the Journal of Clinical Psychiatry*, Vol. 10, No. 3, (June 2008), pp. 182-186, ISSN 2150-1319

Valenstein, M., Klinkman, M., Becker, S., Blow, F.C., Barry, K.L., Sattar, A. & Hill, E. (1999). Concurrent treatment of patients with depression in the community: provider practices, attitudes, and barriers to collaboration. *Journal of Family Practice*, Vol. 48, No. 3, (March 1999), pp. 180-187, ISSN 1091-7527

Van Rijswijk, E., van Hout, H., van de Lisdonk, E., Zitman, F. & van Weel, C. (2009). Barriers in recognising, diagnosing and managing depressive and anxiety disorders as experienced by Family Physicians; a focus group study. *BMC Family Practice*, Vol. 10, (July 2009), pp. 52, ISSN 1471-2296

Vasiliadis, H.M., Lesage, A., Adair, C., Wang, P.S. & Kessler, R.C. (2007). Do Canada and the United States differ in prevalence of depression and utilization of services. *Psychiatric Services*, Vol. 58, No. 1, (January 2007), pp. 63-71, ISSN 1075-2730

Wagner, E., Austin, B.T., Davis, C., Hindmarsh, M., Schaefer, J. & Bonomi, A. (2001). Improving chronic illness care: translating evidence into action. *Health Affairs*, Vol. 20, No. 6, (November-December 2001), pp. 64-78, ISSN 1544-5208

Walters, P., Tylee A. & Goldberg D. (2008). Psychiatry in primary care. In *Essential psychiatry,* Murray, R.M., Kendler, K.S., McGuffin, P., Wessely, S. & Castle, D.J. (Eds.), pp. 479-

497, Cambridge University Press, ISBN 978-0-521-6408-6, Cambridge, United Kingdom

Wang, P.S., Aguilar-Gaxiola, S., Alonso, J., Angermeyer, M.C., Borges, G., Bromet, E.J., Bruffaerts, R., de Girolamo, G., de Graaf, R., Gureje, O., Haro, J.M., Karam, E.G., Kessler, R.C., Kovess, V., Lane, M.C., Lee, S., Levinson, D., Ono, Y., Petukhova M., Posada-Villa, J., Seedat, S. & Wells, J.E. (2007). Use of mental health services for anxiety, mood, and substance disorders in 17 countries in the WHO world mental health surveys. *Lancet*, Vol. 370, No. 9590, (September 2007), pp. 841-850, ISSN 0140-6736

Wang, P.S., Berglund, P., Olfson, M., Pincus, H.A., Wells, K.B. & Kessler, R.C. (2005a). Failure and delay in initial treatment contact after first onset of mental disorders in the National Comorbidity Survey Replication, *Archives of General Psychiatry*, Vol. 62, No. 6, (June 2005), pp. 603-613, ISSN 0003-990X

Wang, P.S., Lane, M., Olfson, M., Pincus, H.A., Wells, K.B. & Kessler, R.C. (2005b). Twelve-month use of mental health services in the United States: results from the National Comorbidity Survey Replication. *Archives of General Psychiatry*, Vol. 62, No. 6, (June 2005), pp. 629-640, ISSN 0003-990X

Wang, P.S., Berglund. P. & Kessler, R.C. (2000). Recent care of common mental disorders in the United States: prevalence and conformance with evidence-based recommendations. *Journal of General Internal Medicine*, Vol. 15, No. 5, (May 2000), pp. 284-292, ISSN 0084-8734

Weinreb, L., Gelberg, L., Arangua, L. & Sullivan, M. (2005). Disorders and health problems: overview, in *Encyclopedia of Homelessness*, Vol. 1, Levinson, D. (Ed), pp. 115-123, Sage Publications, ISBN 0-7619-2751-4, Thousand Oaks, California

Williams, J.J. Jr, Gerrity, M., Holsinger, T., Dobscha, S., Gaynes, B. & Dietrich, A. (2007). Systematic review of multifaceted interventions to improve depression care. *General Hospital Psychiatry*, Vol. 29, No. 2, (April 2007), pp. 91-116, ISSN 1945-4953

World Health Organization (2008). *The World Health Report 2008: Primary Health Care (Now More than Ever)*, World Health Organization, ISBN 13-9789241563734, Geneva, Switzerland

World Health Organization (2006). The World Health Report 2006: Working together for health. World Health Organization, ISBN 92-4-156317-6, Geneva, Switzerland

World Health Organization (2001). *The World Health Report 2001: Mental health: new understanding, new hope*. World Health Organization, ISBN 92-4-156201-3, Geneva, Switzerland

World Health Organization (1978). Declaration of Alma Ata, *Primary Health Care: Report of the International Conference on Primary Health Care, Alma-Ata, USSR, 6-12 September 1978*, Geneva, Switzerland

Wright, M.J., Harmon, K.D., Bowman, J.A., Lewin, T.J. & Carr, V.J. (2005). Caring for depressed patients in rural communities: general practitioners' attitudes, needs and relationships with mental health services. *Australian Journal of Rural Health*, Vol. 13, No.1, (February 2005), pp. 21-27, ISSN 1038-5282

Younes, N., Gasquet, I., Gaudebout, P., Chaillet, M.P., Kovess, V., Falissard, B. & Hardy Bayle, M.C. (2005). General practitioners' opinions on their practice in mental health and their collaboration with mental health professionals. *BMC Family Practice*, Vol. 6, No. 1, (May 2005), pp. 18, ISSN 1471-2296

7

Health Care Under the Influence: Substance Use Disorders in the Health Professions

Diane Kunyk and Charl Els
University of Alberta
Canada

1. Introduction

Substance use disorders are expressed within most age, economic, cultural, gender, and occupational groupings. They come to expression in individuals who may be considered vulnerable on biological, psychological, social, family, or spiritual levels. As with other mental disorders, vulnerability differs between individuals with both nature and nurture influencing their risk. Some health care professionals will also develop these chronic disorders regardless of any special knowledge or experience they may have. When substance use disorders are expressed within the health care professions, the delivery of safe, competent, compassionate, and ethical care is threatened. The health of the health care professional is also at risk as the substance use disorders typically progress in severity and may result in premature death.

This is often a sensitive issue to address yet its importance demands the concerted attention of the health care professions. The following chapter begins with background on the issue of substance use disorders within the health care professions, followed by a discussion of mitigating associated risks, and an exploration of disciplinary and alternative to discipline policies. This chapter is focused primarily on literature on physicians and nurses because of the predominance of research in these disciplines. The argument will be made that creating conditions that encourage early identification, reduce barriers to treatment, and that include long-term monitoring programs provide the best conditions for ameliorating the risks resulting from substance use disorders amongst the health care professions to patient safety and health care professional health.

2. Background

It has been argued that the substance use disorders are the most important illnesses of our time because they are the most prevalent mental disorder, the leading preventable cause of death and disease, and the single greatest contributor to excess health care spending (Els, 2007). Their scope is widespread as they affect the health and wellbeing of individuals, families, and society at large. The substance use disorders are a leading occupation health issue, ranking second as the cause of disability, and affect individuals predominantly in their prime working years.

The substance use disorders are chronic, progressive, and potentially fatal illnesses that are recognized by both the major disease classification systems as bona fide, chronic and relapsing medical conditions (American Psychiatric Association [APA], 2000; World Health Organization [WHO], 2007). Research has demonstrated that repeated exposure to substances over time might alter brain structure, chemistry, and function in susceptible individuals. The American Psychiatric Association's [APA](2000) *Diagnostic and Statistical Manual of Mental Disorders,* 4th edition, text revision (*DSM-IV-TR*) classification of Substance Use Disorders includes the disorders of Substance Dependence and Substance Abuse.

Substance Dependence is described as the continued use of a substance despite significant substance-related problems and a pattern of repeated self-administration that can result in tolerance, withdrawal, and compulsive drug-taking behaviour. Craving, defined as a strong desire to use the substance, is experienced by most individuals. Substance dependence as characterized by a maladaptive pattern of substance use, leading to clinically significant impairment or distress, and manifested by three (or more) of the following occurring at any time in the same 12-month period:

- Tolerance as defined by either of the a need for markedly increased amounts of the substance to achieve intoxication or desired effect, or markedly diminished effect with continued use of the same amount of the substance,
- Withdrawal as manifested by the characteristic withdrawal syndrome for the substance, or by the ingestion of the same (or a closely related) to relieve or avoid withdrawal symptoms,
- Taking of the substance in larger amounts, or over a longer period, than was intended,
- Persistent desire or unsuccessful efforts to cut down or control substance use,
- Spending a great deal of time in activities to obtain the substance, use the substance, or recover from its effects,
- Reduction or abstinence of important social, occupational, or recreational activities because of substance use,
- Continued substance use despite knowledge of having a persistent or recurrent physical or psychological problem that is likely to have been caused or exacerbated by the substance (APA, 2000).

Substance Abuse is described as a maladaptive use of chemical substance(s) leading to clinically significant outcomes or distress (i.e.. recurrent legal problems, failure to perform at work/home/school, and physically hazardous behaviour). The criteria do *not* include tolerance, withdrawal, or a pattern of compulsive use. Instead it includes the harmful consequences of repeated use. It is pre-empted by the diagnosis of Substance Dependence at any point in the individual's life, and for that specific class (or classes) of substances. Substance Abuse is manifested by one (or more) of the following occurring within a 12-month period:

- Recurrent substance use resulting in a failure to fulfill major role obligations at work, school, or home (e.g., repeated absences or poor work performance related to substance use; suspensions from school; neglect of children),
- Recurrent substance use in situations in which it is physically hazardous (e.g., driving an automobile impaired by substance use),
- Recurrent substance-related legal problems (e.g., arrests for substance-related disorderly conduct),

- Continued substance use despite having persistent or recurrent social or interpersonal problems caused or exacerbated by the effects of the substance (e.g., arguments with spouse about consequences of intoxication) (APA, 2000).

It has been proposed that the substance use disorders will have different criteria in the upcoming American Psychiatric Association DSM-5. Under the new classification of Substance Use and Addictive Disorders, the proposed revision collapses the existing division between dependence and abuse, and lists the existing indicators together (for a total of 11 indicators). Severity of the disorder will be described as moderate with the presence of 2-3 positive criteria and severe for 4 or more positive criteria. The term 'Physiological Dependence' will refer to evidence of tolerance and/or withdrawal (American Psychiatric Association [APA], 2011).

Individuals in the *pedestal professions* are also potentially vulnerable to developing substance dependence or substance abuse, and some health care professionals will be affected regardless of any special knowledge, skills, or insights they may have due to their education and professional experience. The health care professional might have entered their career with a family history of members with these disorders or other vulnerabilities that place them at risk (Kenna & Wood, 2005). There is evidence suggesting health care professionals may be placed at increased risk for developing these disorders because of work related factors such as high job strain, disruption and fatigue related to shift work and long hours, ease of access to medications in the workplace, self-treatment of pain and emotional problems, working in certain specialties, and knowledge of the benefits of medications (Lillibridge et al., 2002; McAuliffe et al., 1987; Trinkoff & Storr, 1998; Trinkoff et al., 2000; Wright, 1990).

Since the late 1970's, numerous studies have examined the use of substances among health care professionals. Methodological inconsistencies between these studies do not allow for direct comparisons or conclusions. In general, however, it appears that health care professionals are affected at rates similar to the general population with possibly higher patterns of use for substances they may have access to within the workplace (Brewster, 1986; Collins, 1999; Hughes et al., 1992; Kenna & Wood, 2004; Kunyk, 2011; Storr et al., 2000; Trinkoff & Storr, 1998; Tyssen, 2007). If this conclusion is accurate, then approximately 8.5% of health care professionals will have an alcohol use disorder (Hasin et al., 2007), and a further 2% (Compton et al., 2007) will experience a drug use disorder within the next 12 months.

3. Mitigation of risk

Substance use disorders within the health care professions is a serious and complex issue for the individual with the disease as well as their families, patients, colleagues, professional body, employer, and society at large. The health of the health care professional is threatened as these disorders typically progress in severity and may result in premature death (Kleber et al., 2006). Health care professionals are in a safety-sensitive positions; their occupational functioning impacts public safety. Patient safety may be placed at risk when health providers practice with active, untreated substance use disorders as alertness, attention, concentration, reaction time, coordination, memory, multi-tasking abilities, perception, thought processing, and judgment can be compromised (Graham et al., 2003).

When substance use disorders are expressed in health care professionals, the goal is for early identification, treatment, documentation, and monitoring of ongoing recovery prior to the illness impacting the care of patients or the health of the health care provider with the disorder. Achieving this goal also reduces the risks of these disorders to the health of the health care professional. The global and chronic shortage of health care professionals (World Health Organization [WHO], 2006) confirms that early identification, recovery, and return to work are critical goals for society. As a group, however, health care professionals often ignore our collective responsibility for identifying, treating, and supporting our colleagues when a substance use disorder comes to expression (Talbot & Wilson, 2005).

3.1 Early Identification

Early identification of health care professionals affected by substance use is necessary to protect the safety of patients and to achieve the best possible outcomes for the health of the health provider. This is a challenging goal as early evidence of the disease may be difficult to identify. Research suggests that the order in which the effects of substance use disorders in physicians are first observed starts with the family, then the community, next is financial, spiritual, emotional and physical health, after which job performance is finally impacted (Talbott & Wilson, 2003).

As the work area is the last place where substance use by the health care professional is apparent, identification may occur late in the progression of the Substance Use Disorder. Identification of concerns about the use of substances by a health care professional on their practice, or on their health, may be self-identified, identified by their colleagues or through a formal complaint to the employer or regulatory body. These will now be discussed.

3.1.1 Self-identification

Health care professionals are ethically required to ensure their fitness to practice by withdrawing, restricting, or accommodating their practice if unable to safely perform essential functions of their role. This responsibility can be interpreted to necessitate self-removal from the work setting if the health care professional questions his/her use of alcohol and/or drugs. For the purposes of ongoing registration, health care professionals may be required to self-identify whether the use of alcohol and/or other drugs may impair their ability to practice upon their initial registration as well as on their annual practice permit application.

There is some evidence to suggest that nurses may be more cognizant of the need to access treatment for their substance use, and more engaged in treatment, when compared with the general population. Within a sample of 129 registered nurses self-identified with substance dependence in the last 12 months, 27 (22.3%) had sought help for their use of alcohol and/or drugs within the last 12 months. Slightly more (28; 23.2%) thought they should seek help but had not done so. Most of this subset (23; 82.0%) indicated they did not get help because they were too embarrassed to discuss it with anyone. The next most cited reason (18; 53.2%) was they did not think anyone could help (Kunyk, 2011). That almost one quarter of nurses with substance dependence were receiving some help is a positive finding. As almost one quarter aware of their need for assistance with their alcohol and/or drug use but had not done so suggests there is a tremendous opportunity to mitigate the risks associated with substance use.

Reducing the barriers to self-identification and treatment seeking is one measure to mitigate risks associated with substance use disorders in the health care professions. Stigma is a key barrier for anyone impacted by the substance use disorders. Stigma is not confined to the general public; it also occurs among health professionals (Standing Senate Committee on Social Affairs, 2006). Some nurses have acknowledged delaying treatment seeking because of stigma felt within the workplace, and this procrastination prolonged their recovery (Lillibridge et al., 2002). Darbro (2005, p.179) noted that a 'culture of mistreatment of addicts in the workplace by health care professionals' was listed as a reason for concealing their illness from colleagues, and that this procrastination prolonged their recovery. In this sense, the environment in which the health care professional works can be a part of the problem.

Confidentiality provides a level of protection from stigma and, for this reason, is considered an essential precondition to successful treatment for individuals with substance use disorders (Roberts & Dyer, 2004). Confidentiality may be placed at risk when health care professionals with substance use disorders seek treatment when their employer is also their health care professional. Confidentiality is also not afforded when health care professionals are subject to formal investigations, open hearing tribunals, and publication of discipline decisions.

"Wearing Two Hats": When the Employer is the Treatment Provider

---

In some situations, health care professionals may be placed in the position of receiving treatment from their employer for their substance use disorder. As the substance use disorders are highly stigmatizing illnesses, confidentiality by the treatment provider is a critical necessity for the individual seeking treatment. However, the employer is also responsible for assuring the provision of safe care by their employees. What are the responsibilities when a treatment provider learns that their health care professional-employee has a substance use disorder?

The Alberta Office of the Information and Privacy Commissioner (Order H2011-001) made a ruling on this question when a complaint was lodged against Alberta Health Services' (AHS) collection, use, and disclosure of the health information of an employee with a substance use disorder. In this case, the health care professional (an employee of AHS) attended addiction counseling through AHS Mental Health and Addiction Services. The counselor provided the information obtained to the AHS human resources department. This information was then used to conduct an investigation that resulted in suspension from employment. The health information was also disclosed to the regulator/professional body.

In examining the case, the Adjudicator raised a number of important questions and conclusions:

- Why would subjecting an individual to a human resource investigation be necessary for promoting and protecting the public health (Section 52),
- Why would an employee receiving treatment for a relapse pose a threat to public health (Section 530),
- Disciplining health professionals rather than treating them is not in the best interests of either health care professionals or their patients given the risk that health care professionals will not seek treatment to avoid professional repercussions. To better protect patients, the privacy of health care professionals should be protected. Patient confidentiality is key to providing reasonable healthcare. Employees/health care

professionals are entitled to the same level of reasonable health care (and confidentiality) as other Albertans (Section 59),

- There is nothing in the Health Information Act that suggests that patients who are also health care professionals should have less protection in relation to their health information than anyone else seeking health services has (Section 71), and
- The AHS interpretation would have *'the extremely deleterious chilling effect of discouraging health care professionals with health problems which could be seen as adversely affecting their ability to perform their employment duty from seeking treatment in order to avoid these problems from coming to light. This approach would have the effect of exacerbating the problems to patient care that the provision is seeking to avoid* (Section 72).'

The Arbitrator concluded that when individually identifying health information was transferred between the addictions counselor and the acting manager and employees of human resources for the purpose of conducting a human resources investigation, this was an internal use of health information, and that the disclosure of health information and also that the professional body contravened the Health Information Act. The employer was ordered to cease collecting, using and disclosing health information in contravention of the Health Information Act.

This decision provides clarification regarding the protection of confidentiality for the health care professional who is receiving treatment, and the boundaries between the role of treatment provider and employer. It is consistent with the American Medical Association (2008) statement that *'as patients, physicians are entitled to the same right to privacy and confidentiality of personal medical information as any other patient'*.

Source: Alberta, Office of the Information and Privacy Commissioner, Order H2011-001, July 29, 2011, Alberta Health Services, Case File Number H3350 (www.oipc.ab.ca)

3.1.2 Peer identification

Perhaps one of the more difficult challenges health care professionals may have to confront in their careers is to determine their obligations when they suspect substance use is affecting the performance of a colleague. Taking action may feel overwhelming when faced with uncertainty about how to proceed, the knowledge that raising concerns in such situations is often difficult at best, and the awareness that any action may permanently risk the reputation of the colleague under concern. There is also the reality that the health care professionals involved in this situation may continue to work together and that action (or inaction) will impact on their ongoing relationship.

Health care professionals are morally, and often legally, compelled to address threats to the delivery of safe, competent, compassionate, and ethical care, as may be the case when the practice of their colleagues may be impaired by the use of substances. Moral obligations are also raised when health care professionals develop substance use disorders, as they would be for any other health care professional with an illness, but particularly when the high stress of caring work and access to substances has placed them at risk (Kunyk & Austin, 2011). For any health care professional having concerns about a colleague, their professional and ethical requirement is to report these.

The urgency of patient safety in the immediate situation is clearly of utmost priority and health care professionals are obliged to intervene when they perceive patient risk. If harm is not imminent, health care professionals are obligated to address their concerns as directly as possible in ways that are consistent with the good of all parties. When appropriate and feasible, actions may include:

- Directly seek input from the colleague whose behaviour or practice has raised concern,
- Maintaining a high level of confidentiality about the situation and actions,
- Seek information from relevant authorities (e.g. supervisor or manager) on expected roles and responsibilities for all of the parties, and
- Consult the relevant professional association and/or regulatory body for guidance and/or to assist in addressing and resolving the problem.

With these initial steps, the colleague may be approached, and advice and direction sought, without revealing the identity of the colleague with the suspected problem (Canadian Nurses Association [CNA], 2008, p. 41).

There are members of the health care community who do not believe they have the able to recognize or to assist when the practice of a colleague may be impaired by the presence of an active and untreated substance use disorder. In an Internet survey of 4064 registered nurses, 98% nurses understood the importance of identifying impaired practice. But only 53% were confident in their abilities to recognize or intervene when it occurs (Kunyk, 2011). Health care professionals must learn about, and become sensitive to, signs of substance use affecting the professional performance of their colleagues. As the substance use disorders are potentially fatal, and impaired practice places patient care at risk, early detection may save their colleagues' or a patients' life.

The manifestations of impaired practice tend to be varied and non-specific. Early on, patterns of high alcohol intake at social events or generalized irritability might be observed. Later they may be as overt as intoxication, with symptoms of ataxia and dysarthia, while at work (Berge et al., 2009). Behaviours associated with physicians might include late rounds, unavailability or inappropriate responses to calls, and prolonged or failure to respond to paging (Talbott & Wilson, 2003). It has been noted that nurses may volunteer to give pain relief to their colleagues patients, wait until alone in the medication room before opening the narcotics cabinet, and consistently sign out more narcotics that their peers (Quinlan, 2003). When the substance of choice is diverted from the workplace, the health provider may show up at work when not scheduled or work longer hours. For health care professionals, alcohol is the most common drug of choice followed by opioids, and multiple drug use is not uncommon (Glasser et al., 1986. Gossop et al., 2001; Reading, 1992). Berge, Seppela and Schipper (2009) have identified specific behaviours suggestive of alcohol dependence and opiate dependence in health care professionals (Table 1).

When concerns about substance use on their professional practice are addressed, the health care professional may reject the possibility. Others may be relieved that they were approached. The identification of the problem by a nurse colleague can be the turning point for recovery (Lillibridge et al., 2002). Recovered nurses have reported that they felt let down when other nurses failed to recognize or confront their substance problem, and some recovered colleagues feel that the intervention probably saved their lives (Lillibridge et al., 2002). In fact, having the support of colleagues is perceived as one of the most important factors in a successful recovery (Hughes, 1998).

When addressing concerns, the objectives are for the health care professional to immediately discontinue work and directly proceed to have a comprehensive assessment to determine the presence of a substance use disorder. With a compassionate, non-confrontational approach, an assessment and discontinuation of work is strongly advised because concerns have arisen without pressing the issue of whether or not there is a bona fide problem. If this is refused, then the individual is advised that the alternative is to refer the matter to the regulatory board (Skipper, 2009). Referral options and an action plan should be in place so that the health care professional-patient will be enabled to follow the recommended assessment and/or treatment. Arguments have been made for a chain-of-custody transfer of the health care professional-patient to the area where the assessment will occur to decrease the risk of a tragic outcome (Berge et al., 2009).

Signs Suggestive of Alcohol Dependence

- Alcohol on breath
- Slurred speech
- Ataxia
- Erratic performance or decrement in performance
- Tremulousness
- 'Out of control' behavior at social events
- Problems with law enforcement
- Hidden bottles
- Poor personal hygiene
- Failure to remember events, conversations or commitments
- Tardiness
- Frequent hangovers
- Poor early morning performance
- Unexplained absences
- Unusual traumatic injuries
- Mood swings
- Irritability
- Sweating
- Domestic/marital problems
- Isolation
- Leaving the workplace early on a regular basis

Signs Suggestive of Opioid Dependence

- Periods of agitation (withdrawal) alternating with calm (drug was just taken)
- Dilated pupils (withdrawal) or pinpoint pupils (side effect of opiate)
- Excessive sweating
- Wearing long sleeves
- Frequent bathroom breaks
- Unexplained absences during the workday
- Spending more hours at work than necessary
- Volunteering for extra call / work
- Volunteering to provide extra breaks or refusing breaks
- Volunteering to clean operating rooms
- Volunteering to return waste drugs to pharmacy

- Rummaging in sharps container
- Slopping record keeping or discrepancies between charted dose and actual dose delivered
- Excessive narcotic use charted for patients
- Assay of waste drug returned showing evidence of dilution
- Never returning any waster at the end of a case
- Patients reporting pain out of proportion to charted narcotic dose

Source: Berge, K.H., Seppela, M.D., Schipper, A.M. (2009). Chemical dependency and the physician. *Mayo Clinical Proceedings 84*(7): 625-631.

Table 1. Possible Signs Suggestive of Substance Dependence in a Health Care Professional

3.1.3 Formal complaint

Both health organizations and regulatory bodies have responsibilities to ensure their patients are receiving safe and ethical care. For regulatory bodies, their mandate is to assure their members are practicing according to their professional standards. But there are also organizational responsibilities to health care professionals with substance use disorders. Human rights legislation in Canada recognizes addiction as a disability. As a result, there exists a duty to accommodate for both the employer and the regulator. Health care professionals with substance use disorders may come to the attention of their regulator and/or employer through formal complaints filed by colleagues, public members, or other individuals. When this occurs, these organizations are required to respond according to their policy directions.

Their options for action will be discussed in section 4.0 on policy alternatives.

3.2 Comprehensive assessment

When concerns about the effects of substance use are identified, the objectives are for immediate withdrawal from practice until a comprehensive assessment may take place. The purpose of this assessment is to establish whether or not the individual has a substance use disorder. One or more medical professionals experienced in the evaluation of substance use disorders and its concomitant problems in health care professionals may perform the assessment (Talbott & Earley, 2003). Certified addiction medicine specialists (American Board of Addiction Medicine [ABAM], 2011) are trained to identify and treat the medical consequences of alcohol and / or substance abuse. These specialists perform a detailed history and examination, and order the appropriate diagnostic and confirmatory testing, to determine the medical diagnosis and recommendations for a range of addiction medicine treatments.

An assessment can determine, with a reasonable degree of medical certainty, if the health professional in question is impaired[1] or potentially impaired because of their use of alcohol and/or other substances. A comprehensive assessment should also determine any coexisting physical or mental problems, and make recommendations for the individual's treatment needs. The assessment team must also determine whether issues involving public

---

[1] The American Medical Association [AMA] Guides to the evaluation of Permanent Impairment, Sixth Ediction (2011) refers to impairment as *'a significant deviation, loss, or loss of use of any body structure or body function in an individual with a health condition, disorder, or disease'.*

health and safety, or violations of ethical standards, require that the health care professional be reported to their regulatory body, if not already aware (Talbott & Earley, 2003).

With a positive diagnosis for a substance use disorder, the first ethical obligation of the health care professional is to remove himself/herself from practice and engage in treatment. Many regulators have a requirement that the member self-report when they have an illness that may possibly impair their ability to practice.

3.3 Detoxification, medical stabilization and treatment

The Substance Use Disorders are widely considered to be amenable to treatment. The outcomes to evidence-based interventions are similar to other chronic disease conditions including hypertension, asthma, and Type 2 diabetes (McLellan et al., 2000). Most persons with a substance use disorder will have one or more relapses (the return to substance use after a drug-free period) during their ongoing process of recovery.

Early intervention with tailored, multi-modal and long-term treatment is generally acknowledged as providing the most beneficial treatment outcomes. These outcomes may include abstinence from, or reduction in, the use of substances, reduction in the frequency and severity of relapse to substance use, improvement in psychological and social functioning, and increased life expectancy (Kleber et al., 2006). For health care professionals, the primary goal is to achieve abstinence and maintain long-term remission of his or her substance use disorder (Talbot & Wilson, 2003).

Comprehensive treatment is aimed at reducing denial, increasing self-care, treating the coexisting family, medical, and psychiatric problems, and helping the health care professional learn to protect himself/herself from the substance use disorder. Safe and effective evidence-based treatments for individuals with substance use disorders requires matching treatment to include the modalities available for the particular disorder and comorbidities, as well as follow-up on a longitudinal basis. Evidence-based treatments for these disorders recognize their chronic and relapsing nature, and this frames recovery as a process as opposed to an event. With this approach, stand-alone interventions such as detoxification and residential treatment are considered as only one component to comprehensive treatment. The National Institute on Drug Abuse [NIDA] has identified thirteen principles for addiction treatment (Table 2).

Comprehensive treatment often includes detoxification, medical stabilization, individual and group therapy, Twelve Step programs, medication as required, written assignments, psychoeducation, family education and therapy, and workplace/lifestyle restructuring. A longitudinal approach to management of this chronic disease is ideal and, in general, the iterative goals of treatment are first to engage, assess, motivate, and help to retain the health care professional-patient in a safe and effective evidence-based treatment setting. Treatment retention and adherence to mutually agreed-upon goals generally maximize potential benefits of treatment and improve outcomes (Kunyk, Els & Robinson Hughes, 2010).

1.	**Addiction is a complex but treatable disease that affects brain function and behavior.** Drugs of abuse alter the brain's structure and function, resulting in changes that persist long after drug use has ceased. This may explain why drug abusers are at risk for relapse even after long periods of abstinence and despite the potentially devastating consequences.
2.	**No single treatment is appropriate for everyone.** Matching treatment settings,

interventions, and services to an individual's particular problems and needs is critical to his or her ultimate success in returning to productive functioning in the family, workplace, and society.

3. **Treatment needs to be readily available.** Because drug-addicted individuals may be uncertain about entering treatment, taking advantage of available services the moment people are ready for treatment is critical. Potential patients can be lost if treatment is not immediately available or readily accessible. As with other chronic diseases, the earlier treatment is offered in the disease process, the greater the likelihood of positive outcomes.

4. **Effective treatment attends to multiple needs of the individual, not just his or her drug abuse.** To be effective, treatment must address the individual's drug abuse and any associated medical, psychological, social, vocational, and legal problems. It is also important that treatment be appropriate to the individual's age, gender, ethnicity, and culture.

5. **Remaining in treatment for an adequate period of time is critical.** The appropriate duration for an individual depends on the type and degree of his or her problems and needs. Research indicates that most addicted individuals need at least 3 months in treatment to significantly reduce or stop their drug use and that the best outcomes occur with longer durations of treatment. Recovery from drug addiction is a longterm process and frequently requires multiple episodes of treatment. As with other chronic illnesses, relapses to drug abuse can occur and should signal a need for treatment to be reinstated or adjusted. Because individuals often leave treatment prematurely, programs should include strategies to engage and keep patients in treatment.

6. **Counseling—individual and/or group—and other behavioral therapies are the most commonly used forms of drug abuse treatment.** Behavioral therapies vary in their focus and may involve addressing a patient's motivation to change, providing incentives for abstinence, building skills to resist drug use, replacing drug-using activities with constructive and rewarding activities, improving problemsolving skills, and facilitating better interpersonal relationships. Also, participation in group therapy and other peer support programs during and following treatment can help maintain abstinence.

7. **Medications are an important element of treatment for many patients, especially when combined with counseling and other behavioral therapies.** For example, methadone and buprenorphine are effective in helping individuals addicted to heroin or other opioids stabilize their lives and reduce their illicit drug use. Naltrexone is also an effective medication for some opioid-addicted individuals and some patients with alcohol dependence. Other medications for alcohol dependence include acamprosate, disulfiram, and topiramate. For persons addicted to nicotine, a nicotine replacement product (such as patches, gum, or lozenges) or an oral medication (such as bupropion or varenicline) can be an effective component of treatment when part of a comprehensive behavioral treatment program.

8. **An individual's treatment and services plan must be assessed continually and modified as necessary to ensure that it meets his or her changing needs.** A patient may require varying combinations of services and treatment components during the course of treatment and recovery. In addition to counseling or psychotherapy, a

patient may require medication, medical services, family therapy, parenting instruction, vocational rehabilitation, and/or social and legal services. For many patients, a continuing care approach provides the best results, with the treatment intensity varying according to a person's changing needs

9. **Many drug-addicted individuals also have other mental disorders.** Because drug abuse and addiction—both of which are mental disorders—often co-occur with other mental illnesses, patients presenting with one condition should be assessed for the other(s). And when these problems co-occur, treatment should address both (or all), including the use of medications as appropriate.

10. **Medically assisted detoxification is only the first stage of addiction treatment and by itself does little to change long-term drug abuse.** Although medically assisted detoxification can safely manage the acute physical symptoms of withdrawal and, for some, can pave the way for effective long-term addiction treatment, detoxification alone is rarely sufficient to help addicted individuals achieve long-term abstinence. Thus, patients should be encouraged to continue drug treatment following detoxification. Motivational enhancement and incentive strategies, begun at initial patient intake, can improve treatment engagement.

11. **Treatment does not need to be voluntary to be effective.** Sanctions or enticements from family, employment settings, and/or the criminal justice system can significantly increase treatment entry, retention rates, and the ultimate success of drug treatment interventions

12. **Drug use during treatment must be monitored continuously, as lapses during treatment do occur.** Knowing their drug use is being monitored can be a powerful incentive for patients and can help them withstand urges to use drugs. Monitoring also provides an early indication of a return to drug use, signaling a possible need to adjust an individual's treatment plan to better meet his or her needs

13. **Treatment programs should assess patients for the presence of HIV/ AIDS, hepatitis B and C, tuberculosis, and other infectious diseases as well as provide targeted risk-reduction counseling to help patients modify or change behaviors that place them at risk of contracting or spreading infectious diseases.** Typically, drug abuse treatment addresses some of the drug-related behaviors that put people at risk of infectious diseases. Targeted counseling specifically focused on reducing infectious disease risk can help patients further reduce or avoid substance-related and other high-risk behaviors. Counseling can also help those who are already infected to manage their illness. Moreover, engaging in substance abuse treatment can facilitate adherence to other medical treatments. Patients may be reluctant to accept screening for HIV (and other infectious diseases); therefore, it is incumbent upon treatment providers to encourage and support HIV screening and inform patients that highly active antiretroviral therapy (HAART) has proven effective in combating HIV, including among drug-abusing populations.

From National Institute on Drug Abuse [NIDA]. (revised April 2009). Available at:
http://www.drugabuse.gov/PODAT/PODATIndex.html

Table 2. Principles of Addiction Treatment

3.4 Continuing care

As the substance use disorders are conceptualized as chronic diseases, detoxification, medical stabilization, and addiction treatments are only the beginning disease management. Upon successful completion of residential care, if necessary, and primary treatment, the health care professional is challenged with sustaining their recovery while returning to work.

After completion of primary treatment, a comprehensive medical assessment by one or more professionals experienced in the evaluation of addiction and its concomitant problems in health care professionals can provide an independent opinion regarding the scope of continuing care required by the recovering health care professional. Total abstinence is the treatment goal and adherence to this goal is assessed repeatedly throughout the ensuring prolonged monitoring programs (Section 3.5). Continuing care plans are individualized but may include specifics regarding:

- Abstinence from all drugs of abuse,
- Frequency of reassessment,
- Addiction medicine physician,
- Required therapy,
- Attendance at mutual help group meetings e.g. *Caduceus,*
- Random urine screening with observed micturition,
- Modifications in practice,
- Workplace surveillance,
- Additional continuing care assignments,
- Protocols to be followed should mood-altering drugs be required for a medical reason,
- Primary care physician,
- Family therapy,
- Contingencies should a relapse to substance use occur, and
- Names of individuals who will support the health care professional in his or her ongoing recovery.

Not all health care professionals receive similar or optimal treatment programs and return-to-work options. An exploratory study compared initial clinical presentations, service utilization patterns, and post-treatment functioning of physicians and nurses with substance use disorders who received services in an addiction treatment program (Shaw et al, 2004). Members of both professions showed comparable results. Prior to participating in the program, nurses showed less personality disturbance than physicians but did tend to work and live in environments with more triggers to relapse. Following their initial hospitalization, nurses received less primary treatment, worked longer hours, and were more symptomatic than physicians. Furthermore, nurses in this study reported more frequent and severe work-related sanctions. The authors conclude that, although in most areas of study, nurses and physicians demonstrated comparable results but that these significant differences suggest these groups may have different clinical needs.

3.5 Monitoring programs

The purpose of monitoring programs are to support the health care professional, monitor their success and intervene with difficulties during the recovery period and, in so doing, protect the public (FSPHP, 2000). Monitoring programs provide the active case management and supervision system for health care professionals who have signed formal, binding contracts for their participation. Health care professionals who refuse to enter into a contract agreement are usually reported to their regulator, if not previously aware.

Monitoring of recovering health care professionals provides a sensitive and specific mechanism for ensuring treatment occurs and for early detection of relapse, and may be a licensing requirement. Much of the work in the area of monitoring programs has been with physicians. There are several designations for these programs such as physician health programs, physician aftercare, physician recovery networks, diversion, alternative to discipline, impaired physician, and physician health effectiveness programs.

The Federation of State Physician Health Programs guidelines require long-term monitoring of physicians after successful completion of treatment with reporting to the appropriate regulatory body any instance of a physician who is not able to cooperate with indicated treatment and monitoring or who becomes impaired (FSPHP, 2008). Through their experience and research, they have concluded that long-term recovery from the substance use disorders are routinely achieved after five years of successful monitored recovery. They further recognize that, after 5 years of monitored recovery, physicians usually are successful in managing further problems in their recovery through the use of their extensive support network while recognizing that some may benefit from shorter or lengthier periods (FSPHP, 2000).

Monitoring includes substance use detection and compliance with specifics of the monitoring contract plan. With random alcohol and drug testing, participating health care professionals call a telephone number daily during the working week to see if they are to be tested that day. A computer is used to randomly assign the decision as to who gets tested that day. The frequency of testing is more often earlier in the beginning of the contract period and less frequent towards the end of the five years.

When contracted, supervised care and monitoring of the health care professional occurs, regulators often defer disciplinary action with the stipulation that evidence of failure to adhere or relapse under patient care conditions will lead to referral of the health care professional back to the regulator (Dupont et al., 2009). A relapse includes the use of alcohol or other drugs non-medically, and also includes failure to adhere to treatment session or other signs of noncompliance.

Monitored care may start with residential or intensive outpatient care in a specially treatment program. Health care professionals commonly withdraw from practice at this time. The choice of treatment provider may be limited to specific programs with which the monitoring program has had extensive, successful experiences, and is known to provide excellent care. Monitoring is initiated or continues when the recovering healthcare professional moves into continuing care.

The evidence suggests that physicians have high rates of recovery when involved in long-term continuing care and monitoring programs. In a five-year, longitudinal cohort study, 904 physicians in 16 state physician health programs in the United States were followed (McLellan, Skipper, Campbell & Dupont, 2007). The outcome measures were program completion, alcohol and drug use, and occupational status at five years. Of the 80.7% of physicians who had completed treatment and resumed practice under supervision and monitoring, alcohol or drug misuse was detected by urine testing in 1.9% over the five years. At the five-year follow-up, 78.7% were licensed and working. The authors concluded that programs with an appropriate combination of treatment, support, and sanctions to manage addiction among physicians are effective.

There is evidence to support this model for a range of populations but its implementation is not consistent across the health care professions. Talbot (2005), in reiterating his earlier work, postulates that the factors that appear to have predictive value in assessing successful recovery include:

- The number of 12-step (or reasonable alternatives) meetings attended per week.
- A working relationship with a sponsor and frequent sponsor contact.
- Random drug screening.
- Monitoring milestones in each stage of recovery.
- Monitoring for the effects of the emergence of compulsive behaviours.
- Evaluation of the status of current therapies, treatments, and medications.
- Assessment of family relationships.
- Physical health status.
- Number of leisure activities per week.
- Compliance with monitoring activities, timely attendance at recommended therapies, and 12-step (or reasonable alternatives) meetings.
- Amount of time spent exercising per week.
- Evaluation of work-related stressors.
- Monitoring of changes in financial status.
- Additional training and/or continuing medical education.
- Self-rated quality of recovery programs.
- The identification of the soft parts of the physician-patient recovery program.

Physicians in continuing care and monitoring programs receive an optimal treatment model that assumes primary medical responsibility for the disease. These programs combines empathic support with the highest level of structure of close monitoring, and sanctions matched according to need. Physicians with substance use disorders treated within this framework have the highest long-term recovery rates recorded in the treatment outcome literature: between 70% and 96% (Brewster et al., 2008; Domino et al, 2005; Gastfriend, 2005; Gold & Aronson, 2005; McLennan et al., 2007; Smith & Smith, 1991, Talbott et al., 1987).

4. Policy alternatives

Organizations including employers, regulators, professional associations, and unions are obliged to respond when they become aware of their health care professionals whose practice may be impaired by use of substances. The purpose of intervening is to protect the public from harm and not to punish the health care professional (CNA, 2009). Responsibilities for ensuring the provision of safe, ethical care meeting the standards of practice for the profession requires the enactment of comprehensive policies. There are two dominant organizational policy responses to substance use disorders among the health professions: discipline and alternative to discipline. Considerable variation exists within each of these groupings due to legislation, structuring of responsibilities, and professional standards.

In general, disciplinary (punitive) policies are designed to penalize health care professionals and prevent them from practicing for the purpose of protecting the public (Monroe, Pearson, & Kenaga, 2008). Disciplinary measures include actions such as termination, probation, practice restrictions, and suspension or revocation of practice licenses (Corsino, Morrow, & Wallace, 1996). Some disciplinary programs may include aftercare, case management, and assistance for re-entering the workforce (Quinlan, 1994).

In the disciplinary model, upon the receipt of a formal complaint (e.g. pharmaceutical theft from the employer, failure to provide analgesics to patients, or falsification of records), a formal investigation may be launched. This may incorporate, among other powers, access to the health care professionals' workplace including interviewing colleagues, managers, and other individuals connected to the nurse under investigation (*Health Professions Act*, 2000, section 63). If supported by sufficient evidence, the complaint proceeds to an open hearing tribunal that may include a lawyer representing the regulator, another for the health care professional in question, and an independent counsel to advise the tribunal panel members of peers. When the health care professional in question is found guilty of unprofessional conduct, sanctions vary but may include:

- A reprimand that the behavior falls below the expected standards for practice,
- Loss of licensure,
- Suspension,
- Restrictions on the practice permit,
- Requirement of supervised practice,
- Ongoing documentation of specified treatment modalities,
- Random drug screening, and
- Publication of the discipline decision with identification of the health care professional by name or license number.

It has been estimated that the process of investigation followed by a formal hearing to determine disciplinary action may take from eight months to three years for resolution and, as the focus is on discipline, there is little attempt to advocate for the individual, provide treatment or rehabilitation services, or follow outcomes (Sullivan, Bissell, & Leffler, 1990).

With alternative to discipline responses, when there is reason to believe that the use of substances are affecting professional performance, the authority (e.g. employer or regulator) requires the health care professional to submit to specified physical and/or mental examinations and withdrawal from providing professional services pending the report. If the presence of an illness is determined (e.g. a substance use disorder), the authority would direct the health care professional to engage in treatment until their addiction treatment team determines readiness to return to work. If the examination does not detect the presence of an illness, the authority may choose to instigate a formal investigation and, when warranted, an open hearing before a tribunal of peers to determine a decision (*Health Professions Act*, 2000).

Alternative to discipline policies focus on early detection of illness, provisions for adequate treatment, and re-entry to practice without prejudice along with measures to protect the public (Monroe et al., 2008). These objective are achieved through:

- A focus on rehabilitation,
- Protection from public disclosure,
- Disclosure to the employer, and
- Long-term monitoring (aftercare) programs upon return to work.

Alternative to discipline policies provide a mechanism for impaired health care professionals to be moved into treatment within hours or days of detection (Monroe et al., 2008). Long-term monitoring reduces risk to patient safety through early detection of relapse while provide support and affording confidentiality and dignity for the health care professional in recovery.

Regardless of the policy approach taken, both the regulator and the employer have the duty to accommodate the individual with a diagnosed substance use disorder.

Comparisons between discipline and alternative policies are complicated by the degree of variation in the approach, time required for treatment and aftercare, and definitions of success. In a review of comparisons of discipline and alternative to discipline approaches among nurses, it was concluded that alternative to discipline seems to be more compassionate and caring about the welfare, treatment, and recovery of nurses as well as being more effective at retaining nurses in the profession (Monroe et al., 2008). Furthermore, the typical cost savings for aftercare programs are considered substantial compared with the costs of investigation and disciplinary action (Darbro, 2003). Some contend that a non-disciplinary atmosphere of support might be a life-saving first step for nurses with substance use disorders as well as for those in their care (Monroe & Kenaga, 2011).

The policy approach has been noted to impact other nurses in their responsibilities regarding their nurse-colleagues with substance use disorders. Hood and Duphorne (1995) examined the reporting strategies used by nurses confronted with making the decision to report substance abuse among their peers. Nurses who believed that reporting would result in punitive consequences were deterred from making formal reports when they suspected nurse-colleagues of impaired practice, while nurses who believed that rehabilitative consequences would result were more likely to report them. As nurses are the primary source of identification of the problem of substance abuse by their colleagues (Monohan, 2003), the policy approach to nurses with substance use disorders has salience for early detection.

When substance use disorders occur amongst health care professionals, the goals are to protect the public from possible harm and to engage the individual health care professional into treatment. Fear of disciplinary action is an obstacle for the ill health care professional seeking care and a disincentive for reporting by their concerned peers. This raises questions about the effectiveness of disciplinary environments in identifying and monitoring their health care professionals with substance use disorders. When early referrals are not made, health care professionals with substance use disorders often remain without treatment until overt impairment is manifest in the workplace (FSPHP, 2008). After noting their members with addiction were not receiving the same opportunities for treatment as the general public because they were held to a different, disciplinary standard, the American Medical Association and the American Nursing Association advocated for non-public, alternative to discipline responses (Quinlan, 2003).

There are counterarguments to the alternative to discipline focus on rehabilitation, monitoring and confidentiality. Some jurisdictions with disciplinary responses have identified their reluctance to incur expenses involved with monitoring programs (Monroe et al., 2008). There are disciplinary jurisdictions that spend substantive resources on formal investigations and public hearings. A direct comparison of costs between the disciplinary and alternative responses does not appear to be available. A review of disciplinary action on 52,297 registered and licensed practical nurses between 1996 and 2006 in the U.S. determined that 24% were for drug-related violations (Kenward, 2008). A ruling in Alberta determined the costs of one Hearing to be $70,000 without including staff time or salaries (Appendix A). If this contribution is indicative, regulators following disciplinary approaches incur substantive financial burdens.

This conundrum cannot be settled by legislation alone. In Alberta, with health care professionals regulated under the same Health Professions Act (Province of Alberta, 2010), there are different approaches. In this setting, complaints dispositions for physicians feature a confidential, rehabilitative approach and registered nurses with an open, disciplinary one (Els & Kunyk, 2011).

Regulators and employers are, most likely, not addiction treatment specialists. When they impose conditions for treatment and monitoring, these may not be the most appropriate ones for unique needs of the health care professional in question. Nor are the addiction treatment providers for the health care professional because they are required to advocate on behalf of their health care professional patient (Please see the chapter in this textbook, 'Workplace Functional Impairment due to Mental Disorders' by Els, Kunyk, Hoffman & Wargon). In neither of these conditions, is there an external body to evaluate the quality of care delivery.

Concerns about the quality of treatment, and the neutrality of return to work decisions, can be addressed by the introduction of a neutral and independent intermediary. A neutral body with experts in addiction medicine can provide independent medical assessments, and determine the necessary treatments, continuing care, and conditions for return to work. This neutral body can also monitor that these conditions are met, and notify regulators and/or employers when they are not. An 'arms length' relationship between the treatment providers and the monitoring program appears to be important. If there is slippage in the performance of a particular treatment program or other service provider, it can be removed from the list of approved providers (Dupont et al., 2009).

Case Scenario: Lost Opportunities for Monitoring in a Disciplinary Environment

Outcome studies on physicians engaged in long-term monitoring programs demonstrate the effectiveness of this approach in maintaining recovery, supporting return to work, ensuring ongoing treatment, and providing for early detection of relapse. Due to the success of this model, the goal must be to ensure that recovering health care professionals with substance use disorders are directed into similar programs. When an employer or regulator becomes aware of their employees/members with addiction, they have the authority to ensure that compliance with continuing care and monitoring programs occurs.

Fear of disciplinary action is an obstacle for the ill health care professional seeking care and a disincentive for reporting by their concerned peers. This raises questions about the effectiveness of disciplinary environments in identifying when their health care professionals practice while impaired by the use of substances.

The province of Alberta, Canada provides a unique opportunity for study as the registered nurses belong to one provincial regulator, and one health authority provides most of their employment. Complaints received by the regulator regarding behaviours related to substance use are handled through formal investigations (CARNA, 2008a) and, if supported by sufficient evidence, the complaint proceeds to an open hearing tribunal. When the nurse in question is found guilty of unprofessional conduct, sanctions may include a reprimand advising that their behaviour falls below the expected standards for nursing practice, suspension and/or restrictions on their practice permit, requirement of supervised practice, ongoing documentation of specified treatment modalities, random drug testing paid for by the nurse in question, conditions required for return to practice, and publication of the discipline decision in its newsletter *Alberta RN* (CARNA, 2008a, p. 10). The nurse may also be directed to pay a contribution toward the costs of the investigation).

In a study in Alberta, 100 registered nurses who had self-identified with substance dependence in the last 12 months who were currently working in nursing. Within this sample, there were 2 nurses who had been reported to their regulator and 3 that were known by their employer. This left 95 registered nurses unknown to an authority that could have required ongoing monitoring (Kunyk, 2011).

Jurisdictions with disciplinary policies often claim that they are mandated to protect the public (Quinlan, 1994) and do not advocate for the health of the health care professional (Monroe et al., 2008). This approach may be counterproductive. The findings from this study suggest that with a disciplinary approach, the public is minimally protected from the risks associated with substance use. A recommendation for future research is to ask a similar question in a jurisdiction that follows an alternative to discipline approach.

5. Conclusions

Substance use disorders among the health care professions is a complex professional and occupational health issue. It is one that will likely affect every one of us, either directly or indirectly, at some point in our careers. The serious nature of its threats to patient care, health care professional health, and our professional image demands that we deal well with the issue.

For the purposes of mitigating such risks, fitting organizational policies need to take into consideration the implications of the broader environment in contributing to the situation. Effective treatments for health care professionals with substance use disorders include provisions for early detection, tailored, multi-modal, effective, affordable and affordable interventions. Aftercare programs are considered an essential component as they enhance the recovery of affected health professionals while also reducing the risk to the public through the early detection of relapse.

How can we best deal with substance use disorders amongst health care professionals? The heterogeneity between jurisdictions, individual situations, social environments, and responsibilities suggests that there is not one solution that is appropriate for all and under every circumstances. However, the evidence presented in this chapter, particularly the mature models employed with physicians in their interventions and aftercare, suggest there are some guiding principles for reducing the risks to patient care and to health care professional health. These include:

1. **Policy.** The substance use disorders will affect some members within the health care professions. This inevitability demands that the health professions, and their employers, prepare for dealing well with the situation through the development of evidence-based policies.

2. **Health values.** Following the principle of think globally, act locally, the manner in which this issue is understood and dealt with has global implications not only for health care professionals but also for the individuals in their care in similar situations. Consistency with health values and beliefs will enhance our professions and health care organizations in our respective missions. Health values include respect for health care professional - patient confidentiality, the recognition of disease conditions, and the need for evidence based care.

3. **Confidentiality.** The substance use disorders are highly stigmatizing illnesses. Health care professionals should be afforded the same confidentiality that is required for other patients.
4. **Chronic disease model.** The substance use disorders are chronic, relapsing conditions. Their treatment involves a continuum of care and a long-term perspective based on the chronic disease model that includes provision for relapse prevention and early detection of relapse. Provision for detoxification, medical stabilization and treatment is only the beginning of the intervention this chronic, relapsing disease. Continuing care with monitoring for five years is advisable.
5. **Evidence-based care.** The substance use disorders are highly responsive to multi-modal, evidence-based treatment based on the needs of the individual. Policy development must take into consideration access to comprehensive and high quality addiction treatments that incorporate the NIDA Principles of Addiction. Policy development must also outline provisions for coverage of care in the same manner as it would for other medical conditions.
6. **Comprehensive intervention.** The objective for intervention when impaired practice occurs is to minimize the risks to patient care and practitioner health through early identification, comprehensive assessment, detoxification, medical stabilization and treatment, and continuing care with long-term monitoring.
7. **Monitoring programs.** Long-term monitoring of recovering health care professionals is effective for supporting recovery and protection of the public when relapses happen. Monitoring requires a contractual agreement signed by the recovering health care professional with provisions for referral to the regulator should a risk of impaired practice occur. These monitoring programs are best performed by a party considered 'arms length' and neutral rather than the treatment provider or regulator.
8. **Decision-making.** Assessment, treatment and continuing care decisions are best made by a health care team specialized in addiction management, and not the regulator or employer.
9. **Minimize discipline.** Health care professionals who voluntarily seek recommended treatments, successfully complete their treatment, and contract to participate in a monitoring program should not receive punitive sanctions. This would encourage both self and peer identification.
10. **Early identification.** Employers and regulators need to create conditions that require fitness for duty, and encourage self and peer identification. This would include minimizing the use of discipline and ensuring the right of confidentiality.
11. **Environmental change.** As the conditions of being a health care professional may have contributed to the development of substance use disorders, the environment is also a part of the solution. The empirical findings that errors made by health professionals reflect system and organizational issues (Baker et al., 2004) may have some transferable learning to this situation. A body of research is required to determine aspects of psycho-dynamically healthy workplaces for the purposes of preventing the expression of substance use disorders amongst health care professionals, their early detection, as well as for their return to work upon recovery.
12. **Consistent between disciplines.** As the standards developed with physicians' health programs have produced the highest documented long-term recovery rates recorded in

the treatment outcome literature, these should be the standards for the other health professions.

13. **Return to work.** Confidentiality is the privilege of the individual with the disease, and disclosure must ultimately be a decision they make. The need to know is restricted to those necessary to meet the conditions for return to work.

14. **Human rights.** The health care professional with a substance use disorders should be afforded the same rights and privileges, including the duty to accommodate, as other individuals in society.

In conclusion, when substance use disorders are expressed amongst some members of the health care professions, there are serious implications for risk to the public and to the health of the health care professional with the disease. There are many unanswered questions regarding management of the substance use disorders amongst health care professionals. Research is required on transferability of knowledge between the health care professions, outcomes of the effectiveness of specific approaches, unique needs of the professions and their specialties, and creating conditions to optimize early identification and ongoing recovery. The existing evidence supports creating conditions that encourage early identification, reduce barriers to treatment, and that include long-term monitoring programs provide the best conditions for mitigating the risks resulting from substance use disorders amongst the health care professions to patient safety and health care professional health.

6. Appendix A: CARNA Decision on Registration #62,312

During the hearing the Tribunal was presented with an exibit (41) detailing the cost in total of this hearing up to February 10, 2010 of $63,174.96 with an additional estimate of costs for February 26 of $7,275.

This totalled approximately $70,000. The costs did nit include costs such as staff time or salaries. These were out of pocket expenses as detailed in Exhibit 41. These were expenses that CARNA had to pay from its resources, which are in effect the resources of the membership.

American Board of Addiction Medicine [ABAM](2011). American Board of Addiction Medicine Certification. http://www.abam.net/become-certified

7. References

American Medical Association [AMA](2008). AMA statement on Physician Health Programs. Attributed to R.J. Patchin. Retrieved from http://www.fsphp.org/Publications.html

American Psychiatric Association (2011). DSM-5: The Future of Psychiatric Diagnosis. http://www.dsm5.org/ProposedRevision/Pages/proposedrevision.aspx?rid=431

American Psychiatric Association [APA] (2000). *Diagnostic and Statistical Manual of Mental Disorders* (4th ed., text revision). Arlington, VA: Author.

Berge, K.H., Seppela, M.D., Schipper, A.M. (2009). Chemical dependency and the physician. *Mayo Clinical Proceedings 84*(7): 625-631.

Brewster, J. (1986). Prevalence of alcohol and other drug problems among physicians. *Journal of the American Medical Association, 255*(14), 1913–1920.

Brewster, J., Kaufmann, M., Hutchison, S., & MacWilliam, C. (2008). Characteristics and outcomes of doctors in a substance dependence monitoring programme in Canada: Prospective descriptive study. *British Medical Journal, 337*, a2098.

Canadian Nurses Association (2009). *Position Statement: Problematic Substance Use by Nurses.* Retrieved from
http://www.cna-aiic.ca/CNA/issues/position/protection/default_e.aspx

Canadian Nurses Association (2008). *Code of Ethics for Registered Nurses.* Retrieved from http://www.cna-aiic.ca/CNA/practice/ethics/code/default_e.aspx

Collins, R., Gollnisch, G., & Morsheimer, E. (1999). Substance use among a regional sample of female nurses. *Drug & Alcohol Dependence, 55*(1/2), 145-155.

Compton, W.M., Thomas, Y.F., Stinston, F.S., Grant, B.F. (2007). Prevalence, correlates, disability, and comorbidity of *DSM-IV* drug abuse and dependence in the United States: results from the National Epidemiologic Survey on Alcohol and Related Conditions. *Archives of General Psychiatry* 64(5): 566-576.

Corsino, B., Morrow, D., & Wallace, C. (1996). Quality improvement and substance abuse: Rethinking impaired provider policies. *American Journal of Medical Quality, 11*(2), 94-99.

Darbro, N. (2005). Alternative diversion programs for nurses with impaired practice: Completers and non-completers. *Journal of Addictions Nursing, 16*(4), 169-185.

Domino, K.B., Hornbein, T.F., Polissar, N.L., Renner, G., Johnson, J., Alberti, S., Hankes, L. (2005). Risk factors for relapse in health care professionals with substance use disorders. *Journal of the American Medical Association, 293*, 1453-1460.

DuPont R. L., McLellan T., White W. L., Merlo, L., & Gold, S. G. (2009). Setting the standard for recovery: Physicians' health programs. *Journal of Substance Abuse Treatment, 26*, 159-171.

Els, C. (2007). Addiction is a mental disorder, best managed in a (public) mental health setting - but our system is failing us. *Canadian Journal of Psychiatry* 52(3): 167-169.

Els, C., Kunyk, D. (2011). Differential Treatment of Impaired Health Professionals Under the HPA in Alberta.

Els, C., Kunyk, D., Hoffman, H., Wargon, A. (2011). Workplace Functional Impairment due to Mental Disorders. In L. L'Abate (Ed.). INTECH.

Federation of State Physician Health Programs [FSPHP]. Goals of the FSPHP. Retrieved from http://www.fsphp.org

Federation of State Physician Health Programs [FSPHP]. Public Policy Statement: Physician Illness vs. Impairment. Retrieved from http://www.fsphp.org

Gastfriend, D.R. (2005). Physician substance abuse and recovery. What does it meant for physicians—and everyone else? *Journal of the American Medical Association* 293: 1513-14.

Glasser, F.B., Brewster, J., Sisson, B.V. (1986). Alcohol and drug problems in Ontario physicians: characteristics of the physician sample. *Canadian Family Physician. 32*, 993-9.

Gold, M.S., Aronson, M. Physician health and impairment. *Psychiatric Annals, 34*, 736-740.

Gossop, M., Stephens, S., Stewart D., Marchall, J., Beam, J., Strang, J. (2001). Health care professionals referred for treatment of alcohol and drug problem. *Alcohol and Alcoholism, 36*, 160-4.

Graham, A., Schultz, T., Mayo-Smith, M., Ries, R., & Wilford, B. (Eds.). (2003). *Principles of Addiction Medicine* (3rd ed.). Chevy Chase, MD: American Society of Addiction Medicine.

Haack, M., & Yocom, C. (2002). State policies and nurses with substance use disorders. *Journal of Nursing Scholarship, 34*(1), 89–94.

Hasin DS, Stinson FS, Ogburn E, Grant BF. (2007). Prevalence, correlates, disability, and comorbidity of *DSM-IV* alcohol abuse and dependence in the United States: results from the National Epidemiologic Survey on Alcohol and Related Conditions. *Arch Gen Psych.* 64(7):830–842.

Hood, J., Duphorme, P. (1995). To report or not report: Nurses' attitudes toward reporting co-workers suspected of substance abuse. *Journal of Drug Issues* 25(2): 313-339.

Hughes, P., Brandenburg, N., Baldwin, D., et al (1992). Prevalence of substance use amongst U.S. physicians. *Journal of the American Medical Association 267*: 2333-2339.

Kenna, G. A., & Wood, M. D. (2005). Family history of alcohol and drug use in health care professionals. *Journal of Substance Use, 10*(4), 225–238.

Kenna, G.A., & Wood, M. D. (2004). Substance use by pharmacy and nursing practitioners and students in a northeastern state. *American Journal of Health-System Pharmacy, 61*(9), 921–930.

Kenward, K. (2008). Discipline of nurses: A review of disciplinary data 1996–2006. *JONA's Health careLaw Ethics Regulation, 10*(3), 81–85.

Kleber, H., Weiss, R., Anton, R., George, T., Greenfield, S., Kosten, T., … Connery, H. (2006). *Practice guidelines for the treatment of patients with substance use disorders* (2nd ed.). Arlington, VA: American Psychiatric Association.

Kunyk, D. (2011). *Nursing under the influence: Understanding the situation of Alberta nurses.* Electronic Theses and Dissertations. Retrieved from http://hdl.handle.net/10048/2043

Kunyk, D., & Austin, W. (2011). Nursing under the influence: A relational ethics perspective. *Nursing Ethics, 18*(5).

Kunyk D, Els C, Robinson Hughes J (2010). Substance-related disorders. In *Psychiatric Nursing for Canadian Practice. 2nd. Ed.* W. Austin (Ed). Philadelphia: Lippincott, Williams & Wilkins.

Lillibridge, J., Cox, M, and Cross, W. (2002). Uncovering the secret: giving voice to the experiences of nurses who misuse substances. *Journal of Advanced Nursing, 39*(3): 219-29.

McAuliffe, W.E., Santangelo S., Magnuson E., et. al.(1987). Risk factors of drug impairment in random samples of physicians and medical students. International Journal of Addiction 22(9): 825-841.

McLennan, T., Skipper, G., Campbell, M., DuPont, R. (2008). Five year outcomes in a cohort study of physicians treated for substance use disorders in the United States. *BMJ:* 337: a2038.

Monohan, G. (2003). Drug use / misuse among health professionals. *Substance use and Misuse 38:* 1877-1881.

Monroe, T., & Kenaga, H. (2011). Don't ask don't tell: Substance abuse and addiction among nurses. *Journal of Clinical Nursing, 20*(3–4), 504.

Monroe, T., Pearson, F., & Kenaga, H. (2008). Procedures for handling cases of substance abuse among nurses: A comparison of disciplinary and alternative programs. *Journal of Addictions Nursing, 19*, 156–161.

Province of Alberta (2010). Health Professions Act: Revised Statutes of Alberta 2000 Chapter H-7. Edmonton: Alberta Queen's Printer.

Quinlan, D. (2003). Impaired nursing practice: A national perspective on peer assistance in the U.S. *Journal of Addictions Nursing, 14*(3), 149-153.

Reading, E.G. (1992). Nine years experience with chemically dependent physicians: the New Jersey experience. *Maryland Medical Journal.* 41, 325-9.

Roberts, L., & Dyer, A. (2004). Health care ethics committees. In *Concise guide to ethics in mental health care* (pp. 295-318). Washington, DC: American Psychiatric Publishing.

Shaw, M.F., McGovern, M.P., Angres, D.H., and Rawal, P. (2004). Physician and nurses with substance use disorders. *Journal of Advanced Nursing, 47*(5): 561-71.

Skipper, G.E. (2009). Confrontational approach has no role in addressing physician addiction. *Mayo Clinic Proceedings 84*(11): 1042.

Smith, P.C., Smith, J.D. (1991). Treatment outcomes of impaired physicians in Oklahoma. *Journal o- Oklahoma State Medical Association, 84,* 599-603.

Standing Senate Committee on Social Affairs, Science and Technology. (2006). *Out of the shadows at last: Transforming mental health, mental illness and addiction services in Canada.* Chair, M. Kirby. Retrieved from http://www.parl.gc.ca/39/1/parlbus/commbus/senate/com-e/soci-e/rep-e/pdf/rep02may06part1-e.pdf.

Storr, C., Trinkoff, A., Anthony, J. (1999). Job strain and non-medical drug use. *Drug and Alcohol Dependence 55*: 45-51.

Sullivan, E., Bissell, L., & Leffler, D. (1990). Drug use and disciplinary actions among 300 nurses. The International Journal of the Addictions, (25)4, 375-391.

Talbott, G.D. (1995). Reducing relapse in health providers and professionals. *Psychiatry Annals. 23*(11): 669-672.

Talbott, G.D., Earley, P.H. (2003). Physician Health Programs and the addicted physician. In *Principles of Addiction Medicine,* 3rd ed. A.W. Graham, T.K. Schultz, M.F. Mayo-Smith, R.F. Ries, B.B. Wilford Eds. Chevy Chase MD: American Society of Addiction Medicine.

Talbott, G.D., Wilson, P.O. (2005). Physicians and other health professionals. *In Substance Abuse: A Comprehensive Textbook.* 4th ed. J. Lowinson, P. Ruiz, R. Millman, J. Langrod Eds. Philadelphia: Lippincott, Williams & Wilkins.

Trinkoff, A. M., & Storr, C. (1998). Substance use among nurses: Differences between specialties. *American Journal of Public Health, 88*(4), 581-585.

Trinkoff, A. M., Zhou, Q., Storr, C.L., & Soeken, K. L. (2000). Workplace access, negative proscriptors, job strain, and substance use in registered nurses. *Nursing Research, 49*(2), 83-90.

Tyssen, R. (2007). Health problems and the use of health services by physicians: A review article with particular emphasis on Norwegian studies. *Industrial Health* (45): 599-610.

World Health Organisation. (2007). International Statistical Classification of Diseases and Related Health Problems. 10th Revision Version. Geneva. World Health Organisation.

World Health Organization [WHO] (2006). *The World Health Report 2006: Working Together for Health.* ISBN 92 4 156317 6.

Wright, C. (1990). Physician addiction to pharmaceuticals: personal history, practice setting, access to drugs and recovery. *Maryland State Medical Journal (39)*: 1021-1025.

8

Coping and Meaning in Everyday Life: Living with Mental Disabilities in Late-Modern Society

Bengt Eriksson[1,2] and Jan Kåre Hummelvoll[1]
[1]Hedmark University College
[2]Karlstad University
[1]Norway
[2]Sweden

1. Introduction

Studies of the living conditions of vulnerable groups often focus on their actual situation. There is often a description of the way the circumstances of the group in question differ from those of others with respect to health, finances, and their ability to support themselves or make and develop social contacts, i.e., their ability to participate in social life in a similar way to other groups. There is less often a discussion of how long-term changes in the structure and organisation of society affect the living conditions of individuals and groups. Yet long-run societal changes influence everyone's possibilities and limitations and it seems likely that vulnerable groups such as people with mental disabilities are affected to a greater extent than others. There is a risk that groups of people who have a weaker buffer than others with regard to health, social contacts or finances find it more difficult to cope with changes, and are hit harder when changes occur. Organisational changes in health and medical care[1], economic recessions and structural changes in working life are examples of such changes.

In this chapter, longitudinal societal changes and the everyday conditions of people with mental disabilities are coupled. Recent researchers in social sciences have described how changes in the way individuals are regarded – such as the development of technology and changes in administration and logistics – have together had a great impact. Life today differs from that of 50 years ago in important respects. By means of what has been named 'the process of individualisation', the individual has gradually become the significant social unit. Each and everyone has to a larger extent the possibility to make his or her own choices, but is also responsible for the consequences of the decisions made, whether positive or negative. Previously unknown elements of insecurity have developed, and society has sometimes been characterised as a 'risk society'. Concepts like 'post-modernism' or 'late modernity' attempt to describe this distancing from, but at the same time connection with, the society that developed with the industrial revolution[2].

---

[1] Studies of changes in psychiatric care, for example, show a class gradient in the changeover from traditional hospital-based institutional care to open, sectorised psychiatry: The latter favoured primarily people from the middle class, while patients with a working-class background found it more difficult to get adequate help (Eliasson & Nygren 1981).

[2] At the same time, these and similar concepts express uncertainty about the new by not giving it a name of its own (Harste 1999).

An empirical study was carried out to relate these longitudinal societal changes to the everyday life situation of people with mental disabilities. In collaboration with members of a Norwegian user-organisation (Mental Health) multistage focus group interviews were conducted to explore and discuss whether concepts like 'late modernity' and 'risk society' appeared relevant and meaningful.

The way of regarding, and society's support of, people with mental disabilities have changed in a radical way during the last few decades. We describe these changes briefly in the continuation of this chapter and then give a more detailed picture of the long-term and radical, but sometimes fairly invisible, social changes that have been mentioned above. After that we give an account of the empirical work the chapter is based on, first by describing the research model – Co-operative Inquiry – that has been used for data collection and analysis, and then by reporting the participants' experiences of living with mental disabilities in today's society. In a following section the empirical results are discussed in relation to the change in society, on the basis of the following questions: *Have concepts like 'late modernity' and 'risk society' explanation value for the understanding of everyday life for a person with a mental disability? Can the characteristics of social change be identified and – if so – how can they be handled? Can development towards a 'risk society' be both positive and negative, imply both (new) possibilities and obstacles? How, in that case, can negative consequences be minimized and new, positive possibilities be taken advantage of and developed?* At the end of the chapter the discussion is summed up and we indicate some possible ways of acting in 'late-modern' society.

This chapter thus aims to report and discuss experiences of people who themselves suffer from mental disabilities. By way of conclusion of the chapter we broaden the perspective to some extent to also include professional groups with the task of supporting the mentally disabled, as well as training courses for these groups and research on nursing, support and care. However, here too, the point of departure is the experiences the people concerned have themselves reported. We think that the participation and influence of people with their own experience of mental disabilities should also be a natural and forceful component in professional work, training and research in this field.

2. Historical review: From stigmatisation to social inclusion – a vision with complications

People with mental ill-health, mental disabilities or mental diseases are one of the groups that have been paid attention to in public discussions and social policy in the last few decades. The discussions have been both about society's care and support, and about the participation and integration in society of the mentally disabled – or rather their lack of integration and participation. In the 1960s and 1970s a wave of intense criticism of the established psychiatry swept over Europe and the USA (Svensson 2005). Its forms of treatment were described as inhuman, segregating and marginalising. The criticism focused particularly on the ideological function of psychiatry, the tendency to convert an increasing number of human life problems into psychiatric symptoms, as well as its ambition to treat mental suffering on the same basis as physical afflictions, by adopting 'the medical model' (Szasz 1961). According to the critics, mental disabilities were caused by social factors rather than biologically or psychologically based defects in the individual. Scheff (1966) formulated a social-science theory about how mental disabilities develop and consolidate that was based on the labelling and social-role theory.

During the following decades, the radical criticism of psychiatry was replaced by a reformist period of reform, which can still be regarded as going on. The reforms have been characterised by ideas about normalisation, integration and social inclusion. An early and forceful expression of the change was that the big mental hospitals in many European countries were phased out – the great moving-out (Forsberg 1994)[3] – a process that is still going on, not least in Eastern Europe. The patients, often committed against their will, were instead to be able to live in their own homes and 'live like others'. The ambition was that people with mental disabilities, instead of being an out-group, separated from society and everyday life, would live their lives in the local community and on as similar terms as others. Besides having their own, personally furnished homes, the possibilities for work , meaningful activities, and recreation, were important components of the individual's everyday life. To the extent that they could not manage on their own, formal and informal support could be offered, by public or private institutions. Nursing and social care would primarily be formed as an offer, and be available in open and non-stigmatising forms. Institutional care, in psychiatric wards, should be available as a last, and normally short, extra support measure.

Forsberg (1992) describes the situation of the 'long-term mentally ill'[4] in a comparative study between Italy, Poland, England and Sweden. The lack of information on Polish conditions makes it difficult to comment on this country, but in all the other countries he finds that it is largely the same deficiencies in societal support that are complained of: There are insufficient resources for non-institutional care and for various forms of intermediate care, e.g. in the form of alternative forms of accommodation, sheltered workplaces or day-care and rehabilitation facilities. The risk of social isolation, as a result of an insufficient social network, is greater for the 'long-term mentally ill' and there is a lack of resources to break it. Granerud and Severinsson (2006) found the same deficiencies in their Norwegian study just over ten years later. Forsberg (a.a.) also points to the fact that collaboration between the authorities did not function satisfactorily, and that the support for the 'long-term mentally ill' was instead mainly suited to people with mild mental problems.

Purely concretely, the reforms of the last 20 years have thus had the aim of giving mentally disabled people a life in their own home, with or without personal support, instead of, as previously, being obliged to live in an institution or in other strictly regulated forms. For many people this has meant changed and improved conditions, even though there are still shortcomings in many ways. The change has largely followed the same pattern in many European countries, but earlier in certain countries than in others.

3. From a modern to a late-modern society

The society that developed during industrialism had its roots in the Age of Enlightenment of the 18th century, characterised by a belief in reason, the human being and the new science. The 19th century and the early 20th century saw a radical transformation of society, with

---

[3]'The great moving-out' alludes to M. Foucault's concept 'the great locking-up'. In his book *History of Madness (2006)*, Foucault describes how large groups were judged abnormal and interned in various institutions in European countries, from the 17thh century and onwards. A development that was only seriously reversed by the de-institutionalisation that was started in the years after the Second World War.

[4]This expression is used by Forsberg and therefore also in the text that describes his research.

industrialisation and mass production, often according to the principle of 'the conveyor belt'. In many countries an urbanisation process was started, from a poor agrarian society to a more urbanised and richer one. Modern society developed, not least in Europe and the USA. Working life was modernised, housing was improved. Society developed and prosperity increased rapidly. Functionalism, a trend that characterised important fields in social life, agreed well with the prevalent belief in progress, growth and development. The modern project also included welfare. Health and medical care, education, care of the elderly and groups that could not support themselves on account of handicaps/disabilities – it was all an expression of the idea that the general welfare should include the whole population. In many countries, not least in Scandinavia, a strong state apparatus to administer and produce welfare services was developed. In other countries the responsibility was placed on separate organisations, working life or family, but in close co-operation with the public sector.

At all events we have to a certain extent left the society of modernity behind us. The vision of society that lay behind the industrial society and the modernisation process can no longer be completely used as a description model for the stage of development in which we now find ourselves. Modern society's secure anchoring in the belief in growth and increasing material prosperity to share is wavering gravely. We are in a different stage of development. Many researchers think that this differs on such decisive points from the industrial society that it ought to have a different name. It is in this connection that concepts like 'late-modernism', 'post-modernism' or 'the second modernity' have been used. They all aim to describe a change from the previous industrial society, without therefore having to define the coming one, the post-industrial one. The concept of the 'risk society' also refers to the stage of society that we now find ourselves in, but wants to focus on one aspect of this society, namely its connection with the partly new and different risks and insecurities created by the development itself. The fact that we have chosen in this text to use 'late-modernism' is more an expression of our desire for a broad and generally applicable concept than criticism of other, closely related, terms. In our description of the late modernity society we also include quite a few factors that have been paid attention to in the discussion of the risk society – since they have a special relevance to vulnerable groups and their life situation.

The characteristics of the late modernity society include processes like globalisation and an economy that does not know any national or geographical boundaries. Service production increases and a greater and greater proportion of the workforce are occupied with services. The role of the mass media grows. Communication technology is increasingly important and constitutes one of the strongest forces in society – we need only mention the role that mobile phones and the Internet have recently played in national changes in society in North Africa. The big visions of society, the big stories, are challenged – maybe the age of the big stories is over. Power is in many places and more difficult to identify. Society has become more 'invisible'. It is also characterised by the fact that threats and risks affect both society and the lives of individuals to an increasing extent. They can be industrial risks or environmental threats, but also risks produced in and by the abstract, often worldwide, systems that more and more manifestly also influence the everyday life of the individual. The recent accident at the nuclear power station at Fukushima can be seen as an example of such environmental catastrophes. We do not yet know what consequences it will have, and accidents of this kind are of course always unique. But a comparison can be made with the nuclear power accident at Chernobyl in 1986, which had consequences that extend right up to our day. The risks in today's society thus tend to be global. Terror attacks of previously unknown dimensions can strike anyone, in principle anywhere in the world. A society's electricity supply can be knocked out by some abstract fault very far away. Speculation against a country's currency by unknown forces can have disastrous consequences for the finances of the individual.

These and similar new risks cause the term risk society to be used to denote this society – after modernity – a name that was to be established with great impact by Ulrich Beck's epoch-making work *Risk Society – Towards a New Modernity* (1992)[5]. Beck has, however, later himself questioned this term. Perhaps it should rather be said that there is a new kind of insecurity or danger that characterises the society of our time – and perhaps of the future.

The traditional risks of the industrial society were to a much greater extent local, visible and possible to take care of. Modernisation's emphasis on reducing and eliminating risks in working life, social life and private life, for example by means of work-environment measures, traffic-safety work and an extensive social policy, were intended to realise the vision of "the good society". In a certain sense the industrial society's emphasis was on "conquering nature" ("the end of nature"), for example by converting natural resources into useful products. The fight was between man and nature. The insecurity involved in being exposed to unpredictable nature would gradually be overcome by means of technology and science.

In the society of our time, it is instead – to a certain extent – man's own products, the results of development, that constitute threats. The threats are man-made; Beck and Giddens speak about "manufactured uncertainty" (Beck, 1998; Giddens, 1996). It is these "cultural products" – results of the technical and economic development itself – that create risks and make society vulnerable. The uncertainty that unpredictable nature could constitute has largely been overcome – human beings have tamed nature – but has been re-created in the unpredictability of the culture. Beck (1994) speaks about "the return of uncertainty to society". Modernisation's faith in science's ability to solve global, national and individual problems, to create the good life, has struck back: Science solves many problems but also creates new ones. The optimism of the industrial society has been replaced by reflexive modernisation.

In this society the individual has been made distinct in a completely different way than previously – a process that has gone on for a long time. Nowadays we must as individuals continually create and re-create our social existence – one speaks about social reflexivity. While collectively steering traditions and rituals in the previous society often also functioned as direction guidance for the various attitudes of the individual, these must nowadays to a far greater extent be formed by the individuals themselves. These choices are now instead guided by reflexive consciousness, considerations and consequence assessments in the light of their own lives. Guidance is not taken from over-individual beliefs but from people's own life history. To "realise one's life project" or to "pin one's faith on oneself" have become established slogans that in the spirit of individualisation express social reflexivity in terms of positive possibilities. At the same time, it is evident that distinctions between individuals and groups are tending to increase even more, for example between social classes or groups with different educational backgrounds. Individuals are

---

[5]Original title: Risikogesellschaft: Auf dem Weg in eine andere Moderne (1986).

quite simply left more to their own resources in the form of material assets, social networks, knowledge, social competence and image of themselves.

Security and safety were to pervade the modern society, closely connected to high-technological production, an efficient economy and a positive view of the possibilities of science. The society that is now developing, the second modernisation (Beck, 1992), means that the question of society's possibilities to create security and safety, and to inspire confidence in important respects has changed.

Questions of trust and confidence are thus closely connected to the successive transition from an industrial society to a late-modern society characterised by global movements, technical and economic as well as political and cultural. Trust based on spatial closeness, personal acquaintance and cultural similarity is replaced by trust in anonymous expert systems that the individual has very little knowledge of but is nevertheless obliged to trust. Giddens (1996) speaks here about the "transformation of intimacy" from trust based primarily on personal acquaintance – trust in a person – into trust in relation to abstract systems – trust in a system. He uses the term "disembedding" to describe this change in social relations. Disembedding means that the relations are removed from their ontological connection and become abstract and impersonal. Living in late-modern society involves demands for acceptance and trust without (always) being able to view the whole situation and comprehend. The individual is obliged to trust the competence of the expertise just in its function of expertise. Trust is established for abstract systems rather than for individual and well-known people. Abstract systems like bank services, telecommunications, electricity supplies or booking systems for train tickets, for example, are what first come to mind, but it is not too far-fetched to also exemplify with the expert systems for nursing and care that are built up within the framework of social policy. As representatives of the systems, nursing and care staff have a central task to re-create trust in these abstract systems. Giddens (1996) speaks here of re-embedding, which implies that the abstract expert systems are re-connected to the local connection. This re-connection, which is of decisive importance for the establishment of a new form of trust, under the conditions of late modernity, is of two kinds (Giddens, 1996): facework commitments and faceless commitments. An ordinary visit to the doctor can serve as an example of both forms of contact: the doctor represents a facework commitment, a personal contact, but is at the same time a representative of the unsurveyable field of experts that medical care today constitutes for the individual. The medicine order that can be the consequence of the visit to the doctor is controlled by an administration, logistics and dispatch that are not represented by any individual person that the patient can establish a relationship with (as is the case in some sense with the doctor). The handling of the medicine can therefore be regarded as a faceless commitment.

Against this background, it is of great interest to investigate how a group that is considered exposed, people with mental disabilities, experience, think and behave in a late-modern society such as for example the Norwegian.

4. Method: Creating knowledge in co-operation

The aim of the study was to investigate whether the theory of 'risk society' was considered relevant when related to the experiences of everyday life of a group of persons with mental health disabilities who regularly attended a user-run centre (the Centre) in a middle-sized Norwegian town. The research questions dealt with the following themes: In what way are the 'risk society', and the underlying process of individualisation materialised in everyday life? How can the consequences of this societal development be handled and mastered both individually and collectively?

We chose co-operative inquiry as our research design. This mode of inquiry has its roots in action research and has a holistic and humanistic basis (Rowan, 2006). Co-operative inquiry emphasises the active influence and participation of all partners in the research process, from the beginning to the end of the research. Researchers and co-researchers (i.e. participants) constitute a 'community of inquiry' with mutual responsibility for development of knowledge. The value basis of this research approach is expressed quite precisely by Peter Reason (1994):

Human inquiry practitioners assert, in contrast to the positivist world-view, that we can only truly do research with persons if we engage with them as persons, as co-subjects and thus as co-researchers: hence co-operative inquiry, participatory research, research partnerships, and so on. And while understanding and action are logically separate, they cannot be separated in life; so a science of persons must be an action science. I use the term human inquiry to encompass all those forms of search which aim to move beyond the narrow, positivistic and materialist world-view which has come to characterize the latter portion of the twentieth century. While holding on to the scientific ideals of critical self-reflective inquiry and openness to public scrutiny, the practices of human inquiry engage deeply and sensitively with experience, are participative, and aim to integrate action with reflection. (p. 10)

Thus, co-operative inquiry is relevant when investigating local knowledge and experience from those who are directly involved, and thereby increases the possibilities of developing relevant knowledge. In can be maintained that there are likenesses between this research strategy when approaching the empirical field and the general development towards a late-modern society characterised by greater elements of individual responsibility, participation and a lesser trust in experts – also concerning research and developmental work.

Data collection and analysis: The dialogical nature of co-operative inquiry fits well with multistage focus group interviews as a method for data collection (Hummelvoll 2008). Therefore, this variant of focus group was chosen in this study. The multistage focus group is characterised by the same group exploring a certain problem, theme or phenomenon through several meetings. The method could be conceived as inquiring knowledge dialogues that focus on experiential material. Through these dialogues, there are possibilities to 'elevate' the participants' experiences to a higher level of abstraction. Thus, the potential utility value of the knowledge exceeds the concrete situation in which it is created.

In multistage focus groups, the researcher functions as moderator and leads the knowledge dialogue throughout the whole process. The researcher decides the theme of inquiry and then successively elaborates on it together with the participants. Compared to traditional focus group interviews, the group feeling establishes itself through both interaction and increased knowledge of each other. A calmer atmosphere than if 'all things' should be said in only one interview session often characterises the inquiry. Consequently, the focused theme is gradually enriched by adding new perspectives and nuances by means of examples from everyday life (or practice) and experiences made in the period between the interviews. Additional meetings contribute to exploring experiences and counter-experiences. This presupposes development of trust amongst the co-researchers (i.e. the participants), appreciation of divergent views and staying open-minded by allowing one's own views to be put to the test.

An essential feature of multistage focus groups is that the persons participating in the first group sometimes change in subsequent meetings. This happens because the inquiry process extends over a period of time and hence some of the original participants may be unable to attend following meetings. Therefore, one or two new members can join the group in the second or third session. This has proved to be an asset because alternative opinions or perspectives of the new members can challenge the group effect marked by more or less pressure against consensus (Hummelvoll 2008). Thus, the group dynamics may be stimulated and the inquiry vitalised by deepening the understanding of the focused theme. However, in order to secure the continuity of the group, it is important to keep the group size so large and stable that the core process of knowledge development is maintained.

In our study the participants consisted of the research group (two researchers and one user representative employed by the University College) and members of the user-organisation Mental Health who regularly attended the Centre. The focus group met three times during the autumn of 2008, with – apart from the research group – eight, five and four participants, of 20 to 60 years of age, both men and women. Each interview lasted about two hours. Immediately following the first two interviews, a summary was made and a preliminary analysis carried out, which were presented and commented upon at the beginning of the following focus group. The interviews were recorded and transcribed verbatim. A qualitative analysis as an empirically led content analysis (Malterud 2003) was carried out: The entire data material was read repeatedly; meaning units were coded and grouped together under preliminary themes, validated in relation to data, and finally the main themes from the inquiry process were created. Then the results of the analysis and interpretation were presented at an open meeting at the Centre. Guided by comments from the participants at this meeting, the analysis was finalised and published as a research report (Hummelvoll, Eriksson & Beston 2009) and later as a peer reviewed article (Eriksson & Hummelvoll 2011 - in press).

Ethical considerations: Ethical aspects were taken care of by presenting the theme and design of the study to the Board of the Centre, from which the research was sanctioned. The written information was discussed with the board members before it was distributed to potential participants. Participation in the focus groups was voluntary and written informed consent was obtained from the participants. None except the research group and the co-researchers had access to the data. The principles of the Declaration of Helsinki (World Medical Association 2002) – autonomy, beneficence, non-maleficence and justice - were taken into account in all parts of the study.

5. Results: Coping and meaning – everyday life in today's society

The thematic analysis of the material from the multistage focus group interviews resulted in five overriding themes, namely, change and uncertainty; mental disabilities and societal obstacles; the technological dominance; individualisation and loneliness; searching for a meaningful everyday life. These themes are described and deepened in the following text and exemplified with quotations from the focus group interviews.

5.1 Change and uncertainty

Society is changing at a fast pace which have impacts on the concrete level as well as on the abstract level. The familiarity of the local community has partly been replaced by a society which is difficult to comprehend and which creates feelings of alienation:

-   *What we are talking of now – the 'risk society' – isn't something new. It has probably to do with a process of alienation...*
-   *There has been a distinct change since I was a kid. Earlier you could pop in to your neighbour for a brief visit. The doors were open. Now this has changed. You have to make an appointment if you are going to visit somebody. Why is it so?*
-   *We are living in a cold society, where the chill is eased with tranquillizers.*
-   *It is demands on efficiency that characterise life in so many areas.*

The emphasis on efficiency and busyness seems to lead to meetings between people being more superficial and anonymous:

-   *There has become a lot of anonymity: We don't meet as people.*
-   *Yes, there is anonymity in society as a whole and in everything official: Quickly in the door and fast out again and as cheap as possible.*

Swift changes and demands for readjustment in a variety of areas create an experience of uncertainty and insecurity. The ongoing changes which we have to face awaken a longing for a safe basis for one's orientation in the world:

-   *Insecurity...it is difficult to make an enduring platform because things are constantly changing... You meet demands to adjust and be able to deal with all the new things that arise.*
-   *Yes, everything goes so quickly – and so quickly in such a wide area: We meet people with different languages; Technology develops and dominates; the village used to be a limited area but now the boundaries are gone – I think of globalisation. The Internet for example – there the language is English.*
-   *The village as a clearly defined and manageable unit has changed now in relation to a world around without boundaries. You can lose your sense of direction.*
-   *Yes, there is nothing you can make a map of...*

One aspect of the societal development is the lack of time and the increase of stress:

-   *Our time is stressed. We have to make the best of the fifteen minutes we get from the doctor, and it is difficult to say all that you have been pondering on for a long time. If you have two things on your mind, then you have to make a new appointment for the second one. It was easier when I could just drop in at the doctor's office. With my problems I have enough with today and tomorrow – I can't plan for a long time ahead.*

A specific phenomenon in our daily life is all the music that encroaches on people in shopping centres or as "waiting music" when making phone calls. This "sound bombardment" may be conceived as difficult to endure for people with mental disabilities:

-   *It is hard to stand all the sound. Hasn't this to do with protection of privacy?*
-   *I love music and make active choices for myself. But music is used everywhere in order to sedate and ease. Is it so that silence is embarrassing? I find quietness good now and then. But many people have hectic days, and these things are forced upon us – music that we don't want to have. Yes, I think we are living in a kind of terror world – and therefore we have things that sedate us everywhere.*
-   *Perhaps music replaces some of the real contacts between people?*

5.2 Mental disabilities and societal obstacles

Mental disabilities are connected with relationships between the individual and society – which defines the individual person's difficulties. Disabilities are experienced in society and in relation to not being able to cope with necessary daily tasks. Thus, disabilities are connected with the individual person's life in the community. However, defining mental disability is not easy. One of the participants highlights two solutions related to well known challenges:

- *If a person chooses to avoid using the bus at times when it is usually crowded, and instead chooses quieter periods of the day – is this then a disability? What about shopping food on Monday morning instead of shopping when it is crowded and busy. Is this then a functional deficit? Does it only become a hindrance when it obstructs you from doing the things you otherwise would have done if you were "free"?*

The participants maintain that many people with mental disabilities have problems related to their weak financial situation:

- *It is expensive to be poor. Lacking means makes you "fall off" and become excluded…*
- *You must do everything in the right way. Then everything works. If you need help, perhaps there aren't people…*
- *Or that information and help cost money. Services cost money and they cost more for those who don't have much!*
- *People with ailing finances and mental health problems are therefore doubly exposed.*

The relationship between society and persons with mental disabilities is often problematic. Societal institutions are experienced as somewhat abstract and impersonal. Mental disabilities may in one aspect be considered as created by society – like "manufactured societal hindrances":

- *We don't get more information than the caseworker tells you. Earlier our rights were not so complicated, and there was personal knowledge. The doctor knew the members of the local rural community.*
- *The officials also don't tell us about all the things that are available. There are so many possibilities for help now. But they are not so quick to inform us. It is the officials that decide what you shall have, and you are dependent on the official … The website of NAV[6] is incomplete. So societal hindrances are produced. We are dependent on the officials and vulnerable.*
- *If your application is incomplete on one point, or there is a paper missing, they send the whole application back instead of pointing out what was missing and asking to get just that.*

One aspect of these hindrances is 'the rule of the red tape", which is about the superfluity of forms that society demands that you know and can handle in order to take care of your rights and to get access to help. In a more abstract meaning this has to do with fitting into the definitions and the right categories.

- *Many people have a phobia about forms, and have great problems to understand the wording and the kind of answers that are expected in the various columns and boxes. It is difficult and embarrassing to ask for help to fill in – and it will have major consequences if you don't do so.*
- *The various services should have a low threshold and not be so run by systems. The waiting time for getting help is quite often long… In acute psychiatry the problem is whether you fit the criteria or not – and if you are so-called 'amendable to treatment' according to the form.*

When meeting the public, trust in the social services is put to the test. Stability and coherence in relationships are needed in order to promote trust, and the caseworker must be worthy of trust. When meeting public representatives, several factors seem to create distrust:

- You don't get trust in eight different people. Trust must be built over time.
- Sometimes I think that "the systems" have shown me very much distrust through letters and threats …you have to fulfil requirements and you must justify and document everything. The whole system is founded on distrust, and then it is difficult for me to show trust in return.

---

[6] NAV is an abbreviation for The Norwegian Labour and Welfare Administration

The possibility of having work and developing work-life integration is part of society's political objectives – also for persons with mental disabilities. However, many have experienced problems when applying for supported employment:

- *We have an official policy about integration and universal arrangements. Nevertheless, there are more persons outside the labour market now than before – even though the Norwegian economy is really thriving...What can the reasons be?*

5.3 The technological dominance
Mastering the new technology – computer technology in particular – contributes to social inclusion, but those who, for various reasons, are unfamiliar with the technology experience themselves as excluded. Authorities and social organisations expect most people to be connected to the Internet – or at least have access to the Internet. Some of the functional obstacles that people experience are therefore related to lack of knowledge concerning how to use computer technology. Consequently, the question is whether one copes with the technology – or feels ruled by it.

- *Things are more accessible – only one press on the button away – but at the same time more closed for those who don't have the knowledge or the facilities.*
- *Try to find your way to the right form on the NAV site... Yes, you must know the name of what you want. You have to know it.*
- *I asked to have a form but was told to go to the Net and fetch it. I felt that it was weak to say " I don't know how" ... so I said thank you and left – without a form.*
- *Yes, knowledge is necessary to make your way in society. If you lack knowledge you will easily be outside and powerless. If you have knowledge, you are inside.*

The participants wish to be involved when public websites are being developed so that they will be user-friendly. It is necessary to get access to relevant information in order to be able to choose. However, help is increasingly needed to find what they are searching for.

There are positive aspects of computer technology as well: personal blogs can be used as a means of building one's identity and to make a profile of interests and competence. One can create one's own identity. The blog may also function as an open diary that many people can follow and stay updated.

- On the Internet you can become who you want. What is different and good is that you can throw out people when you want to, and that is not possible when they are sitting on your sofa at home.
- And you needn't disclose more than you decide on the Web. In personal interactions you disclose more of yourself because we see each other – we notice the facial expressions...

5.4 Individualisation and loneliness
Individualisation is a prominent feature of the societal development. This implies that the responsibility today to a large extent relies on the individual when it comes to questions which in earlier times could be handled within the framework of the family or other collectives. The individual is more free, but at the same time more responsible. There is also a paradox here: On one hand the individual is to create his or her own life and be responsible, while on the other hand one is expected to go with the stream – i.e. to be like others expect 'people' to be:

- *Everybody is supposed to follow the mainstream. This is more important now than before.*

- *Hasn't it always been like this?*
- *Yes, but the problem is that there are so many streams to follow.*
- *Individualisation is focused, but nevertheless you have to fit into social expectations. Consequently, there are no real options if you deviate from the mainstream. You get a loser stigma if you have mental problems or problems with drugs.*

One aspect of individualisation and societal rationalisation is that the concrete contacts between professionals and users are reduced. Thus, when the face-to-face contacts between the parties are replaced by automation, the impersonal feature of daily life becomes even more prominent. When the development is characterised by automation and anonymity instead of personal contacts, the feeling of loneliness arises:

- *I think of the 'terror society' – we are afraid of the neighbours and are sceptical towards them. The 'risk society' is marked by loneliness. This is also shown in user research, using the method "User asks user". In this study the biggest problem was loneliness – and with loneliness other problems followed...*
- *'Risk society' ... yes, we are lonely – and there are constantly new things we have to learn and respond to – simultaneously.*

With individualisation follows increased demand on the ability for self-presentation, i.e. being capable of speaking for oneself and not leaving it to experts or administrators. Being able to express oneself also involves believing that what one says is worth listening to and experiencing acknowledgement from others – and finally being able to realise that this is true. When one is able to participate in the conversation or discussion, a feeling of being significant may grow. But it is also a right to remain silent if the theme of conversation is unfamiliar.

5.5 Searching for a meaningful everyday life

Dealing with daily duties and creating a meaningful life are vital to persons with mental disabilities as well as for others. Societal developments present opportunities in that direction. This presupposes having a network of persons who support you and who you feel a spirit of community with. Adapted work conditions can contribute to mastery and meaning. Possibilities exist, but are not sufficiently utilized:

- *It is up to the individual. A disabled person can participate if the work situation is tailored. Nowadays, people can work at home – the options are multiple and flexible if they are used. But this flexibility isn't utilized.*
- *There are a lot of tasks or jobs which don't require sitting in an office. But it depends on having computer tools and equipment and being trained in computer skills. People with disabilities must be upgraded, they must receive training and they need help...*
- *People want to get into jobs and be part of working life. It is healthy. But people are medicated too quickly, thus covering up the problems. The pills serve as a chemical lid over what is difficult.*

In order to participate in society, e.g. by having a job, the support systems should to a larger extent focus on helping the individual to cope with daily tasks despite problems and disabilities:

- *I think that one should be better at learning how to live with one's shortcomings, and learning to live better with oneself. Everybody has faults, nobody is perfect.*

Belonging to an alternative fellowship: When the public service and support systems cannot provide practical assistance to solve problems, it is important to have access to alternative arenas and fellowships that make it possible to learn from others who are in the same life situation – and to be able to try out new modes of being, new problem-solving strategies in a supportive milieu. The Centre is an example of such a milieu. It constitutes an alternative fellowship characterised by a low threshold service for work and activities – and in addition serves as a competence centre for user involvement. Participating in the community of the Centre gives support to daily coping and provides meaningful experiences. Here one can "be oneself" in an accepting environment:

- *You are yourself when you arrive – you are accepted as long as you don't hurt anybody. You may come and just sit and look around, and you may take part in preparing meals or renovating the house.*
- *The building is being renovated. You can also go on a trip or go for a walk in the town. We also have a football team here, and we go on summer tours. So there is something for everyone …*
- *But the Centre must not contribute to passivity. It is a place for growth and being – a place to be, to learn and to recover when it is needed. It is not meant to be a replacement for school attendance. Here, it is possible to recover – yes, recover – that is the right angle. The basic values of the Centre are trust, user management and appropriate care. It is not treatment– but action focused.*

Expectations and demands: Expectations on the individual are that one contributes "such as one is" and with "what one can". This means on the one hand acknowledgement and recognition, and on the other that fellowship norms are accepted.

- *Your religious belief is not an obstacle to being here either, but it is basically nothing we talk about much. If you want to talk about religion you can do so, but you can't stand and talk in front of the whole assembly. Religion is a private matter. But otherwise people can come as they are.*

In addition to the requirement not to hurt others, there is another demand and a permanent hindrance from using the Centre:

- The requirement for being here and using the Centre is: Not to be drunk or have a hangover. But you are not excluded, but just sent home! "You are warmly welcome back when you are sober".

Trust and care: The Centre is regarded as an addition to other services offered in the local community. This means that the participants can have treatment relations or work/activity offers besides the Centre. Therefore one can come "home" to the Centre – home to a fellowship that is like a good family. In the description of the atmosphere and culture, one participant chooses "greenhouse" as a metaphor. The culture in the greenhouse has been influenced by the fact that it is a different place where basic values are *trust, user management* and *adapted care*. Trust is shown in many ways, but very concretely in that 13 people have been given keys to the house. Importance is attached to there not being guardianship, but user management.

- *People decide themselves whether they feel that the place is something for them. They find out by coming to visit – walking around a bit – seeing how they feel. But it is like that everywhere: Not everyone fits in to every place. The most important thing is that they choose the Centre – or not. There are qualities here that are not experienced in the community.*
- *What are the qualities of the Centre here?*
- *Just look round here: It's the people! Here things are steered by the users.*
- *A low degree of control characterises the relations here – and it is just that which is missing in the public helping services. There – there are agreements and rules and they are stuck in their structures. Here it is different.*
- *I have had some problems with drugs and such things. In other places there has been a focus on negative talk, but here I have been given a golden opportunity for ordinary talk. And I can also*

be here late in the evening, at the weekend – and when I myself may want to. I can work, cook and be together with the other users of the place.

The adapted care, which nobody can manage without, is a question of caring about and caring for others. In the focus group discussions, this finds expression in the following reflections:

- *You don't need treatment when you are taken care of!*
- *No, you feel the caring atmosphere.*
- *Yes, here we are met in a genuine way. For example, we mean it when we ask: How are you now? We understand each other without having to make long explanations.*
- *And if there is a day when you don't see someone who is usually here, you ask how that person is today. It is care that it is a question of.*

The Centre is different and unique because it is not an institution, and because it is a place with a fellowship that each person chooses to be part of. In this way, the Centre constitutes an essential part the participants' network. Here, they get information, understanding and suggestions for how to cope with the challenges and possibilities of everyday living in the local community.

6. Discussion

6.1 Co-operative inquiry – a fruitful way of producing knowledge about everyday life?

The model that was used in this study to increase knowledge about what it is like for people with mental disabilities to live in late-modern society – co-operative enquiry – is characterised by co-operation, flexibility and dynamics. It is a research model where the roles between researchers and those researched are partly dissolved and where knowledge grows in dialogues between the people involved, rather than through information being transferred from information-givers to researchers. The distance between knowledge and action is short – elements of change/action are often combined with development of new knowledge. The model is particularly well suited in studies where experiences from actual life – the life-world – are sought. The collection of data by means of focus group interviews, particularly multistage focus groups, also means that these experiences are shared between the participants and can be the objects of reflection, development and deepening.

In this connection, social science theories on the long-term development of society, and structural concepts like 'risk society', 'disembedding' and 'individualisation' constitute starting points. Concepts that might be expected to be too intangible to be able to be operationalised and identified in an open discussion as in a multistage focus group. However, the main purpose of the study was not to contribute to the theory of late-modernity or the risk society. Instead the focus was on the everyday experiences of the participants and the extent to which they are connected with or differ from the distinctive features that characterize late-modern society. The everyday life of people with mental disabilities was the starting point against which the explanation value of the concepts could be discussed.

In spite of this, it appears that many of the concepts used to characterise late-modern society – or the risk society – can be identified by the participants and correspond well with their everyday life experiences with regard to content. Not surprisingly, the study also shows that other expressions are used to describe these experiences. The content of concepts like 'the disembedded society' could very well be recognised and described, while the concepts themselves could feel unfamiliar. At least two experiences with regard to method can therefore be noted:

- That the study's bases in structural social-science theory can well be combined with the open participant-based and formative element in co-operative inquiry, and
- That structural concepts like these also have a broad explanation value in a discussion on concrete life experiences, i.e. the structural macro-level and the social micro-level could be successfully combined in this study.

We will now proceed to discuss the empirical results in relation to the earlier description of societal changes and changes in the way of regarding people with mental disabilities – and society's support of this group.

6.2 Everyday life in late-modern society

The results of the study have been reported in five comprehensive categories. The first of these – *change and uncertainty* – focuses on the rapid change in society, which means that social relations based on spatial closeness and long-term consideration tend to be replaced by anonymous, 'technified' and shorter-term relations. Giddens (1996) uses the concept 'disembedding' to describe just this process – that the relations are removed from their ontological context. The result tends to be anonymisation and alienation. 'Waiting music', which is common in shopping centres and telephone contacts, for example, can be viewed in the same perspective, as an anonymising sound barrier. For people who are strained by mental disabilities the result can be increased stress and concentration difficulties. One of the participants describes it as a "process of alienation". The rapid pace of change and demands for increased efficiency have the same effect. The conditions for spontaneous and informal meetings are reduced in a world in which membership of a limited local community is weakened.

Mental disabilities and societal obstacles is a category that focuses on the relation between the individual and society, primarily in nursing and medical care. The participants give examples of how their mental disabilities are made evident in various societal contexts, often in contacts with support and treatment professionals. Bureaucratic administrative routines, shortage of time and – once again – lack of a personal and long-term contact make societal contacts difficult and, paradoxically enough, can contribute to accentuating the mental disability instead of mitigating its consequences. "You don't get trust in eight different people. Trust must be built over time." This quotation illustrates Giddens' expression (1996) 'transformation of intimacy'. In contemporary society trust can be built on personal contacts to a lesser extent. But the quotation shows even more clearly the difficulty of trusting a system that seems impersonal and incomprehensible. The problems are also evident in the meeting with a society that in general demands more and more adaptation and streamlining, for example when it is a question of the possibility of getting a job and a reasonable income. Concepts like 'employability' indicate this development – it is the individual that is to be adapted to the labour market, not the other way round. A weak financial situation in combination with a great need of support and service, which often cost money, contribute even more to a feeling of being an outsider: "It is expensive to be poor."

The technical dominance is a prominent feature in late-modern society, as in the discussion about the risk society. Advanced computer technology and communication technology characterise practically every area of social life and for the individual. Knowing how to handle the technology and access to computers and mobile phones are regarded as more or less implicit conditions for a functioning everyday life. The participants in the study see several problems with this. For those who do not have access to a computer of their own and connection to the Internet it can be difficult to handle contacts with authorities and carers. Information via the Internet is often more difficult to understand than necessary, the participants would like to see the participation of users when web pages are set up. If one is familiar with the Internet and has access to modern computer equipment, on the other hand, the technology offers new possibilities. For those who can find face-to-face contacts difficult, particularly meeting groups of people, computer technology makes personal communication possible, but on their own terms; they can be close and distant at the same time. By means of a personal blog they can show the sides of themselves they wish, but at the same time keep other parts to themselves. Computer and information technology mean both limitations and advantages, but the negative aspects outweigh the positive ones. Up-to-date knowledge is decisive – "If you lack knowledge you will easily be outside and powerless. If you have knowledge, you are inside."

The development towards increased individualisation can be traced over a long period of time and is not primarily caused by the rise of late-modern society. Nevertheless, the individualisation process is very clear in today's society, where both possibilities and responsibility rest to such a high degree on the individual. The participants' experiences in this area are summed up in the category *Individualisation and loneliness*. The possibilities to create and form one's own life have never been greater. Globalisation, unbounded technology, a higher level of education and a generally higher material standard of living are important factors here. Paradoxically enough, they also involve greater pressure on the individual to live up to various standards and fashions, at the same time as the demand to 'stand up for what you are' increases. It can be difficult to meet these apparently conflicting demands. A greater feeling of loneliness can therefore go with increased individualisation. The distance between people increases. The participants even think we have created a 'terror society': "... we are afraid of the neighbours and are sceptical towards them – the 'risk society' is marked by loneliness."

As is shown above, the characteristics of late-modern society can to a great extent be found in the everyday experiences of the participants. For the most part it is a question of the change in society involving an increase in problems and stress, which was also the fundamental assumption behind the study. For those who suffer from mental disabilities society has become more anonymous, 'depopulated', inaccessible, demanding and insecure. How much more natural then to seek new ways for fellowship and belonging. In the category *Searching for a meaningful everyday life* the focus is on two of the arenas of the world of life – working life and social network. Through the development of computer and communication technology new possibilities have been opened for adapting working life also to various forms of mental disability. However, for this to be possible those responsible must have the will to do so, and the participants experience that this is not always the case. Instead there is a tendency towards increased medication, something that can be "a chemical lid over what is difficult".

At least as important as having a job or something meaningful to do is belonging to a social community (which can naturally also be connected with a job). The participants in the study come from a user-steered centre connected to the user organisation Mental Health. The Centre provides the possibility of building up a new social network, having the feeling of belonging to a social community. The Centre is a 'free zone', members are met with trust and positive expectations, they support each other and show genuine care – "We mean it when we ask: How are you now?" It is not a question of a get-together without demands, but the demands are adapted to the person and the situation; one of the participants compared the Centre with a 'greenhouse' where everyone has the possibility for personal growth on their own premisses.

The user organisation Mental Health and the activities in the Centre are examples of how people with mental disabilities (as one of several groups) have developed a greater degree of user organisation and user influence in recent years. Late-modern society leaves more freedom of choice and responsibility to the individual but also opens the way to new forms of organisation and support. In one sense this society leaves the individual to his own fate to a greater extent. The vision of the modern – industrial – society, of an all-embracing and united welfare society, can partly be regarded as having cracked. But in the cracks new possibilities open up. The activity at the Centre can be regarded as such an alternative organisation, an answer to the needs that societal development has created, but at the same time made possible.

The participants think that the larger society can learn something important from such alternative fellowships – like what the Centre represents. Some of the special characteristics here are the flexibility both in relation to organisation and content, and the positive balance between individual and collective focusing. Besides, the Centre has something to teach to others about different expressions of trust, mixture of age and gender and the tolerance for diversity which characterise the milieu. Being met with care and trust strengthens personal responsibility and the feeling of community. Such beneficial social relationships seem to promote recovery processes (Schön et al 2009). Public service systems could develop in a more user-friendly way if they were based to a greater extent on trust and shared responsibility instead of distrust accompanied by the need for control systems, namely, a welfare system in alliance with the users "focusing on supporting them to deal with the uncertainty that is a feature of late-modern society" (Börjeson 2005: 23).

7. Possible ways forward, from the perspective of users, professionals, educators and researchers

The purpose of the study was focused on experiences in everyday life of people with mental disabilities. They constitute a group that – like several others – can be regarded as exposed and vulnerable, and thus dependent on support from society, not least from mental health care and social support work. The question of everyday life in late-modern society for people with mental disabilities therefore does not concern only themselves but also several other groups: professionals in care and support activities, teachers and heads of higher education, and people working with research and development (R&D). We therefore conclude the chapter with some ideas – visions - about continued development and the needs of change that can be regarded as called for in a society characterised by late modernity and new uncertainties. The tree groups we deal with are users (and user organisations), professionals and educators, and those working with R&D.

7.1 The role of service users and service users' organisations

The process towards openness and participation in social life for people with mental disabilities that was started in connection with de-institutionalisation in the 1960s will continue. User perspective and user influence can be expected to be far more prominent than today. This is the case with regard to individual users, but to an even higher degree for various forms of organised co-operation between them.

Service users in the area of mental disabilities create and strengthen their own organisations and associations. These organisations consist in certain cases only of service users/former service users, while in others relatives, professionals in the field of mental disabilities and, in certain cases, others who wish to support the work can be members. In certain countries people with mental disabilities have, not least with inspiration from Italian examples, built up co-operative enterprises that provide income but also social support and belonging. Forming organisations of their own and increased user influence are themes that are gaining greater scope. Having experience of functional disorder or social failure oneself is gradually also becoming valued as an important competence from the perspective of society. With a continued and even more pronounced development in this direction, it also seems logical for user-led organisations to establish contacts and be organised over national borders. Service users' voices would then be more united and have a greater impact.

7.2 The role of professionals and educators

The societal changes in the late-modern countries and the development towards a risk society also have consequences with regard to professionals and higher education in this field. Care and support for people with mental disabilities can be expected to involve markedly changed professional roles. Being a professional does not always mean knowing best. The knowledge of service users (knowledge from experience) will in many cases be valued as equal in merit to the knowledge of professionals (theoretical knowledge and experiential knowledge). Definition power and decision power are to be shared between professionals and service users.

Academic programmes should prepare students for work where professionals are in alliance with service users to a far greater extent. Training must also give a preparedness to work together with other professions to a far higher degree than today. Knowledge on everyday-living – with shortcomings due to the mental disability taken into account - will be an increasingly important part of higher education. In mental health care the balance of power shifts from the scientific/medical perspective towards the sociological/humanistic perspective. The growing research on recovery processes points unequivocally to the importance of an ideographic approach to knowledge, where all aspects of a person (physical, mental, social, spiritual) have their justified space. Internationalisation, globalisation, a closer collaboration between countries and harmonisation in an increasing number of fields will demand training courses that add a regional and a European perspective to the local and national perspective.

7.3 The role of Research and Development (R&D)

Research and the production of knowledge play an increasingly important role. The development of a risk society changes knowledge requirements. Research has a greater responsibility for developing and implementing knowledge that can be used in people's everyday lives. Research that is close to practice and linked to life environments and local communities can contribute to knowledge for coping with new risks and uncertainties. It will then also be natural for research and social change to be linked together in action research projects, for example by using the co-operative inquiry research model (Reason & Heron 1986, Hummelvoll 2006). Service users, but also professional welfare workers, are more and more closely involved in research. Increasing needs, in combination with stagnating or diminishing resources, make greater demands on research to develop new forms of care and treatment, but also to point out deficiencies in forms of support that are out of keeping with the times, so that they can be phased out. The responsibility of research to contribute to society's development becomes increasingly clear.

8. References

Beck, U. (1986) *Risikogesellschaft: Auf dem Weg in eine andere Moderne.* Frankfurt am Main: Suhrkamp Verlag.

Beck, U. (1992) *Risk Society. Towards a New Modernity.* London: Sage.

Beck, U. (1994) The reinvention of politics: Towards a Theory of Reflexive Modernization. In U. Beck, A. Giddens & S. Lash (Eds.) *Reflexive Modernisation. Politics, tradition and aesthetics in the modern social order.* Oxford: Blackwell Publishers.

Beck, U. (1998) Politics of Risk Society. I J. Franklin (Red.) *The Politics of Risk Society.* Oxford: Polity Press.

Børjeson, M. (2005) *Vi vet inte vilka metoder vi ska använda – om relationen mellan kunskap, praktik och politik när det gäller det sociala arbetet med hemlöshetsfrågor.* Akademisk avhandling. Institutionen för socialt arbete. Stockholm: Stockholms universitet.

Eliasson, R-M. & Nygren, J. (1981) *Utvärdering av psykiatrisk verksamhet. Del I.* Stockholm: Prisma.

Eriksson, B.G. & Hummelvoll, J.K. (2011) To live as mentally disabled in the risk society. *Journal of Psychiatric and Mental Health Nursing,* In press.

Forsberg, E. (1992) The 'long-term mentally ill'. I P-G. Svensson och B. Starrin (Eds.) *Health policy development for disadvantaged groups.* Oslo: Scandinavian University Press.

Forsberg, E. (1994) *Den stora utflyttningen – studier av psykiatrins omvandling.* Rapport 1994:3.

Foucault, M. (2006) *History of Madness.* London: Routledge.

Granerud, A. & Severinsson, E. (2006) The struggle for social integration in the community – the experiences of people with mental health problems. *Journal of Psychiatric and Mental Health Nursing* 13, 288-293.

Harste, G. (1999) Postindustrialism, kulturkritik och risksamhälle. I H. Andersen & L. B. Kaspersen (red.) *Klassisk och modern samhällsteori.* Lund: Studentlitteratur.

Hummelvoll, J.K. (2006) Handlingsorientert forskningssamarbeid – teoretisk begrunnelse og praktiske implikasjoner. *Norsk Tidskrift for Sykepleieforskning,* 8:1, 17-30

Hummelvoll, J.K. (2008) The multistage focus group interview - a relevant and fruitful method in action research based on a co-operative inquiry perspective. *Norsk Tidsskrift for Sykepleieforskning,* 10(1): 3-14.

Hummelvoll, J.K., Eriksson, B.E. & Beston, G. (2009) *Mennesker med psykiske funksjonshindringer i risikosamfunnet - en hverdagsnær tilnærming.* Elverum: Høgskolen i Hedmark, Rapport no. 13.

Malterud, K. (2003) *Kvalitative metoder i medisinsk forskning. En innføring.* Oslo: Universitetsforlaget.

Reason, P. (1994) Three Approaches to Participative Inquiry. In: N.K Denzin & Y.S. Lincoln (eds.). *Handbook of Qualitative Research.* London: Sage Publications.

Reason, P. & Heron J. (1986). Research with people: The paradigm of co-operative experiential inquiry. *Person Centered Review,* 1: 456-475.

Rowan, J. (2006) The Humanistic Approach to Action Research. In: P. Reason & H. Bradbury (eds.). *Handbook of Action Research.* London: SAGE Publications. pp 106-116.

Scheff, T. J. (1966) *Being Mentally Ill: A Sociological Theory.* Chicago: Aldine.

Schön, U-K., Denhov A. & Topor A. (2009) Social relationships as a decisive factor in recovering from severe mental illness. *International Journal of Social Psychiatry* 55, 336-347.

Svensson, T. (2005) Psykiatri eller inte? Radikal psykiatrikritik undere 1960 och 1970-talen. I
    L-C. Hydén (Red.) *Från psykiskt sjuk till psykiskt funktionshindrad.* Lund:
    Studentlitteratur.

Szasz, T. (1961) *The Myth of Mental Illness.* New York: Hoerber-Harper.

World Medical Association (2002) *The Declaration of Helsinki* (document 17C). Retrieved
    15.11.04, 2004.

Part 3

Conclusion

9

The Future of Mental Health Care Toward an Integrative Paradigm

James Lake
University of Arizona College of Medicine
USA

1. Introduction

The future of mental health care will be both daunting in its challenges and filled with the promise of new and better ways of understanding, preventing and treating serious mental illness. Novel approaches for assessing and treating mental illness are being shaped by advances in neuroscience, genetics and the scientific validation of ancient healing traditions in the social context of a growing range of expert resources and services that are becoming possible through rapidly increasing global access to the internet. Future models of mental health care will be determined by demographic trends and economic necessity as well as changing social norms and increasingly holistic values among both physicians and patients.

In the coming decades advances in conventional biomedicine will take in place in parallel with growing insight into the mechanisms underlying non-conventional therapies. Complementary and alternative medicine will evolve from the use of "herbs and vitamins" to a sophisticated research-driven model of integrative medicine based on individualized treatments incorporating biological, mind-body, informational and energy therapies targeting complex multi-factoral causes of mental illness. Improvements in the pharmacological management of mental illness and advances in manufacturing and quality assurance of vitamins, herbals, amino acids and other natural products will result in more efficacious and safer conventional and alternative treatment choices for psychiatric disorders. Treatment protocols incorporating validated mind-body and energy therapies will become widely used preventive therapies for maintaining optimal mental functioning in healthy populations and will be more frequently "prescribed" for the treatment of depression, anxiety, psychosis and other mental health problems.

Following a brief overview of the perspectives and limitations of biomedical psychiatry, emerging paradigms in the basic sciences and medicine that are changing the way we think about and treat mental illness are concisely described. Important recent research advances that will impact mental health care in the coming decades are summarized. Core principles and practical clinical methods of an emerging paradigm, integrative mental health care, are then discussed. In the coming decades advances in the basic sciences will transform biomedicine into a more robust and more *complete* paradigm that will reconcile modern Western scientific theory with the World's great healing traditions. A near term benefit will be more effective person-centered mental health care. The emerging paradigm of *integrative mental health care* is an important step in this evolutionary process. The chapter concludes with a forecast of important advances that will transform mental health care in the first decades of the 21st century.

2. Framing the problem

Conventional biomedicine – also called allopathic medicine – is based on an enormous body of research and is often very effective however conventional biomedicine has failed to adequately address medical and psychiatric illnesses in the United States and the world at large. In the U.S. 15% of the GNP (approximately $1.6 trillion) is spent on healthcare, yet drug reactions, infections, surgical errors or other complications of conventional medical care are among the leading causes of death and morbidity (Starfield 2000; Zhan 2003). Broad economic issues that interfere with the capacity of allopathic medicine, including the specialty branch called biomedical psychiatry, to meet health care needs include restrictions of treatments covered under managed care, Medicare, and private insurance contracts, growing dissatisfaction with the quality of conventional medical care because of concerns over efficacy and safety, and the increasing cost of care for the average consumer (Astin 1998a).

The shortcomings of conventional treatments suggest that biomedicine does not fully explain the causes of mental illness while inviting rigorous consideration of novel explanatory models of symptom formation and studies on promising non-conventional treatment modalities. Growing acceptance of non-allopathic healing traditions in Western culture is the result of both scientific advances and social trends. Conventional biomedicine is being influenced by the increasing openness of Western culture to non-Western healing traditions in the context of growing demands for more meaningful and more personal contact with medical practitioners – often difficult to find during brief appointments in managed care settings. These issues have led increasing numbers of individuals who see conventionally trained physicians to seek concurrent treatment from alternative practitioners, including Chinese medical practitioners, herbalists, homeopathic physicians, energy healers and others (Barnes 2008).

Recent years have witnessed growing openness to non-conventional therapies among conventionally trained clinicians and researchers. At the same time people who are critical of Western biomedicine as currently practiced are turning increasingly to non-conventional therapies for the treatment of both medical and mental health problems (Rees 2001; Astin 1998a). Approximately 72 million U.S. adults used a non-conventional treatment in 2002, representing about one in three adults (Tindle 2005). If prayer is included in this analysis almost two thirds of adults use non-conventional therapies (Barnes & Bloom 2008). Anyone diagnosed with a psychiatric disorder is significantly more likely to use non-conventional therapies compared to the general population (Unutzer 2000; Unutzer 2002). One third of individuals who report a history of generalized anxiety, mood swings or psychotic symptoms use non-conventional approaches to treat their symptoms (Unutzer 2000). Furthermore, two thirds of severely depressed or acutely anxious individuals use both conventional and non-conventional treatments concurrently, and as many as 90% of these see a psychiatrist or other mental health professional (Kessler 2001). The findings of two large patient surveys suggest that most individuals who have mental health problems use conventional medications and non-conventional approaches at the same time (Unutzer 2000; Eisenberg 1998). According to one large physician survey approximately half of U.S. physicians believe that acupuncture, chiropractic and homeopathy rest on valid medical principles, and frequently refer patients to non-conventional practitioners for these therapies (Astin 1998b).

Mental health care in its present form is at a critical juncture. In spite of enormous industry-funded research efforts over many decades the evidence supporting pharmacologic treatments of major psychiatric disorders is inconsistent and disappointing (Sussman 2004). Billions of dollars of research spending for new drug development have failed to significantly reduce the prevalence rates of serious psychiatric disorders. In fact there is evidence that rates of some disorders are increasing in spite of ongoing advances in biomedical psychiatry. Furthermore, recently published systematic reviews of quality double-blind placebo-controlled trials fail to show strong efficacy for widely used conventional pharmacological therapies used to treat common psychiatric disorders including major depressive disorder, bipolar disorder, schizophrenia, dementia, and others (Moller 2007; Kirsch 2008; Thase 2008; Fournier et al 2010; Fountoulakis 2008; Katzman 2009; Dixon et al 2009; Tajima et al 2009; Birks 2006) In addition to growing concerns about their lack of efficacy psychopharmacologic treatments are plagued by serious safety issues. Many widely used psychotropic drugs are associated with serious adverse effects including weight gain and increased risk of diabetes and heart disease, neurologic disorders, and sudden cardiac death, and increased suicide risk. Furthermore conventional drugs often result in partial response or no response even when recommended treatment protocols are followed. The persistence of serious symptoms of mental illness during treatment results in impairments in occupational functioning with associated losses in productivity. Concerns about the limitations of contemporary biomedical psychiatry including inequalities in delivery of mental health services, the lack of integration of mental health services into other medical specialties, conflicts of interest in relationships with the pharmaceutical industry and other clinical practice issues have been raised by leading figures in academic psychiatry (Reynolds et al 2009).

In response to the limitations of conventional mental health care future directions of research and clinical therapeutics are becoming progressively more open to the rigorous examination of novel perspectives. This growing intellectual openness is giving birth to a truly *integrative* model of mental health care that draws from the best evidence in both conventional biomedical psychiatry and alternative modalities. Novel theories are being advanced in response to the conceptual and practical clinical limitations of the orthodox view embraced by conventional biomedical psychiatry in efforts to more adequately explain both normal conscious functioning and the complex factors that contribute to mental illness. These emerging theories will shape the future of mental health care. They are at the heart of a rapidly evolving paradigm called "integrative mental health care" that is leading to innovative new research methods and more effective clinical therapeutics. At the level of individual patients an important result of this evolutionary process will be *more effective* and *more compassionate* "whole person" mental health care that takes into account the complex biological, psychological, social, cultural and possibly also *spiritual* causes and meanings of mental illness.

3. Biomedicine and biomedical psychiatry in overview

At its core, biomedicine or "allopathic" medicine incorporates assumptions about the nature of material existence and identifiable causal relationships between factors in the environment and illness phenomena that can be traced to cultural and philosophical roots of early Western civilization. This ancient philosophical perspective eventually led to the establishment of formal methods of observation and measurement, culminating in modern scientific method. In spite of the recent confirmation of a role of quantum mechanics in complex living systems including the human brain, biomedicine continues to rely exclusively on the tenets of classical Newtonian physics in building its theories and evaluating claims of mechanism and demonstrations of outcomes in its clinical methods. In short, the dominant paradigm of contemporary biomedicine—and by extension biomedical psychiatry—rests on metaphysical assumptions about the properties of phenomena that can have existence according to the classical materialist world-view of the universe—a model that was replaced over a century ago by a more inclusive paradigm informed by quantum mechanics and general relativity theory.

Contemporary biomedical psychiatry—the orthodox perspective in which mental health care is practiced—is based on the assumption that mind is a manifestation of what the brain does. Diverse perspectives on the so-called "mind-body" problem exist in contemporary psychiatry however there is still no consensus on a sufficient explanatory model of mind-body interactions (Kendler 2001; Wright & Potter 2003). Complete understanding of mind-body interactions will probably require a convergence of classical and non-classical paradigms (Shang 2001). For example, light exposure therapy is known to have therapeutic effects on melatonin and neurotransmitter activity and may also interact with brain dynamics on subtle levels possibly consistent with the postulates of quantum mechanics or quantum brain dynamics (Curtis 2004). The human bio-field is probably best described with respect to complex interactions between classical and non-classical kinds of energy and information, including electrical, magnetic, acoustic, and large-scale quantum properties of living systems (Rein 2004). Practitioners of conventional biomedicine frequently regard "energy" treatments as examples of the placebo effect because of the assumption that postulated forms of energy or information on which energy treatments rest simply do not exist. Rigorous research designs investigating "energy" medicine are difficult to achieve and findings on the effectiveness of directed intention and putative non-classical energy effects on human health remain inconclusive (Abbott 2000). Nevertheless, accumulating research evidence shows that beneficial effects of some energy treatments can be replicated under controlled conditions, suggesting that non-classical forms of energy or information influence outcomes in some cases.

The reductionist perspective implicit in Western science informs the central dogma of biomedical psychiatry, namely neurotransmitter theory, which holds that discrete correspondences exist between symptoms of mental illness and *deficiencies* or *dysfunction* at the level of specific neurotransmitters (Lopez-Munoz 2009). To date the neurotransmitter theory has failed to provide an adequate explanatory model of the causes of mental illness or to consistently predict responses to treatments targeting specific neurotransmitters (Lopez-Munoz 2009). In addition to problems related to the questionable validity of core assumptions on which biomedical psychiatry is based, the orthodox paradigm is limited by numerous practical issues. Biomedical psychiatry prioritizes pharmacological and psychotherapeutic treatment of acute symptoms of serious chronic mental illnesses over prevention and maintaining wellness. While pharmacological treatments often result in rapid, dramatic stabilization of severe symptoms, many so-called *maintenance* therapies of common psychiatric disorders have marginal efficacy compared to placebos (Sussman 2004). Furthermore, significant unresolved safety issues and the high cost of many psychotropic drugs significantly limit the potential reach of biomedical psychiatry in Western culture and render them inaccessible and often irrelevant in less developed world regions. On a practical vein mental health care as practiced in North America, and the EU is typically limited to brief impersonal appointments emphasizing "medication management" under cost constraints of "managed care" that fail to take into account the complex medical, psychosocial, cultural or spiritual factors that frequently contribute to mental illness.

4. Biomedical psychiatry is an evolving paradigm

Recent discoveries in neuroscience and genetics suggest that contemporary models of human consciousness and, by extension, understandings of mental illness are incomplete. Theories describing neurochemical mechanisms underlying normal brain functioning continue to evolve at a rapid rate pointing to the limitations of the neurotransmitter theory. This still-current model advanced in the early 1960s characterizes neurotransmitters as substances that are invariably synthesized and released by neurons, act on post-synaptic receptors, and mediate both normal and abnormal states of consciousness in relationship to specific activity levels or dysregulations at the level of their synthesis or receptor binding affinities. In contrast to the above model in which dysregulations of specific neurotransmitters correspond to discrete symptoms, certain recently characterized neurotransmitters and neuropeptides are not stored in synaptic vesicles or released by exocytosis and do not act at receptor sites on post-synaptic vesicles, thus they do not fulfill criteria for neurotransmitters. D-serine is an example of such "atypical" neurotransmitters. This molecule is synthesized and stored in neuroglia and binds to NMDA receptors whose dysregulation has been implicated in the pathogenesis of schizophrenia and other psychotic disorders. Other "atypical" neurotransmitters that may play significant roles in psychiatric disorders include nitric oxide, carbon monoxide, and possibly hydrogen sulfide. It has been suggested that nitric oxide (NO) may play an important role in learning and memory. (Snyder 2000).

When mental health care is most effective it addresses symptoms of mental illness at their root psychological, social, cultural, biological and spiritual causes. The contemporary biomedical model of mental health care is limited in its capacity to alleviate the root causes of suffering because its theoretical foundations and clinical methods address only some of the complex causes and meanings of mental illness. This is largely due to the fact that the root causes of mental illness are still poorly understood resulting in numerous poorly substantiated models of mental illness causation and a corresponding multiplicity of therapies that do not adequately address or correct the root psychological, cultural or spiritual meanings or biological causes of symptoms (Wright & Potter 2003). At a basic theoretical level the causes of symptom formation in psychiatric illness are poorly understood because of the absence of research methods needed to examine and elucidate the roles of disparate external and internal factors that cause or exacerbate cognitive, affective or behavioral symptoms. This has led to multiple biological and psychodynamic theories whose premises are often contradictory or mutually exclusive. In the broader context of the history of medicine it is not surprising to find that psychiatry lacks a unifying body of theory or universally endorsed standards of clinical practice. Factors contributing to the ambiguous position of psychiatry have been discussed at length in two important works (Grof 1985; Wilber 2001) Among psychiatrists, the dominant view is an extension of contemporary biomedicine, which equates mental health problems to discrete functional abnormalities at the level of neurotransmitters. According to this model, successful "treatment" entails "correcting" a presumed neurochemical abnormality with the goal of restoring to normal a corresponding dysregulation in cognitive, emotional, or behavioral functioning. While psychiatrists often use cognitive-behavioral approaches or "talk" therapies directed at changing maladaptive interpersonal dynamics, depth psychological approaches examining existential or spiritual themes are typically regarded as incidental to "more serious" psychotherapeutic or pharmacological treatments informed by the dominant biomedical paradigm. Agreeing on a "most relevant" theory or a "most appropriate" treatment is even more problematic for psychologists for whom numerous theories of symptom formation have yielded disparate and frequently contradictory explanations of the underlying causes or meanings of psychopathology. Because of the multiplicity of theories and clinical practices that comprise contemporary psychology and psychiatry there is no theory-neutral method for evaluating the relative merits and weaknesses of disparate treatments. Subsequently consensus is lacking on the "most appropriate" or "best" conceptual framework or practical clinical methods when approaching a specific mental health problem. In addressing this dilemma Wilber has systematically reviewed divergent psychological theories of mind-body, and has proposed guidelines for the creation of an "integral psychology" that takes into account core psychological and spiritual features of many dominant theories of mind-body (Wilber 2001). An important practical goal of this work is the elaboration of a series of integrative psychotherapeutic strategies that are ideally suited for specific symptoms of mind-body, psychological or spiritual distress.

In a more practical vein contemporary biomedical psychiatry is constrained by ambiguous research evidence supporting its various theoretical claims. This stands in contrast to biomedicine in general, in which discrete unambiguous relationships have been confirmed to take place between identifiable disease-causing factors and discrete disorders. Novel assessment and treatment approaches in biomedical psychiatry will emerge from on-going advances in the basic neurosciences, brain imaging, immunology and genetics. Future models of mental illness causation will not depend exclusively on empirical verification of strictly biological processes and will postulate both classically described kinds of biological and biophysical causes (eg, genetic factors and neurotransmitter dysregulation) as well as non-classical kinds of phenomena (eg, non-linear brain dynamics and quantum-level processes). Future studies will used advanced functional imaging technologies to examine the role of complex non-linear dynamic relationships between neural circuits and the immune system and specific psychiatric disorders, as well as the postulated role of quantum "entanglement" associated with large-scale coherent macroscopic quantum field effects in both normal consciousness functioning and psychiatric symptom formation.

5. Important advances are taking place in the theory and practice of psychiatry

In contrast to the limitations of the clinical practice of biomedical psychiatry steady advances in medical research are contributing to a more robust paradigm of mental health care that will translate into improvements in patient care in the coming decades. On-going advances in the neurosciences, psychopharmacology and brain imaging research will soon yield novel assessment approaches, more effective and safer conventional treatments including drugs based on novel mechanisms of action and new therapeutic uses of light, weak electrical current and magnetic fields. Collectively, these advances are transforming the theoretical foundations and clinical therapeutics of contemporary Western mental health care. Novel theories in biomedical psychiatry promise significant advances in understanding of the nature and causes mental illness. For example, it has been suggested that non-linear dynamics (ie chaos theory) may help explain mood changes associated with the menstrual cycle on the basis of postulated complex influences of hormones and neurotransmitters, as well as social and psychological variables on mood (Rasgon 2003). Substantiation of this model by research findings may eventually lead to effective preventive strategies addressing hormone-mediated mood disturbances. There is significant emerging evidence that complex interactions between immune functioning, neurotransmitters and hormones are important in depressed mood, anxiety, and other disorders (Miller 2004).

Improved understanding of genetic factors that mediate mental illness will continue to accrue from analysis of the genetic library available in the Human Genome Project. Biomedical psychiatric research is increasingly taking into account the significance of genetic and biochemical variability in mental illness. For example, the high degree of individual variability in response to conventional drugs suggests poorly characterized differences in neurotransmitter deficiencies or imbalances associated with major depressive disorder, generalized anxiety and other psychiatric disorders (Delgado 2000). Studies on the effects of neurotransmitter depletion on mood are consistent with the view that changes in brain serotonin or norepinephrine activity levels *alone* do not fully explain the causes of depressed mood or observed differential responses to antidepressants which are probably related to complex biological and social factors including genetic variability (and thus ethnicity), diet, and culturally determined expectations. Genetic, cultural and social variability translates into differences in effective dosing strategies using conventional drugs and commensurate differences in susceptibility to adverse effects (Lin 2004). The high degree of biological variability may be especially problematic for patients of African or Asian ethnicity potentially causing safety issues or poor outcomes (Lawson 2004; Edmond 2004). The AmpliChip CYP450™ test, recently introduced by Roche Pharmaceuticals, incorporates two DNA amplification and detection technologies that screen for genetic mutations. The polymerase chain reaction (PCR) is used to amplify or make copies of genetic material, and a high-density microarray technology is subsequently used to capture and scan the amplified DNA. The device will enable physicians to determine when variations or mutations are present in the CYP450 cytochrome system providing clinically relevant information about individual differences in prescription drug metabolism. In the near future psychiatrists will routinely order outpatient laboratory studies using this technology to determine the most appropriate drugs and doses to use for a given patient while minimizing the risk of adverse effects (Amanda, Meyers and Nemeroff 2010).

In biomedical psychiatry classically established forms of energy are used as probes to provide information about brain activity associated with symptoms. Normal brain functioning is characterized by complex bio-magnetic and electrical activity that can be measured using functional brain imaging techniques including positron emission tomography (PET), single photon emission computed tomography (SPECT), functional magnetic resonance imaging (fMRI), magneto-electroencephalography (MEEG) and quantitative electroencephalography (QEEG). Advances taking place in functional brain imaging will permit studies on discrete neurotransmitter/receptor systems underlying normal conscious functioning as well neural and molecular processes involved in the pathogenesis of specific psychiatric disorders. This will result in improved diagnostic accuracy of neurologic and psychiatric disorders with commensurate improvements in the efficacy of treatments targeting discrete neurotransmitter systems and neural circuits (Bandettini 2009). Emerging evidence suggests that consistent relationships exist between specific patterns of electrical brain activity and discrete psychiatric disorders (John 2007; Bares 2007; Venneman 2006; Brinkmeyer 2004) however it is often difficult to determine whether energetic "abnormalities" in the CNS are causes or effects of pathology. Electrical currents and pulsed electromagnetic fields are established conventional treatments in contemporary biomedical psychiatry. Electrical current and focused magnetic fields probably have real-time effects on the biomagnetic properties of brain functioning in addition to long-term effects at the level of neurochemical and biomagnetic changes in the activity of brain circuits associated with the regulation of affect, cognition and behavior (Liboff 2004).

Important technological innovations that will become more widely used treatments of mental illness in the first half of the 21st century include transcranial magnetic stimulation (TMS), EEG biofeedback and virtual reality exposure therapy (VRGET). Biofeedback techniques addressed at modifying autonomic activity include galvanic skin resistance (GSR), electromyography (EMG), and electroencephalography (EEG) training techniques are widely used in outpatient clinic settings to treat phobias and other anxiety disorders. Emerging findings suggest that biofeedback training based on heart rate variability (HRV) significantly reduces stress and improves general feelings of emotional well-being in individuals who are subjected to acute job-related stress (McCraty 2001). Continued rapid growth in broad-band internet access will soon result in widespread use of these biofeedback techniques by patients at home and at work environments using portable devices based on existing computer technology. Chronically anxious patients, and especially those with panic disorder or agoraphobia, are frequently too impaired by their symptoms to seek professional care. Others are geographically isolated and cannot obtain conventional cognitive-behavioral therapy (CBT) or pharmacological treatment for severe anxiety syndromes. Broad-band videoconferencing using internet technology is being explored as a cost-effective alternative mode of treatment delivery to these home-bound patients. It has been established that an effective therapeutic alliance can be achieved between therapist and patient when CBT is done by videoconference (Manchanda 1998; Bouchard 2000). Although CBT can be done by telephone (telepsychiatry), videoconferencing has the advantage of permitting the therapist to demonstrate behavioral exercises to the patient, and both therapist and patient are able to accurately observe non-verbal behaviors during sessions creating an authentic sense of "presence" that simulates face-to-face interactions in conventional psychotherapy settings. A large controlled study showed that CBT is equally effective for a range of anxiety symptoms when done in conventional out-patient therapy settings or via broad-band videoconferencing (Day 2002). CBT delivered via videoconferencing is as effective as face-to-face CBT in patients with both panic disorder and agoraphobia (Bouchard 2004). This is a significant finding in that it provides a viable and affordable alternative to routine CBT for this severely impaired population who might otherwise not utilize mental health services. In the coming decades advances in artificial intelligence will lead to the creation of therapist "avatars" that will interact with patients in virtual environments, will be capable of optimizing psychotherapeutic interventions in response to each unique patient's needs, and will be capable of simulating both expert factual knowledge and therapeutic interventions.

Controlled studies confirm that virtual reality graded exposure therapy (VRGET) (sometimes called *experiential cognitive therapy* or "ECT" in European countries) is more effective than conventional imaginal exposure therapy (using mental imagery to provoke the feared object or situation), and is comparable to in vivo exposure therapy (Pertaub 2001; Emmelkamp 2001). Many VRGET tools are already available over the internet, permitting mental health professionals to guide patients in the use of these computer-based advanced exposure protocols through real-time videoconferencing anywhere high-speed internet access is available (Botella 2000). Within the next few decades treatments of phobias, panic attacks, and other severe anxiety disorders will combine VRGET with biofeedback, cognitive-behavioral therapy (CBT) or mind-body practices in outpatient settings or in the patient's home via real-time interactions permitting authentic "presence" between the patient and the therapist or a therapist "avatar" via broadband internet connections. Research progress in all of these technology-based therapies will soon yield effective, safe non-pharmacological treatments for major depressive disorder, bipolar disorder, anxiety disorders and other serious psychiatric disorders.

Brain-computer interface (BCI) is a frontier technology that is emerging from the new field of neural engineering that will soon enable paralyzed individuals to regain use of their limbs. This technology permits direct communication between brain centers that control movement and robotized prosthetic devices. In the coming decades continued evolution of this technology will lead to neuroprosthetic devices that will permit individuals diagnosed with psychiatric disorders to regulate behaviors, mood or cognitive problems to enhance functioning in all of these areas (Krusianski 2011). By the year 2050 non-invasive neuroprosthetic devices will be widely used to effectively and safely treat serious psychiatric disorders that are poorly responsive to psychotropic drugs including bipolar disorder, severe depressed mood and dementia.

In addition to advances in psychoparmacology, genetics and technology-based therapies, natural product research is yielding significant findings of beneficial effects when a specific vitamin, mineral or herbal is used as a monotherapy to treat a specific psychiatric disorder (Sarris et al., 2009). An important trend that is pushing the evolution of contemporary biomedical psychiatry toward increasing integration with other healing traditions comes from the use of synergistic combinations of synthetic drugs and select natural products (Sarris et al., 2009). This principle has been demonstrated in many studies showing increased antidepressant efficacy when SAMe, folic acid, L-tryptophan or omega-3 fatty acids are combined with antidepressants in the treatment of depressed patients. (Sarris et al., 2009); and increased efficacy when n-acetyl cysteine, magnesium, folic acid or amino acids are combined with conventional mood stabilizers in bipolar patients (Sarris et al., 2010b). Future studies will examine such synergistic combinations of synthetic drugs and natural products to determine optimal formulas addressing common psychiatric disorders. The use of natural products including nutrients or botanicals in combination with pharmacotherapeutic agents holds the potential for improving outcomes while reducing adverse effects by permitting reductions in effective doses of psychotropics and commensurate reduction of adverse effect risks.

6. Novel paradigms are shaping the future of medicine and mental health care

In conventional biomedicine, mainstream concepts from chemistry and biology provide the theoretical foundations for current explanatory models of illness phenomena. Conventional biomedicine posits that health and illness can be adequately characterized in terms of established theories in biology and physics. Some novel approaches in medicine and psychiatry do not radically depart from assumptions embedded in the orthodox views of conventional biomedicine. For example psychoneuroimmunology (PNI) is a synthetic model that starts from established theories in psychiatry and biomedicine and postulates complex dynamic relationships between stress, immunological status and psychiatric or neurological symptom formation (Irwin 2008; Muller & Schwarz 2007; Muller & Schwarz 2006). There is a rich discussion of PNI and other emerging paradigms in the peer-reviewed journal literature including emerging models in physics, biology and information science describing structure-function relationships in complex living systems. However, in general the day to day clinical practice of biomedicine takes place without regard to these novel ideas. Non-classical paradigms including complexity theory and quantum field theory (QFT) may eventually lead to novel research methodologies that will elucidate subtle inter-relationships between "healing intention," immune status and psychiatric symptom formation. Phenomena regarded as legitimate subjects of inquiry in non-Western healing traditions have been largely ignored in biomedical research including, for example, the role of prayer and intention in health and healing; and putative beneficial effects of so-called "subtle energy" on immunological or neurobiological functioning as postulated by practitioners of QiGong, "healing touch" or other forms of "energy medicine."

Although many non-allopathic therapies meet conventional scientific criteria for efficacy and effectiveness they have not been endorsed as mainstream treatments largely because of entrenched conservative beliefs in Western medicine and strong academic biases against novel ways of understanding illness. Non-allopathic treatments based on biological mechanisms of action have been more thoroughly investigated in controlled studies compared to mind-body or "energy" therapies. St. John's Wort (Hypericum perforatum), SAMe, 5-HTP and folic acid are examples of non-conventional biological modalities that have been thoroughly evaluated. Mind-body therapies and treatments based on established or postulated forms of energy or information have not yet been carefully evaluated in Western-style research studies. For example, Reiki, qigong, and homeopathy are based on postulated forms of energy or information that have not been verified and may in fact not be potentially verifiable by Western science. While some non-allopathic therapies are probably no more effective than placebos, the same argument can be applied to conventional biomedical treatments. The placebo effect is widely accepted among conventional Western medical practitioners as playing a significant treatment role in both medical and mental health problems (Dixon 2000). Meta-analyses of controlled trials suggest that conventional drugs used to treat major depression and other psychiatric disorders are no more effective than placebos (Kirsch 2002; Thase 2002; Sussman 2004). Unanswered questions about the role of placebo effects in treatment response are shared concerns for both conventionally trained and alternative medical practitioners. The controversy over placebo effects is complicated by the more recently described "nocebo" effects—adverse effects associated with placebos—which may affect as many as 40% of individuals who take placebos (Tangrea 1994). These findings suggest that many treatments probably have non-specific effects that are either beneficial or detrimental to health, including general effects on the body's immune, endocrinologic, and central nervous system. There is no agreed on theory that fully explains placebo and nocebo effects however personal, social and cultural factors that are difficult to quanitfy may facilitate "self-healing" when patients undergo any kind of medical or psychiatric treatment.

Disparate systems of medicine postulate the existence and involvement of different forms of energy and information in health, illness and healing. Some assessment approaches rely on the accurate characterization of classically described biological, energetic or informational processes that constitute the presumed causes of a particular symptom or symptom pattern. A more complete and accurate understanding of the role of consciousness in health and healing may require a convergence of biomedicine and non-biomedical paradigms. Some non-allopathic treatment approaches are based on classical forms of energy including electromagnetic energy and sound. Examples include Western herbal medicine, functional medicine, EEG biofeedback, music and patterned binaural sounds, full spectrum bright light exposure, micro-current brain stimulation, and dim light exposure at selected narrow wavelengths. It has been established for decades that all living organisms emit ultra-weak photons and under certain conditions such biophotons are emitted as highly ordered or "coherent" light (Bajpai 2003; Popp 2003). Research on biophoton emissions from the human body have led to speculation about "light channels" that regulate energy and information transfer within the body, biological rhythms associated with the intensity and patterns of biophoton emissions, and diseases related to energetic "asymmetries" between the left and right sides of the body (Cohen 2003; Wijk 2005). Studies on biophoton emissions associated with acupoints suggest that subtle differences in count, wavelength and coherence may correspond to energetic "imbalances" in yin and yang elements that, according to Chinese medical theory, are associated with neurologic and psychiatric disorders (Yang 2004).

Treatment approaches based on classically accepted forms of energy can have both direct energetic effects and indirect informational effects on biological or energetic processes associated with health and illnesses. The latter can be described as "informational" effects of classical forms of energy. In contrast treatments based on postulated non-classical models of energy or information, including quantum mechanics, quantum information, and quantum field theory may have both direct and subtle effects on brain functioning and physiology (Curtis 2004; Hankey 2004). Functional medicine is an important emerging paradigm that views health and illness in relationship to informational changes in complex intercellular communication processes. Functional medicine rests on conventional biomedical understandings of pathophysiology in the context of assumptions of biochemical and genetic individuality (Bland 1999). According to this model health and illness result from interactions between the unique genetic constitution of each individual and many different internal and external factors including infection, trauma, lifestyle, diet or environmental influences that can modify genetic expression and alter intercellular communication manifesting as complex physical or psychiatric symptom patterns. Disparate molecules serve as cellular mediators, including neuropeptides, steroids, inflammatory mediators and neurotransmitters. Functional assessment approaches identify informational changes in intercellular communication associated with symptoms, and effective treatments modify the informational basis of illness taking into account complex interactions between mediators and different cell types. Preliminary findings suggest that immunological dysregulation plays a significant causative role in the pathogenesis of affective disorders, schizophrenia, Alzheimer disease, and other degenerative neurological disorders (Sperner-Untewegger 2005). The relationship between immunity and mental illness is complex and poorly understood and the same immunological dysregulation is sometimes found in patients with disparate symptoms (Irwin 2008). Recent studies suggest that nonspecific over-activation of the immune system involving T-helper cells takes place in subgroups of persons with schizophrenia (Strous & Shoenfeld 2006). The immune-mediated dysregulation of both dopamine and glutamate neurotransmission has also been implicated in the pathogenesis of schizophrenia (Muller & Schwarz 2006). In response to these findings, anti-inflammatory and immune-modulating therapies are being investigated as future treatments for affective disorders and schizophrenia. Horrobin (Horrobin 1996; Horrobin 1998) proposed a "membrane phospholipid" model of schizophrenia which posits that abnormal metabolism of phospholipids resulting from genetic and environmental factors manifests as a chronic, severe constellation of symptoms typically diagnosed as a variant of schizophrenia or schizoaffective disorder. The membrane phospholipid hypothesis posits that a spectrum of psychiatric disorders is associated with abnormalities in neuronal membranes and the type and severity of symptoms are functions of the magnitude and specific type of metabolic errors resulting in abnormal phospholipid metabolism.

Some established and emerging non-allopathic assessment approaches postulate that illness phenomena can be more completely described in terms of non-classical forms of energy. Examples include analysis of the vascular autonomic signal (VAS) (Ackerman 2001), Chinese meridian diagnosis (Hammer 2001; Zhang 2002; Langevin et al 2004), homeopathic constitutional assessment, and Gas Discharge Visualization (GDV) (Korotkov, Williams and Wisneski 2004). Because disparate factors contribute to mental illness it is often difficult to accurately and reliably assess the causes of symptoms and to identify the most efficacious treatments. The integrative mental health care of the future will include sophisticated assessment approaches capable of evaluating the causes of mental illness at biological, informational and "energetic" levels of body-brain-mind. On-going research studies of non-allopathic assessment approaches will validate some as clinically useful in mental health care while others will become marginalized. The increasing use of novel assessment approaches in clinical psychiatry will gradually lead to more comprehensive and more cost-effective treatment planning. Promising emerging approaches in psychiatric assessment include:

- Testing of the urine and blood to reveal dysregulation at the level of neurotransmitters and immune factors associated with mental illness
- Quantitative electroencephalography (QEEG) to quantify differences in brain electrical activity for clarifying psychiatric diagnosis and predicting treatment response
- The use of micro-array "chips" to analyze genetic differences in drug metabolism associated with individual differences in the P450 cytochrome system
- The use of advanced semiconductor devices to measure ultra-weak biophotons providing clinically useful indicators of the causes of mental illness at subtle neurochemical and"energetic" levels of brain function
- The use of pulse diagnosis as used in Chinese medicine, Ayurveda, and Tibetan medicine and scientific studies to validate energy assessment in the context of novel paradigms in physics including quantum mechanics

Like emerging assessment approaches many non-allopathic treatment approaches are also based on postulated non-classical forms of energy or information including for example acupuncture, homeopathic remedies, Healing Touch, Qigong and Reiki. In Chinese medicine "Qi" is regarded as an elemental energy that cannot be adequately described in the language of contemporary science, but may have dynamic attributes that are consistent with quantum field theory (Chen 2004). Quantum brain dynamics (QBD) is an example of a non-classical model which invokes quantum field theory to explain certain dynamic characteristics of brain functioning, including possibly the influences of non-classical forms of energy or information on mental health. It has been suggested that healing intention operates through non-local "subtle" energetic interactions between the consciousness of the medical practitioner, and the physical body or consciousness of the patient (Zahourek 2004). In contrast, energy psychology assumes that highly developed energetic techniques, including acupuncture, acupressure and healing touch, are required to affect energetic balance and health. "Mind energetics" is a recently introduced conceptual model that postulates the exchange of "energy" through language and intention during therapeutic encounters, and claims that "energy" transforms psychological defenses in beneficial ways (Pressman 2004). Widespread interest in the role of spirituality and religion in mental health has resulted in increasing research in this area and the inclusion of a special V code in the DSM-IV for religious or spiritual problems (Turner 1996).

7. Complex systems theory will expand the paradigm of biomedical psychiatry

Contemporary biomedical theory argues that medical or psychiatric disorders are attributable to discrete "causes" that are biological in nature and take place at the level of interactions between molecules or cells. An implicit assumption underlying this reductionist view is that for any *disorder* a particular biological marker corresponds to an underlying "cause" in a simple linear fashion. A corollary of this view is that a treatment is "effective" when it adequately addresses and ultimately "corrects" the discrete underlying biological cause of a specific (medical or psychiatric) symptom or disorder by repairing abnormal functioning at a cellular or molecular level. This is in fact the basic logic supporting the neurotransmitter theory as an explanatory model in biomedical psychiatry (see above). The complex systems model stands in contrast to the conventional view of linear causality that is implicit in biomedical theory (Auyang 1998; Bell 2002). Biomedicine is beginning to incorporate concepts from emerging theories in physics, biology, and information science describing structure-function relationships in complex living systems including the human brain. Complex systems theory invites an increasingly integrative perspective in the social sciences, biology and medicine. Important advances will take place in the conceptual foundations of biomedical psychiatry when the research dialog includes complex systems theory, which argues that dynamic non-linear energetic or informational states at multiple levels in the brain and body manifest as symptoms (Morowitz & Singer 1995). This view implies that although a particular symptom may have one apparent "primary" or discrete cause, complex dynamic cause(s) can vary significantly between individuals reporting similar symptoms as a consequence of each person's unique biochemical, genetic, social, psychological, and energetic makeup. For example, light exposure therapy is known to have therapeutic effects on melatonin and neurotransmitter activity that result in improved mood—but emerging research evidence suggests that light interacts with brain dynamics on subtle energetic levels consistent with the predictions of quantum mechanics. In contrast to the orthodox view of empiricism and linear causality many traditional healing systems conceptualize illness, health, and healing in terms of subtle non-linear processes at multiple hierarchic levels of body-mind-spirit within each unique human and between humans and their environments.

In the framework of complex systems theory, a symptom or symptom pattern (ie, a "disorder") is viewed as an emergent property of multiple factors interacting at multiple hierarchical levels. Practical differences in assessment and treatment approaches in the world's healing traditions can be viewed as reflecting basic differences in assumptions underlying contemporary biomedicine and complex systems theory. Biomedicine assumes that linear causality operates in the dynamic interactions between natural phenomena and, by extension, discrete causal relationships exist between identifiable causal factors and disease states in a system that can be adequately characterized using existing empirical research methods. In contrast to the linear view, the complex systems model posits that dynamic non-linear relationships exist between multiple factors in a hierarchical web and dynamic emergent properties of body-brain-mind experienced as physical or mental symptoms (Strogatz 2001). In some cases, for example in the management of infectious diseases, discrete symptoms are correlated with an identifiable viral or bacterial infection, and the linear biomedical model probably yields a relatively accurate description of symptom formation, and is therefore an adequate basis for effective treatment planning. However in mental illness, causes, conditions or meanings associated with a symptom pattern are typically more complex and change over time. Even in cases where conventional biomedical assessment yields clinically useful information, it is reasonable to approach assessment of multiple interacting factors associated with mental illness within the framework of complex systems theory and to regard discrete biological markers (eg, thyroid hormone levels, electrolytes, immune factors) as important elements of a complex dynamic web of factors associated with mental illness.

Conventional biomedicine tacitly acknowledges the validity of the complex systems model by employing pharmacological or other kinds of biological treatments targeting disparate metabolic or cellular functions when addressing a particular disorder. The same logic supports the use of integrative approaches using modalities that combine to yield synergistic effects when addressing disparate causal factors underlying psychiatric disorders. Although a particular symptom pattern may have one or few primary causes, each patient's unique biochemical, genetic, social, psychological, and possibly also energetic or spiritual constitution translates into unique differences at all of these levels in individuals diagnosed with the same psychiatric disorder. The situation becomes even more complex when taking into account that in any individual the psychological, biological, energetic, informational and possibly spiritual causes of a disorder may fluctuate over time in relation to both dynamic internal and environmental factors. Conventional biomedical psychiatry argues that persisting cognitive, affective and behavioral symptoms in the same individual are associated with varying levels of activity in neurotransmitters and receptors—or dysfunction at either level—over time however reasons for such variability remain unclear. It follows from this observation that an assessment or treatment approach that is appropriate for a particular psychiatric disorder at one time for a particular patient may not be the most appropriate approach with respect to another individual diagnosed with the same disorder, or even the same individual diagnosed with the same disorder at a future time. Because complex systems theory does not inform contemporary biomedical psychiatry clinical methods used in assessment and treatment planning do not take into account the complex and highly variable nature of factors associated mental illness at the level of each unique patient. Starting from complex systems theory and assuming that dynamic symptom patterns that comprise psychiatric disorders are associated with multiple factors and multiple *kinds* of factors that change over time, it is reasonable to assume that using two or more assessment approaches will more adequately *capture* multiple causes as well as different kinds of causes. It follows from the complex systems model that the most appropriate and effective treatment plan will include disparate modalities targeting disparate causal factors identified through history or formal assessment. Different approaches are being used to model complex variables that operate in non-conventional healing approaches including path analysis and the analysis of latent variables (Schuck 1997; McArcle 2009). The latter approach has been used to assess quality of life in psychotic patients (Mercier 1994).

8. Emerging understandings of "energy" and information will contribute to future mental health care

Some "alternative" treatments not currently endorsed by biomedical psychiatry are based on well described forms of energy such as electromagnetism and sound. Examples include EEG biofeedback, music and patterned binaural sounds, full spectrum bright light exposure, micro-current brain stimulation, and high-density negative ions. Treatment approaches based on such classically described forms of energy and information have specific or general beneficial effects at the level of neurotransmitter systems or brain circuits. In contrast, treatments based on postulated non-classical kinds of energy or information, including quantum mechanics and quantum field theory, may have both direct and subtle effects on brain function and mental health. Non-conventional modalities based on concepts that are presently outside of the tenets of biomedicine include acupuncture, homeopathic remedies, Healing Touch, qigong, and Reiki. Ancient healing traditions and accumulating modern research evidence suggest that prayer and other forms of directed intention may help alleviate symptoms of physical and mental illness. This is the domain of energy medicine (Chen 2004).

In contrast to the materialist philosophy implicit in contemporary biomedicine and by extension biomedical psychiatry, Indo-Asian philosophy is based on the premise that the nature of reality, including both inanimate matter and living systems, is best understood in terms of fundamental properties of a postulated "vital energy" (Di Stefano, 2006). The meaning and role of causality in non-Western systems of medicine is not constrained by physical processes interacting in a world ordered by linear time flow. According to this view states of both living and non-living systems are regarded as secondary manifestations of more primary energetic states. By extension "energetic" factors are believed to play important roles in the manifestations of all living systems including changes in functioning associated with illness and health. Although "Qi" in Chinese medicine and "Prana" in Ayurveda cannot be directly observed or measured using Western style research methods professional practitioners of Chinese Medicine and Ayurveda can infer the roles of specific energetic "imbalances" when particular illness phenomena are present. Because of the philosophical difference between the Western medical tradition and Indo-Asian medicine proponents of contemporary biomedicine often regard methods used in non-Western systems of medicine as subjective or arbitrary. By the same token, non-Western healing traditions often place little emphasis on the empirical methods of Western science that attempt to "reduce" subjective symptoms into mechanistic descriptions of discrete underlying biological "causes." Indeed, from the perspectives of traditional Chinese medicine (TCM) and Ayurveda, attempts to empirically verify relationships between energetic phenomena are regarded as unnecessary because a fundamental energetic principle is assumed to be immanent throughout the universe.

Novel understandings of energy and information are also coming from recent theoretical developments in quantum physics. A fundamentally new direction in our understanding of consciousness and by extension the causes of mental illness—will come from an emerging theory that regards brain functioning from the perspective of quantum mechanics and quantum field theory (Naeqau & Kafatos 1999; Elitzur 2005; Lorimer 2004). Quantum brain dynamics attempts to explain subtle characteristics of brain functioning in terms of non-classical forms of energy and information (Jibu and Senta 2001). Pending further confirmation through advanced functional brain imaging studies quantum brain dynamics may eventually help explain reports of therapeutic benefits achieved through non-local interactions between the consciousness of the medical practitioner and the patient (Schlitz & Braud 1997; Astin 2000; Standish 2001; Wackerman 2003; Standish 2003). This work will eventually yield a testable hypothesis about the role of prayer and intention in health and healing clarifying therapeutic mechanisms associated with spiritual and mind-body practices including meditation, yoga and energy medicine.

9. Possible future pathways of medicine and psychiatry and a forecast

Within the first decades of the 21st century psychiatrists will embrace assessment and treatment approaches now excluded by orthodox Western medicine. Novel diagnostic and treatment modalities will emerge in the context of on-going research on non-conventional modalities. Future explanatory models of mental illness will take into account established Western scientific theories, emerging paradigms, and non-Western healing traditions. In this process Western psychiatry will become a truly integrative paradigm yielding more complete understandings of biological, informational and "energetic" processes associated with mental illness. A future more integrative psychiatry will emerge from a synthesis of disparate explanatory models of mental illness. More complete understandings of complex dynamic relationships between biological, somatic, energetic, informational, and possibly also spiritual processes associated with symptom formation will lead to more effective assessment and treatment approaches addressing causes or meanings of symptoms at multiple inter-related hierarchic levels. Future studies on meditation, healing intention, meditation and prayer will elucidate the role of consciousness in health and healing.

It is likely that the theories and methods that comprise conventional biomedicine and biomedical psychiatry in the early 21st century will follow one of two possible future evolutionary pathways resulting in either continued conservative growth or radical change. Although it will not be necessary to go outside the established paradigm of contemporary biomedicine in order to develop a conceptual framework for integrative medicine, the empirical validation of novel assessment and treatment approaches will require the rigorous evaluation of novel concepts in physics, chemistry and biology. This conservative pathway does not assume or require the violation of orthodox scientific models of reality based on implicit assumptions of linear causal interactions between discrete particles in order to explain illness and health. However the conservative model does assume that important future directions in medical research will not be completely determined by currently entrenched economic, institutional or intellectual dogma influencing beliefs and research studies in academic centers. A more radical pathway is conceivable in which an increasingly eclectic framework of conventional biomedicine will progressively embrace novel ideas in physics and neuroscience as well as concepts from non-conventional systems of medicine that rest on assumptions currently outside of the orthodox paradigm (Rubik 1996; Liboff 2004; Jonas & Crawford 2004). If intellectual, institutional and economic trends favor the more radical pathway in the coming decades it is likely that conventional biomedicine—and along with it biomedical psychiatry—will gradually transform into a fundamentally new paradigm that will have little resemblance to mental health care of the early 21st century.

Regardless of whether future mental health care undergoes gradual conservative changes or radical transformation, practical clinical advances tracking the conceptual evolution of medicine will result in an increasingly "whole person" systems approach that will more adequately address the underlying causes and meanings of mental illness. This systems approach will incorporate the broad range of both conventional and alternative therapies. By employing individually tailored treatments integrative mental health care will will more adequately address unique needs and concerns of each patient including their physical and psychological well-being, social relationships, and spiritual values. Novel scientific models of complex relationships between biological, energetic, and informational processes associated with mental illness will lead to more effective integrative assessment and treatment strategies addressing the causes or meanings of symptoms at multiple hierarchical levels of body-brain-mind. This evolutionary process will result in an increasingly integrative perspective in conventional biomedicine and novel explanatory models of illness and healing that address the assumptions underlying contemporary Western science and medicine. This trend will accelerate in the first half of the 21st century in response to increasing intellectual openness in Western culture to non-biomedical systems of medicine and ongoing advances in the basic sciences resulting in evolution of the conceptual foundations and clinical therapeutics of conventional biomedical psychiatry into a more sophisticated model of care incorporating both scientific and intuitive understandings of normal psychological functioning and the complex psychological, biological, energetic and informational factors contributing to mental illness.

In the coming decade mental health care will emerge as a more eclectic and more open paradigm responding to research advances in both biomedicine and alternative medicine. Congressionally mandated reforms will progressively restrict the influence of the pharmaceutical industry on research in both academic psychiatry and the private sector. Quality manufacturers of select CAM modalities will become established players in an increasingly diversified healthcare marketplace in which private insurance and Medicare will cover select alternative therapies that will have parity with conventional biomedical treatments. Under reforms in health care policy that will come into effect in this decade, government, industry and academic research centers will work in a more coordinated fashion to develop systematic research programs on a wide range of assessment and treatment modalities resulting in more effective and more cost-effective treatment choices addressing urgent unmet needs of mental health care in the U.S. and other western countries. Increased collaboration between researchers and clinicians in the U.S. and internationally will help advance and accelerate evolution towards integrative mental health care.

The first decades of the 21st century will bring a gradual transition away from psychopharmacology as the dominant mode of treatment toward increasing reliance on advanced technologies for alleviating serious mental illness. Growing global access to broadband internet services will permit patients to benefit from psychotherapy through "tele-presence," advanced biofeedback techniques and virtual reality exposure therapy, and therapist "avatars" in the comfort of their homes. By the year 2050 psychiatrists and other mental health practitioners will routinely use a scientifically validated integrative "tool kit" incorporating the most advanced biomedical technologies together with empirically validated traditional healing practices. The more integrative mental health care of the future will permit more accurate assessment of biological, energetic and informational factors associated with symptoms and lead to individualized multi-level treatment strategies addressing the unique pattern of biological, energetic and informational factors associated with each patient's unique symptoms. The transformation of biomedical psychiatry to integrative mental health care will result in deeper understandings of mental illness, improved and more rapid treatment response, and reduced costs.

By mid-century a new paradigm will be solidly established and will inform the theories and clinical therapeutics of mental health care. Biomedical theory will be informed by complexity theory, novel theories in physics and information science and accumulating findings from the basic sciences and consciousness research. There will no longer be a rigid dichotomy between biomedical and alternative modalities. By mid-century advances in the genetics and neurobiology of mental illness will have yielded more specific, more effective and more individualized pharmacological, genetic and energetic therapies for major psychiatric disorders. Rigorously designed Western-style research studies will have verified the mechanisms of action of some non-conventional biological, mind-body and so-called "energy" modalities and validated their therapeutic claims. By the same token many contemporary conventional and alternative modalities will have been discredited as lacking efficacy by well designed studies and will no longer be used. Treatments that will be abandoned in the coming decades will include many conventional pharmacological therapies and psychotherapeutic treatments in current widespread use as well as natural products from diverse healing traditions. In parallel with these changes on-going advances in functional brain imaging will permit studies on postulated roles of magnetic fields, biophotons, and macroscopic highly coherent quantum field effects on normal brain functioning and mental illness.

10. Concluding remarks

Mental health care as practiced today is in urgent need of new ideas, better, safer, more affordable and more compassionate approaches to the prevention and treatment of mental illness. The future of mental health care is being shaped by emerging paradigms in the basic sciences, increasing openness to non-Western systems of medicine, changing clinicians' attitudes, but most of all by our patients' demands for better, more personalized and more compassionate care.

The theoretical foundations and clinical practices of mental health care will continue to evolve as biomedicine begins to explore perspectives that recognize complex inter-relationships in brain-body-mind, for example, the field of psychoneuroimmunlogy, an integrative paradigm which reconciles non-biomedical systems of medicine with contemporary biomedicine has been emerging for some time now and yield significant improvements in the day to day practice of mental health care (Irwin 2008). A more robust theory of mental illness causation will require novel research methodologies to adequately address complex psychological, neurochemical, immunological and energetic mechanisms associated with both normal brain functioning and mental illness. The new paradigm that is emerging from advances in functional brain imaging, genetics, and molecular biology will be capable of elucidating complex relationships between the biological and electromagnetic (possibly also quantum-level) activity of the brain and body in healthy individuals, as well complex factors underlying cognitive, affective and behavioral symptoms. The new paradigm will be highly integrative taking into account both classically described biological factors including neurophysiological and immunological functioning as well a non-classical phenomena, including the postulated role of macroscopic coherent quantum fields in neuronal activity associated with human consciousness (Pizzi 2004; Thaheld 2001). The disparate viewpoints of biomedicine and non-Western healing traditions call for conceptual bridges between different systems of medicine and practical strategies for integrating therapeutics used in different cultures. Future technologies may eventually result in empirical validation of "Qi" or other non-Western concepts of "energy" however important differences will probably persist between the theories and clinical practices of biomedicine and non-conventional healing traditions.

11.

Dr. Lake chairs the International Network of Integrative Mental Health www.INIMH.org You may contact Dr. Lake at www.IntegrativeMentalHealth.net.

12. References

Abbot N. Healing as a therapy for human disease: a systematic review. *J Altern Complement Med*. 2000;6:159-169.

Ackerman J The biophysics of the vascular autonomic signal and healing Frontier Perspectives Fall 2001, 10:2, 9-15

Amanda J. Myers, Ph.D., and Charles B. Nemeroff, M.D., Ph.D. New Vistas in the Management of Treatment-Refractory Psychiatric Disorders: Genomics and Personalized Medicine, Focus 8:525-535, Fall 2010

Astin, J. Why Patients use alternative medicine, JAMA May 20, 1998a, 279:19, 1548-1553.

Astin, J., Harkness, E., and Ernst, E. (2000) the efficacy of "Distant Healing": A systematic review of randomized trials. *Annals of Internal Medicine*. 13(11:903-910.

Astin, J., Marie, A, Pelletier, K. et al A review of the incorporation of complementary and alternative medicine by mainstream physicians, Arch Intern Med, 158: Nov 23, 1998b, 2303-10.

Astin, J., Marie, A, Pelletier, K. et al A review of the incorporation of complementary and alternative medicine by mainstream physicians, Arch Intern Med, 158: Nov 23, 1998b, 2303-10.

Auyang S Foundations of complex-system theories in economics, evolutionary biology, and statistical physics Cambridge Univ. Press, Cambrdige, England 1998.

Bajpai RP. Quantum coherence of biophotons and living systems. Indian J Exp Biol. 2003 May;41(5):514-27.

Bandettini, P. A. (2009) What's new in neuroimaging methods? Ann N Y Acad Sci, 1156, 260-93.

Bares M, Brunovsky M, Kopecek M, Stopkova P, Novak T, Kozeny J, Höschl C. Changes in QEEG prefrontal cordance as a predictor of response to antidepressants in patients with treatment resistant depressive disorder: a pilot study. J Psychiatr Res. 2007 Apr-Jun;41(3-4):319-25. Epub 2006 Aug 4.

Barnes P Powell-Griner E McFann K Nahin R Complementary and alternative medicine use among adults: United States, 2002 Seminars in Integrative Medicine 2:2; 54-71, 2004.

Barnes PM, Bloom B. Complementary and Alternative Medicine Use Among Adults and Children: United States 2007. National health statistics reports: no 12, Hyattsville, MD: National Center for Health Statistics 2008.

Bell I Caspi O Schwartz G Grant K Gaudet T et al Integrative medicine and systemic outcomes research Arch Intern Med 2002;162:133-140.

Birks J. Cholinesterase inhibitors for Alzheimer's disease Cochrane Database Syst Rev. 2006 Jan 25;(1)

Bland J New functional medicine paradigm: dysfunctional intercellular communication Int Jour Integrative Medicine 1:4;July/Aug 1999;11-16.

Blankert B, Tangermann M, Vidaurre C, Fazli S, Sannelli C et al The Berlin brain–computer interface: non-medical uses of BCI technology, Neuroprothesis (add volume, date)

Bolwig TG, Hansen ES, Hansen A, Merkin H, Prichep LS. Toward a better understanding of the pathophysiology of OCD SSRI responders: QEEG source localization. Acta Psychiatr Scand. 2007 Mar;115(3):237-42.

Bouchard, S Paquin B Payeur R Allard M Rivard V Fournier T Renaud P Lapierre J Delivering cognitive-behavior therapy for panic disorder with agoraphobia in videoconference Telemedicine Jour and e-Health 10:1, 2004; 13-25.

Bouchard S Payeur R Rivard V Allard M Paquin B Renaud P Goyer L Cognitive behavior therapy or panic disorder with agoraphobia in videoconerence: preliminary results. Cyberpsychol Behav 2000;3:999-1008.

Botella C Banos R Guillen V et al Telepsychology: public speaking fear treatment on the Internet Cyberpsychol Behav 3:6;959-968, 2000.

Brinkmeyer J, Grass-Kapanke B, Ihl R. EEG and the Test for the Early Detection of Dementia with Discrimination from Depression (TE4D): a validation study. Int J Geriatr Psychiatry. 2004 Aug;19(8):749-53.

Chen, K. an analytic review of studies on measuring effects of external Qi in China, Review Article, Alt. Therapies July/Aug 2004 10:4 38-50

Cohen S, Popp FA. Biophoton emission of human body. Indian J Exp Biol. 2003 May;41(5):440-5.

Curtis B Hurtak J Consciousness and quantum information processing: uncovering the foundation for a medicine of light JACM 10;1:2004, 27-39.

Day S Schneider P Psychotherapy using distance technology: story and science J Counseling Psychol 2002; 49:499-503.

Delgado PL, Moreno FA. Role of norepinephrine in depression J Clin Psychiatry 2000;61 Suppl 1:5-12

Deslandes A, Veiga H, Cagy M, Fiszman A, Piedade R, Ribeiro P. Quantitative electroencephalography (qEEG) to discriminate primary degenerative dementia from major depressive disorder (depression). Arq Neuropsiquiatr. 2004 Mar;62(1): 44-50. Epub 2004 Apr 28.

Di Stefano V. Holism and complementary medicine: origins and principles. Crows Nest, NSW: Allen & Unwin; 2006.

Dixon M Sweeney K The human effect in medicine: theory, research and practice Radcliffe Medical Press, Oxford, 2000.

Eisenberg, D., Davis, R., Ettner, S, et al, Trends in alternative medicine use in the United States, 1990-1997: results of a follow-up national survey, JAMA November 11, 1998, 280:18, 1569-75.

Elitzur A Dolev S Kolenda N Eds., Quo Vadis Quantum Mechanics? Springer New York and Berlin, 2005.

Emmelkamp P Bruynzeel M Drost L Van der Mast C Virtual reality treatment in acrophobia: a comparison with exposure in vivo Cyberpsychology Behav 4:3; 335-339 2001.

Fountoulakis KN, Vieta E. Treatment of bipolar disorder: a systematic review of available data and clinical perspectives. Int J Neuropsychopharmacol. 2008 Nov;11(7):999-1029.

Fournier JC, DeRubeis RJ, Hollon SD, Dimidjian S, Amsterdam JD, Shelton RC, Fawcett J. Antidepressant drug effects and depression severity: a patient-level meta-analysis. JAMA. 2010 Jan 6;303(1):47-53.

Grof S Beyond the brain: birth, death and transcendence in psychotherapy State Univ. of New York Press, Albany, NY 1985.

Hammer L Qualities as signs of psychological disharmony, Ch 15 pp. 539-594, in Chinese Pulse Diagnosis: a contemporary approach Eastland Press, Seattle, WA. 2001.

Hankey A Are we close to a theory of energy medicine? JACM 10;1:2004, 83-86.

Horrobin D. Schizophrenia as a membrane lipid disorder which is expressed throughout the body. *Prostaglandins Leukot Essent Fatty Acids.* 1996;55:3-7.

Horrobon D. The membrane phospholipid hypothesis as a biochemical basis for the neurodevelopmental concept of schizophrenia. *Schizophr Res.* 1998;30:193-208.

Irwin MR. Human psychoneuroimmunology: 20 years of discovery. *Brain Behav Immun.* 2008;22:129-139.

Irwin MR. Human psychoneuroimmunology: 20 years of discovery. Brain Behav Immun. 2008 Feb;22(2):129-39. Epub 2007 Oct 29

Jibu M and Yasue K Quantum brain dynamics and consciousness: an introduction, Vol. 3 in Advances in consciousness research Eds. Stamenov M and Globus G, John Benjamin Publishing Company, Philadelphia, PA., 1995.

John ER, Prichep LS, Winterer G, Herrmann WM, diMichele F, Halper J, Bolwig TG, Cancro R. Electrophysiological subtypes of psychotic states Acta Psychiatr Scand. 2007 Jul;116(1):17-35.

Jonas, W Crawford C eds., Healing, Intention and Energy Medicine: science, research methods and clinical implications, Churchill Livingstone New York, N.Y. 2003.

Katzman MA. Current considerations in the treatment of generalized anxiety disorder CNS Drugs. 2009;23(2):103-20.

Kendler, K. A Psychiatric Dialogue on the Mind-Body Problem, [Perspectives: Reviews and Overviews] J. Am Psych Assn 158:7 July 2001 989-1000.

Kessler R Soukup J Davis R Foster D Wilkey S et al The use of complementary and alternative therapies to treat anxiety and depression in the United States Am J Psychiatry 158:289-294; 2001.

Kirsch I Moore T Scoboria A Nicholls S The emperor's new drugs: an analysis of antidepressant medication data submitted to the U.S. Food and Drug Administration. Prevention & Treatment 5:Article 23, 2002. available at www.journals.apa.org/prevention/volume5/toc-jul15-02.html.

Kirsch I. Challenging received wisdom: antidepressants and the placebo effect. Mcgill J Med. 2008 Jul;11(2):219-22.

Kleinman A. Rethinking psychiatry: from cultural category to personal experience The Free Press, New York City, N.Y. 1988.

Korotkov K Williams B Wisneski L Assessing biophysical energy transfer mechanisms in living systems: the basis of life processes JACM 10;1:2004, 49-57.

Krusienski DJ, Grosse-Wentrup M, Galán F, Coyle D, Miller KJ, Forney E, Anderson CW. Critical issues in state-of-the-art brain-computer interface signal processing J Neural Eng. 2011 Apr;8(2):025002

Langevin, H., Badger, G, Povolny, B, Davis, R, Johnston A, et al Yin and Yang Scores: A new method for quantitative diagnostic evaluation in traditional Chinese Medicine Research JACM 10:2 2004 389-395.

Liboff A toward an electromagnetic paradigm for biology and medicine JACM 10;1:2004, 41-47.

Lin K Ethnicity, pharmacogenetics and psychopharmacotherapy, [abstract 44A], Symposium 44: culture, ethnicity, race and psychopharmacology: new research perspectives, 2004 Annual APA Meeting, New York, N.Y.

Lopez-Munos F, Alamo C., Historical Evolution of the Neurotransmission Concept, J Neural Transm. 2009 May;116(5):515-33. Epub 2009

Lorimer D Science, consciousness and ultimate reality Imprint Academic, Exeter, England 2004.

Manchanda M McLaren P Cognitive behavior therapy via interactive video J Telemed Telecare 1998;4 (Suppl 1):53-55.

McArdle JJ. Latent variable modeling of differences and changes with longitudinal dataAnnu Rev Psychol. 2009;60:577-605.

McCraty, R Atkinson M Tomasino D Science of the Heart: Exploring the role of the heart in human performance—an overview of research conducted by the Institute of HeartMath, Publication 01-001, HeartMath Research Center, Boulder Creek, CA 2001.

Mercier C King S A latent variable causal model of the quality of life and community tenure of psychotic patients Acta Psychiatr Scand 1994;89:72-77

Miller A Advances in psychopharmacology: immune system pathology in psychiatric disease, p. 331 [abstract in "Advances in psychopharmacology," May, 2004 APA New York, N.Y.)

Miller D Homeodynamics in consciousness Advances Fall/Winter 2003, 19;3/4:35-46.

Möller HJ, Maier W. [Problems of evidence-based medicine in psychopharmacotherapy: problems of evidence grading and of the evidence basis for complex clinical decision making]. [Article in German] Nervenarzt. 2007 Sep;78(9):1014-27.

Morowitz H, Singer J Eds., The mind, the brain, and complex adaptive systems Vol 22, proceedings of the Santa Fe Institute studies in the sciences of complexity, Addison-Wesley Publishing Co., Menlo Park, CA. 1995.

Muller N, Schwarz M. Schizophrenia as an inflammation-mediated dysbalance of glutamatergic neurotransmission. *Neurotox Res.* 2006;10:131-148.

Müller N, Schwarz MJ. The immune-mediated alteration of serotonin and glutamate: towards an integrated view of depression. Mol Psychiatry. 2007 Nov;12(11):988-1000. Epub 2007 Apr 24.

Nadeau R Kafatos M The non-local universe: the new physics and matters of the mind, Oxford Univ. Press, Oxford, England 1999.

Nemeroff C Kilts C Berns G Functional brain imaging: twenty-first century phrenology or psychobiological advance for the millennium? Am J Psychiatry 156:5, May 1999, p. 671-673

Penrose R Shadows of the mind: a search for the missing science of consciousness Oxford Univ. Press, Oxford, England 1994.

Pertaub D Slater M Barker C An experiment on fear of public speaking in virtual reality In: Medicine Meets Virtual Reality 2001, Vol 81 Westwood J Hoffman H Mogel G Stredney D eds. Amsterdam IOS Press 2001.

Pizzi R Non-local correlation between human neural networks on printed circuit board, abstract presented at Tucson Conf. on Consciousness, April 2004 (pizzi@dti.unimi.it) NOTE: get final citation and final paper.

Popp FA. Properties of biophotons and their theoretical implications. Indian J Exp Biol. 2003 May;41(5):391-402.

Rasgon N Pumphrey L Prolo P Elman S Negrao A et al Emergent oscillations in mathematical model of the human menstrual cycle CNS Spectrums 2003;8(11):805-814.

Rees, L Integrated medicine: imbues orthodox medicine with the values of complementary medicine BMJ, 2001, 322: 119-120

Rein G bioinformation within the biofield: beyond bioelectromagnetics JACM 10;1:2004, 59-68.

Reynolds C, Lewis D, Detre T, Schatzberg A, Kupfer D. The future of psychiatry as clinical neuroscience, Acad Med 2009 April; 84(4):446-450.

Rubik B Ch. 5 "toward an emerging paradigm for biology and medicine," in *Life at the Edge of Science*, The Inst for frontier science, Oakland, CA. 1996

Rubik B Life at the edge of science: an anthology of papers by Beverly Rubik, The Institute for Frontier Sciences Oakland, CA. 1996.

Sarris, J., Goncalves, D., Robins Wahlin, T.-B. & Byrne, G. (2010a) Complementary Medicine Use by Middle-aged and Older Women: Personality, Mood and Anxiety Factors Journal of Health Psychology, In press.

Sarris, J., Kavanagh, D. & Byrne, G. (2010b) Adjuvant use of nutritional and herbal medicines with antidepressants, mood stabilizers and benzodiazepines. J Psychiatr Res, 44, 32-41.

Sarris, J., Schoendorfer, N. & Kavanagh, D. (2009) Major depressive disorder and nutritional medicine: a review of monotherapies and adjuvant treatments. Nutr Reviews, 67, 125-31.

Schlitz, M., and Braud, W. (1997) Distant intentionality and healing: Assessing the evidence. Alternative Therapies in Health and Medicine. 3(6): 62-73.

Schuck J Chappell T Kindness G Causal modeling and alternative medicine Alt Therapies March 1997;3:2, 40-47.

Shang C Emerging paradigms in mind-body medicine JACM 7;1:2001, 83-91.

Snyder S Ferris C Novel neurotransmitters and their neuropsychiatric relevance Am J Psychiatry 2000;157:1738-1751).

Sperner-Unteweger B. Immunological aetiology of major psychiatric disorders: evidence and therapeutic implications. Drugs. 2005;65:1493-1520.

Standish, L.J. , Johnson, L.C., Kozak, L., and Richards, T. (2003) Evidence of correlated functional magnetic resonance imaging signals between distant human brains. Alternative Therapies in Health and Medicine. 9(1): 128-(need last page)

Standish, L.J., Johnson, L.C., Kozak, L., and Richards, T. (2001) Neural energy transfer between human subjects at a distance. Paper presentation at: Bridging worlds and filling Gaps in the Science of Healing. Kona, Hawaii.

Starfield B Is U.S. health really the best in the world? JAMA 2000 July 26;284(4):483-5.

Strogatz S Exploring complex networks Nature 410;2001:268-276.

Strous RD, Shoenfeld Y. Schizophrenia, autoimmunity and immune system dysregulation: a comprehensive model updated and revisited. *J Autoimmun.* 2006;27:71-80.

Sussman N The "file-drawer" effect: assessing efficacy and safety of antidepressants Primary Psychiatry July 2004 p. 12.

Tajima K, Fernández H, López-Ibor JL, Carrasco JL, Díaz-Marsá M. Schizophrenia treatment. Critical review on the drugs and mechanisms of action of antipsychotics. Actas Esp Psiquiatr. 2009 Nov-Dec;37(6):330-42.

Tangrea J Adrianza E Helsel W Risk factors for the development of placebo adverse reactions in a multicenter clinical trial Annals of Epidemiology 1994;4:327-331.

Thaheld F Proposed experiment to determine if there are EPR nonlocal correlations between two neuron transistors APEIRON 7:3-4, July-Oct 2000 202-205

Thase M Antidepressant effects: the suit may be small, but the fabric is real Prevention & Treatment 5:Article 32, 2002. available at journals.apa.org/prevention/volume5/toc-jul15-02.html.

Thase ME. Do antidepressants really work? A clinicians' guide to evaluating the evidence. Curr Psychiatry Rep. 2008 Dec;10(6):487-94.

Tindle H Davis R Phillips R Eisenberg D Trends in use of complementary and alternative medicine by U.S. adults: 1997-2002 Alt Ther Health Med 2005;11:1;42-49.

Tononi G Edelman G Consciousness and complexity Science 282;1998:1846-1851.

Turner R Lukoff D Barnhouse R Lu F Religious or spiritual problem: A culturally sensitive diagnostic category in the DSM-IV. The Journal of Nervous and Mental Disease, 1996;183(7): 435-443.

Unutzer J Klap R Sturm R Young A Marmon T et al Mental disorders and the use of alternative medicine: results from a national survey Am J Psychiatry 157:1851-1857; 2000.

Unutzer J. et al. Surveys of CAM: Part V–use of alt and comp ther...psychiatric and neurologic diseases JACM 8:1, 93-96, 2002

Unutzer J. et al. Surveys of CAM: Part V–use of alt and comp ther...psychiatric and neurologic diseases JACM 8:1, 93-96, 2002

Venneman S, Leuchter A, Bartzokis G, Beckson M, Simon SL, Schaefer M, Rawson R, Newton T, Cook IA, Uijtdehaage S, Ling W. Variation in neurophysiological function and evidence of quantitative electroencephalogram discordance: predicting cocaine-dependent treatment attrition. J Neuropsychiatry Clin Neurosci. 2006 Spring;18(2):208-16.

Wackermann, J. (2003) Dyadic correlations between brain functional states: Present facts and future perspectives. Mind and Matter. 2(1): 105-122.

Wijk EP, Wijk RV. Multi-site recording and spectral analysis of spontaneous photon emission from human body. Forsch Komplementarmed Klass Naturheilkd. 2005b Apr;12(2):96-106.

Wilber K Integral psychology: consciousness, spirit, psychology, therapy Shambhala Publications, Boston, MA. 2000.

Wilber K Quantum questions: mystical writings of the world's greatest physicists Shambala Press, Boston, MA., 2001.

Wright J and Potter P Psyche and Soma: physicians and metaphysicians on the mind-body problem from antiquity to enlightenment Clarendon Press, Oxford, England 2003.

Yang JM, Choi C, Hyun-hee , Woo WM, Yi SH, Soh KS, Yang JS, Choi C. Left-right and Yin-Yang balance of biophoton emission from hands. Acupunct Electrother Res. 2004;29(3-4):197-211.

Yasue K Jibu M Senta T No Matter, Never Mind Proceedings of "Toward a science of consciousness: fundamental approaches (Tokyo 1999), Vol. 33 in Advances in consciousness research, John Benjamins Publishing Company, Philadelphia, PA., 2001.

Zahourek R Intentionality forms the matrix of healing: a theory Alt Therapies 10;6, 2004: 40-49.

Zhan C Miller M Excess length of stay, charges, and mortality attributable to medical injuries during hospitalization JAMA 2003;290:1868-1874.

Zhang, Chang-Lin, "Skin resistance vs body conductivity: on the background of electronic measurement on skin," Frontier Perspectives, 2002; 11:2, 15-25.

Permissions

The contributors of this book come from diverse backgrounds, making this book a truly international effort. This book will bring forth new frontiers with its revolutionizing research information and detailed analysis of the nascent developments around the world.

We would like to thank Prof. Dr. Luciano L'Abate, for lending his expertise to make the book truly unique. He has played a crucial role in the development of this book. Without his invaluable contribution this book wouldn't have been possible. He has made vital efforts to compile up to date information on the varied aspects of this subject to make this book a valuable addition to the collection of many professionals and students.

This book was conceptualized with the vision of imparting up-to-date information and advanced data in this field. To ensure the same, a matchless editorial board was set up. Every individual on the board went through rigorous rounds of assessment to prove their worth. After which they invested a large part of their time researching and compiling the most relevant data for our readers. Conferences and sessions were held from time to time between the editorial board and the contributing authors to present the data in the most comprehensible form. The editorial team has worked tirelessly to provide valuable and valid information to help people across the globe.

Every chapter published in this book has been scrutinized by our experts. Their significance has been extensively debated. The topics covered herein carry significant findings which will fuel the growth of the discipline. They may even be implemented as practical applications or may be referred to as a beginning point for another development. Chapters in this book were first published by InTech; hereby published with permission under the Creative Commons Attribution License or equivalent.

The editorial board has been involved in producing this book since its inception. They have spent rigorous hours researching and exploring the diverse topics which have resulted in the successful publishing of this book. They have passed on their knowledge of decades through this book. To expedite this challenging task, the publisher supported the team at every step. A small team of assistant editors was also appointed to further simplify the editing procedure and attain best results for the readers.

Our editorial team has been hand-picked from every corner of the world. Their multi-ethnicity adds dynamic inputs to the discussions which result in innovative outcomes. These outcomes are then further discussed with the researchers and contributors who give their valuable feedback and opinion regarding the same. The feedback is then collaborated with the researches and they are edited in a comprehensive manner to aid the understanding of the subject.

Apart from the editorial board, the designing team has also invested a significant amount of their time in understanding the subject and creating the most relevant covers. They scrutinized every image to scout for the most suitable representation of the subject and create an appropriate cover for the book.

The publishing team has been involved in this book since its early stages. They were actively engaged in every process, be it collecting the data, connecting with the contributors or procuring relevant information. The team has been an ardent support to the editorial, designing and production team. Their endless efforts to recruit the best for this project, has resulted in the accomplishment of this book. They are a veteran in the field of academics and their pool of knowledge is as vast as their experience in printing. Their expertise and guidance has proved useful at every step. Their uncompromising quality standards have made this book an exceptional effort. Their encouragement from time to time has been an inspiration for everyone.

The publisher and the editorial board hope that this book will prove to be a valuable piece of knowledge for researchers, students, practitioners and scholars across the globe.

List of Contributors

Rosalinda C. Roberts and Joy K. Roche
Department of Psychiatry and Behavioral Neurobiology, University of Alabama, Birmingham, Birmingham, AL, USA

Shahza M. Somerville
Technical Resources International, Bethesda, MD, USA

Robert R. Conley
Department of Neuroscience, Lilly Technology Center, Indianapolis, IN, USA

Ashok Kumar Jainer, Rajkumar Kamatchi, Marek Marzanski and Bettahalasoor Somashekar
Caludon Centre, Coventry, United Kingdom

Angela Getz, Fenglian Xu and Naweed Syed
University of Calgary, Faculty of Medicine, Department of Cell Biology and Anatomy, Hotchkiss Brain Institute, Canada

Narong Maneeton
Department of Psychiatry, Faculty of Medicine, Chiang Mai University, Thailand

Lindsay G. Oades
University of Wollongong, Australia

Marie-Josée Fleury and Guy Grenier
McGill University, Douglas Hospital Research Centre, Quebec, Canada

Diane Kunyk and Charl Els
University of Alberta, Canada

Bengt Eriksson
Hedmark University College, Norway
Karlstad University, Sweden

Jan Kåre Hummelvoll
Hedmark University College, Norway

James Lake
University of Arizona College of Medicine, USA

Printed in the USA
CPSIA information can be obtained
at www.ICGtesting.com
JSHW011415221024
72173JS00004B/547